Invited papers from the

INTERNATIONAL SYMPOSIUM ON PESTICIDE TERMINAL RESIDUES

INTERNATIONAL UNION OF
PURE AND APPLIED CHEMISTRY

APPLIED CHEMISTRY DIVISION

PESTICIDE SECTION

PESTICIDE
TERMINAL RESIDUES

INVITED PAPERS FROM THE INTERNATIONAL
SYMPOSIUM ON PESTICIDE TERMINAL RESIDUES

held at Tel-Aviv, Israel
17–19 February 1971

Symposium Editor

A. S. TAHORI

Israel Institute for Biological Research

LONDON

BUTTERWORTHS

ENGLAND: BUTTERWORTH & CO. (PUBLISHERS) LTD.
                LONDON: 88 Kingsway, WC2B 6AB

AUSTRALIA: BUTTERWORTH & CO. (AUSTRALIA) LTD.
                SYDNEY: 586 Pacific Highway, Chatswood, NSW 2067
                MELBOURNE: 343 Little Collins Street, 3000
                BRISBANE: 240 Queen Street, 4000

CANADA: BUTTERWORTH & CO. (CANADA) LTD.
                TORONTO: 14 Curity Avenue, 374

NEW ZEALAND: BUTTERWORTH & CO. (NEW ZEALAND) LTD.
                WELLINGTON: 26–28 Waring Taylor Street, 1
                AUCKLAND: 35 High Street, 1

SOUTH AFRICA: BUTTERWORTH & CO. (SOUTH AFRICA) (PTY) LTD.
                DURBAN: 152–154 Gale Street

Published as a supplement to

Pure and Applied Chemistry

Suggested U.D.C. number 632·95·002·68: 54

Suggested additional number 614·7: 632·95·002·68

ISBN: 0 408 70290 7

Printed in Great Britain by Page Bros. (Norwich) Ltd., Norwich

PREFACE

A Symposium on Pesticide Terminal Residues, sponsored by the Pesticide Section of the Applied Chemistry Division of the International Union of Pure and Applied Chemistry, was held in Tel-Aviv, on 17–19 February 1971. The Symposium was attended by 285 scientists from FAO, IAEA, Australia, Belgium, Canada, Cyprus, Denmark, Eire, Finland, France, Germany, Greece, Iran, Israel, Italy, Japan, Jugoslavia, Kenya, Netherlands, New Zealand, Norway, Rhodesia, Rumania, South Africa, Spain, Sweden, Switzerland, Taiwan, Tanzania, United Kingdom, United States of America and Venezuela.

At the Opening Ceremony, greetings were delivered by His Excellency Mr V. Shemtov, Israel Minister of Health, Dr Ch. Resnick on behalf of the Israel Chemical Society, and Dr H. Hurtig, Chairman of the Symposium, on behalf of the Pesticide Section of the Applied Chemistry Division of IUPAC.

Some of the problems studied at the Symposium were further discussed in open Workshops at the Second International Congress of Pesticide Chemistry which took place immediately after the Symposium.

The problems caused by Pesticide Terminal Residues in the environment are becoming more and more acute. The publication of the 24 papers presented at the Symposium aims at making the new information available to as wide an audience as possible. It is hoped that this will help to raise the level of the discussions on the effects of terminal residues on the environment.

A. S. TAHORI, Editor
Israel Institute for Biological Research,
Ness-Ziona, Israel.

ORGANIZING COMMITTEE

Chairman: H. HURTIG (Canada)

Scientific Secretaries: CH. RESNICK (Israel)
K. R. HILL (USA)

Symposium Editor: A. S. TAHORI (Israel)

CONTENTS

THE CHEMISTRY AND METABOLISM OF
ORGANOPHOSPHORUS INSECTICIDES

TERMINAL RESIDUES OF ORGANOPHOSPHORUS INSECTICIDES IN SOIL AND TERMINAL RESIDUES OF ORGANOPHOSPHORUS FUMIGANTS

E. Y. SPENCER

Research Institute, Research Branch,
Canada Department of Agriculture,
University Sub Post Office, London 72, Ontario, Canada

ABSTRACT

The extent of terminal residues of organophosphorus insecticides and fumigants depends on a number of factors. They include chemical and biochemical degradation, temperature, moisture, pH, particle size and type. The soil may assist in the catalytic hydrolysis or stabilize the active toxicant by strong adsorption. Microflora may also accelerate the rate of residue reduction. Two fumigants and a number of organophosphorus compounds used as soil insecticides will be discussed to illustrate the influence of the above-mentioned factors on the type of metabolites and rate of residue disappearance.

The extent of terminal residues of organophosphorus fumigants and insecticides depends on a number of factors. These include chemical and biochemical degradation, temperature, moisture, pH, particle size and type. The residue may be high due to stabilization by strong adsorption on particles or it may be low in another medium where there has been catalytic hydrolysis. In non-sterile soil there is the further possible degradation by microflora, both aerobic and anaerobic. Since organophosphorus insecticides vary in their pH stability, their specificity to enzymatic degradation and surface catalysis and adsorption, predicting residues without carefully defining the system is very precarious. With the gradual replacement of organochlorine insecticides in many cases by carbamate and organophosphorus insecticides a knowledge of their behaviour in soil is of increasing importance. The former will be discussed in another session of the general symposium on terminal pesticide residues. The metabolism of the latter in plants and animals and methods of measurement will be discussed in this symposium along with the organophosphonates, as distinct from the other organophosphorus insecticides.

A knowledge of the ultimate residue in the edible foodstuff, after the application of an organophosphorus insecticide according to 'good agricultural practice', is, of course essential to assure safety from harmful residue levels. Apart from determining the toxic residues remaining after metabolism by the plant or animal, the amount available for uptake by the plant from the soil can also be of significance. There is also the possible interaction between the pesticide and certain microflora whereby the latter are favourably or unfavour-

3

ably affected. However, this aspect will not be considered here. On the other hand microflora, besides reducing residues, can also convert some organophosphorus insecticides into more toxic intermediates.

Before discussing the degradation and terminal residues of individual organophosphorus insecticides in soil the effect of specific factors on stability will be summarized. Chemical hydrolysis, temperature and pH can greatly influence the rate of degradation. To determine the modification of these by other factors such as soil type and microflora, initial measurements in aqueous systems are necessary. Many results have been summarized in a review by Faust and Suffet[1]. For example, the 'half-life' of parathion drops from 1 000 days at 10°C to 15 at 50°C. Although the oxygen analogue of an organophosphorothioate is usually considered to be more reactive and thus more readily hydrolysed than the parent compound, the pH of the medium may reverse this as shown with paraoxon and parathion, above and below pH 5.

In water, Gomaa et al.[2] found that diazinon and diazoxon followed first-order kinetics and half-lives were calculated. Diazinon and diazoxon are most stable near neutrality and at pH 7.4 have a rather long half-life of 185 and 29 days respectively. Although organophosphorus insecticides tend to be more stable in the pH range 5 to 6, non-enzymatic hydrolysis rates can be increased in some cases with certain metal ions. Mortland and Raman[3] showed that cupric ion was the most effective when loosely bound. Hydrolysis was catalysed most rapidly with compounds having a heterocyclic ring structure containing nitrogen as with diazinon and Dursban (O-3,5,6-trichloro-2-pyridyl OO-diethylphosphorothionate) although some hydrolysis did take place with Ronnel (O-2,4,5-trichlorophenyl OO-dimethylphosphorothioate) and to a lesser extent with Zytron. The greatest catalytic effect is possibly due to a bidentate chelation through the heterocyclic nitrogen and the sulphur or oxygen of the phosphorus. By contrast with the relative stability of diazinon in water at pH 7.2, it was found to be fairly unstable in a silty clay amounting to eleven per cent per day as reported in a review by Kearney and Helling[4].

The influence of the introduction of soil was reviewed by Bailey and White[5]. The soil colloids may play a large part depending on the extent of adsorption and desorption. This is affected by pH, temperature, moisture and the structure of the insecticide in relation to the adsorbent. The extent of inactivation by strong adsorption or by catalytic degradation has often been followed by bioassay. If it is the former and the addition of moisture results in desorption, then bioassays will increase, while in the latter, unless a more active intermediate is formed, the bioassay value will decrease.

Moisture can be important in the resulting activity of an organophosphorus insecticide in soil if it competes for the active sites on the soil particles. For example, Harris and Hitchon[6] found that Dursban, bromophos, diazinon and disulphoton were less competitive for the active sites than water and therefore highly active in moist mineral soil. Dursban and bromophos also showed good activity in dry mineral soil as well as muck soil, while disulphoton and diazinon were strongly inactivated in dry mineral soil. On the other hand, disulphoton retained activity in wet muck soil while diazinon was strongly inactivated. The variability of biological persistence in the soil has been strikingly shown by Harris and associates[6, 7]. In sandy loam, 'short residuals'—up to four weeks, included diazinon, phorate, Dursban and parathion; 'moderately residual'—

4

between eight and ten weeks, included Bayer 37289 (O-2,4,5-trichlorophenyl O-ethyl ethyl phosphonothioate) and Dasanit (OO-diethyl O-[p-(methylsulphinyl) phenyl] phosphorothioate)—with aldrin as a comparison, and 'highly residual' —beyond 36 weeks, included AC 47470 (cyclic propylene (diethoxyphosphinyl)dithioimidocarbonate), AC 43064 (the cyclic ethylene derivative) and disyston sulphoxide with dieldrin as a comparison.

The influence of differential interaction between several clays and Ronnel was shown by Rosenfield and van Walkenburg[8] to cause varying rates of molecular rearrangement to the more unstable thiolo derivative. Water bound in the lattice was found to aid in decomposition by assisting in bringing together the toxicant with the decomposition sites; free water actually increased stability by acting as an insulator over capillary surfaces. Thus heat treatment initially increased the catalytic activity by loss of free water, then activity decreased on removal of bound water. Bowman, Adams and Fenton[9] in recent studies with malathion and montmorillonite systems indicated that the hydrogen bonding between groups is not as strong as assumed, since on rehydration the infra-red spectrum shifts showed that water molecules in the primary hydration shell were acting in the complex formation. In either case adsorption was sufficiently strong that no degradation was observed. Current work by Bowman[10] with montmorillonite clays indicates their ability to stabilize other organophosphorus insecticides under varying moisture and temperature conditions. For example, Dasanit was stable for several days, even up to 70°C for 12 h.

Edwards[11] has reviewed the many factors contributing to the final pesticide residue, which include application losses, volatility, leaching and adsorption, degradation (enzymatic and chemical). Although the term 'half-life' has been used to represent the disappearance of an insecticide in the soil, since the decay curve is built from overlapping phases extrapolation beyond a short period of time is often unjustified, as indicated by Polen, Widmark and Sutherland[12], and thus the use of the first-order expression $t_{\frac{1}{2}} = (2.303 \times \log2)/k$ can be precarious and misleading.

Getzin and Rosefield[13] reported that the degradation of diazinon and Zinophos (OO-diethyl O-2-pyrazinyl phosphorothionate) varied in different soil types and did not follow a first-order reaction but best fitted a curvilinear regression equation. However, a recent report by Bro-Rasmussen et al.[14] on eight organophosphorus insecticides in a loam soil under controlled laboratory conditions indicated the possibility of calculating half-lives over an eighty-day period. On the other hand, in field experiments three distinct slopes for June–July, August–September and October–November were found. In spite of this, the compounds examined could be grouped into three classifications: highly persistent (dichlofenthion, trichloronate and chlorfenvinphos), intermediate (bromophos and mecarbam) and rapidly decomposing (diazinon, dimethoate and Aphidan [S-ethylsulphinyl methyl OO-di-isopropylphosphorodithioate]).

In a symposium, Kaufman[15] remarked that the relative contribution of pesticide degradation by microflora and chemical action is often difficult to assess. In addition the degradative systems observed in vitro may not be applicable to systems in vivo. Autoclaved soil may appear to have reduced activity but this may be due to change in soil structure rather than destruction of the microflora.

Getzin and Rosefield[16] used gamma irradiation for sterilizing soil without

5

altering its physical and chemical properties and showed the presence of a heat-labile, non-viable substance(s) which accelerated the degradation of malathion.

Getzin[17] noted that in some diazinon-treated soils greater amounts of hydrolysis products were found in the non-fumigated soil than in the fumigated and that the metabolism of the pyrimidinyl ring occurred more rapidly. Working with submerged soils, Sethunathan and Yoshida[18] showed that the release of the substituted pyrimidinyl ring was slower from the steam-sterilized soil than the controls but under the anaerobic conditions no further degradation was found. By contrast, Trela et al.[19] found, from studies in vitro with micro-organisms isolated from diazinon-treated soil, greatly stimulated cleavage of diazinon. Gunner and Zuckerman[20] made a unique observation on the degradation of diazinon when they found a synergistic action between a *Streptomyces* and an *Arthrobacter* for the metabolism of the pyrimidinyl ring.

To sum up the relative importance of factors that contribute to the rate of disappearance of organophosphorus insecticides in soils the most important are the chemical structure and intrinsic stability along with solubility and volatility. The type of substrate greatly affects the rate of volatilization[21]. The soil type may change the significance of some of the above, as already indicated, along with the moisture level. Temperature has some effect depending on volatility of the compound and the change in moisture content. Microbial populations can be of significance as well as formulation.

Extensive studies on the degradation of several organophosphorus insecticides in soil and identification of the breakdown products have been reported. To obtain sufficient material for identification high dosage levels are sometimes employed in laboratory experiments so that ultimate field conditions are not always exactly comparable. Using clay, loam, sand and peat, treated at 15 p.p.m. with chlorfenvinphos (2-chloro-1-[2',4'-dichlorophenyl]vinyl diethyl phosphate = Birlane), Beynon and Wright[22] reported the major decomposition products as 1-(2',4'-dichlorophenyl)-ethanol, 2,4-dichloroacetophenone, free and conjugates of desethyl chlorfenvinphos and diethyl phosphate with three other components in trace quantities. After four months at 22°C, residues varied from a high of 31 per cent in peat to a low of 7 per cent in loam. The proportion of products varied between soil types but all were present.

In their study of a closely related material, Gardona (2-chloro-1-[2',4',5'-trichlorophenyl]vinyl dimethyl phosphate) in three soil types (clay loam, sandy loam and peat) they found somewhat similar metabolites by cleavage of P—O—C bonds to yield mainly demethyl Gardona, dimethyl phosphate and initially 2,4,5-trichlorophenacyl chloride, which on reduction of the carbonyl group and reductive dechlorination yielded a number of C_8 compounds[23]. However, the rate of degradation was considerably faster than with chlorfenvinphos, as might be expected from a methyl ester derivative.

Another substituted vinyl phosphate, Ciodrin [OO-dimethyl-O-(α-methylbenzyl-3-hydroxy-*cis*-crotonate) phosphate] has an additional ester grouping and therefore has further possible degradative pathways. Konrad and Chesters[24] showed that the final products of degradation in soils were dimethyl-hydrogen phosphate, 3-hydroxy-*cis*-crotonic acid (I) and 1-phenylethanol (II). The dominant pathway involves hydrolysis of the phenyl ethyl ester with (III) as an intermediate. In some soils the subsequent hydrolysis may be rate-limiting so that there is a temporary accumulation of the intermediate (III).

$$(CH_3O)_2P(O)OC(CH_3)=CH-COO-CH(CH_3)-\langle O \rangle \rightarrow$$

$$(CH_3O)_2P(O)OC(CH_3)=CH-COOH \text{ (III)} + HOCH(CH_3)-\langle O \rangle \text{ (II)}$$
$$\downarrow$$
$$(CH_3O)_2P(O)OH + HOC(CH_3)=CH-COOH \text{ (I)}$$

The rates of hydrolysis were first-order in an aqueous system and at pH 6 in soil systems were two orders of magnitude greater.

When azinphosmethyl was applied to a silt loam, Schulz et al.[25] found after one year 13 per cent was recovered as azinphosmethyl and three 1,2,3-benzotriazin-4-one (benzazimide) derivatives in addition to four unknown compounds. At the end of two years there was only a trace of the original material together with benzazimide derivatives, while after four years only a trace of one unknown compound remained.

Parathion, like many others of this group, is considered to be relatively non-persistent. Lichtenstein and Schulz[26] indicated that 97 per cent of the applied dosage had disappeared in three months. Stewart et al.[27] have reported that traces had been found 16 years after application. Heavy annual applications of 15.7 p.p.m. for five years to a sandy loam resulted in a residue of 0.5 p.p.m. in the fall, while 16 years later a residue of 0.06 p.p.m. was found. Although this is small, the more recent improved specificity and analysis has been able to show residues in soils that possibly originated from being strongly adsorbed or occluded material. With two species of Rhizobium, Mick and Dahm[28] found that 85 per cent of the parathion was reduced to the amino derivative, ten per cent hydrolysed and no paraoxon was detected.

The organophosphorus thioether insecticides such as phorate provide the possibility of five oxidative analogues and differ in their adsorption to soil particles. Getzin and Shanks[29] found that phorate and its oxygen analogue were rapidly oxidized, in a silt loam at 25°C, to the corresponding sulphoxide and sulphone. Phorate, the sulphoxide and sulphone persisted beyond 16 weeks and the thiolate analogues degraded to low levels within two to eight days. The strong adsorption of phorate sulphoxide and sulphone to soil constituents was indicated by the lack of contact and fumigant toxicity to the assay organism. Evidence was also found for the conversion of some added phorate sulphoxide into phorate in the soil.

Preliminary information from Harris and Sans[30] demonstrates the effect of moisture and soil type on degradation and biological effectiveness with another 'thioether' derivative, Dasanit (OO-diethyl O-[p-(methylsulphinyl)phenyl] phosphorothioate. In Plainfield sand, Dasanit is converted into the sulphone with a cross-over time at about three weeks. In muck soil, a similar pattern occurs with a cross-over time slightly later. Direct addition of the sulphone to the soil results in degradation but at a slower rate than Dasanit itself. Although the sulphone, as a contact poison, is slightly more toxic to crickets than Dasanit itself, in soil it is less toxic, indicating greater adsorption. However, it is less strongly inactivated in muck soil. The toxicity of Dasanit in soil is more readily affected by soil moisture than the sulphone, indicating again the significance of moisture in influencing the soil–insecticide interaction.

7

With the organophosphorus fumigants, only phosphine and dichlorvos will be discussed, even though there are organophosphorus insecticides that exert a good deal of their action as a fumigant. To trace the fate of phosphine as a fumigant Robinson and Bond[31] labelled it with ^{32}P. Residues of the order of 0.04 to 1.2 p.p.m. calculated as phosphine on flour and wheat were found. However, this residue, not removed after aeration, heating or baking, was largely water-soluble and consisted mainly of hypophosphite and phosphite. The hypothesis concerning the formation of these and ultimately orthophosphate is now under investigation.

Dichlorvos is rapidly lost from stored products after fumigation by evaporation. Residues are readily hydrolysed to dimethyl hydrogen phosphate and dichloroacetaldehyde. The general subject has been reviewed by the Food and Agriculture Organization and World Health Organization Special Committees in 1967, 1968 and 1971[32].

REFERENCES

[1] S. D. Faust and I. H. Suffet. *Residue Revs.* **15**, 44 (1966).
[2] H. M. Gomaa, I. H. Suffet and S. D. Faust. *Residue Revs.* **29**, 171 (1969).
[3] M. M. Mortland and K. V. Raman, *J. Agric. Food Chem.* **15**. 163 (1967).
[4] P. C. Kearney and C. S. Helling. *Residue Revs.* **25**, 25 (1969).
[5] G. W. Bailey and J. L. White. *J. Agric. Food Chem.* **12**, 324 (1964).
[6] C. R. Harris and J. L. Hitchon. *J. Econ. Ent.* **63**, 2 (1970).
[7] C. R. Harris. In *Pesticides in the Soil*, pp. 58–64, International Symposium Michigan State University (February 1970).
[8] C. Rosenfield and W. van Walkenburg. *J. Agric. Food Chem.* **13**, 68 (1965).
[9] B. T. Bowman, R. S. Adams, Jr. and S. W. Fenton. *J. Agric. Food Chem.* **18**, 723 (1970).
[10] B. T. Bowman. Personal communication (1971).
[11] C. A. Edwards. *Residue Revs.* **13**, 83 (1966).
[12] P. B. Polen, G. Widmark and G. L. Sutherland. Report to fifth meeting of the IUPAC Terminal Residues Commission, Erbach, September 1970. *IUPAC Bulletin*, in press.
[13] L. W. Getzin and I. Rosefield. *J. Econ. Ent.* **59**, 512 (1966).
[14] F. Bro-Rasmussen, E. Nødegaard and K. Voldum-Clausen. *Pesticide Sci.* **1**, 179 (1970).
[15] D. D. Kaufman. In *Pesticides in the Soil*, pp. 73–86, International Symposium, Michigan State University (February 1970).
[16] L. W. Getzin and I. Rosefield. *J. Agric. Food Chem.* **16**, 598 (1968).
[17] L. W. Getzin. *J. Econ. Ent.* **60**, 505 (1967).
[18] N. Sethunathan and T. Yoshida. *J. Agric. Food Chem.* **17**, 1192 (1969).
[19] J. M. Trela, W. J. Ralston and H. B. Gunner. *Bact. Proc.* **68**, 6 (1968).
[20] H. B. Gunner and B. M. Zuckerman. *Nature, Lond.,* **217**, 1183 (1968).
[21] E. P. Lichtenstein and K. R. Schulz. *J. Agric. Food Chem.* **18**, 814 (1970).
[22] K. I. Beynon and A. N. Wright. *J. Sci. Food Agric.* **18**, 143 (1967).
[23] K. I. Beynon and A. N. Wright. *J. Sci. Food Agric.* **19**, 250 (1969).
[24] J. G. Konrad and G. Chesters. *J. Agric. Food Chem.* **17**, 226 (1969).
[25] K. R. Schulz, E. P. Lichtenstein, T. T. Liang and T. W. Fuhremann. *J. Econ. Ent.* **63**, 432 (1970).
[26] E. P. Lichtenstein and K. R. Schulz. *J. Econ. Ent.* **57**, 618 (1964).
[27] D. K. R. Stewart, D. Chisholm and M. T. H. Ragab. *Nature, Lond.* (In the press).
[28] D. L. Mick and P. A. Dahm. *J. Econ. Ent.* **63**, 1155 (1970).
[29] L. W. Getzin and C. H. Shanks, Jr. *J. Econ. Ent.* **63**, 52 (1970).
[30] C. R. Harris and W. W. Sans. Personal communication (1971).
[31] J. R. Robinson and E. J. Bond. *J. Stored Prod. Res.* **6**, 133 (1970).
[32] FAO/WHO Special Committee Report on the Residues of some Pesticides in Food. (1967, 1968, 1971).

TERMINAL RESIDUES OF ORGANOPHOSPHORUS INSECTICIDES IN PLANTS

H. FREHSE*

Farbenfabriken Bayer AG, Pflanzenschutz Anwendungstechn. Abteilung, Biologische Forschung, D-5090 Leverkusen-Bayerwerk, Germany

ABSTRACT

Several problems are first discussed which arise out of the presence of residues in plant material and particularly in foods of plant origin. As the metabolism of pesticides in the plant is characterized by the inability of the plant to excrete foreign substances, the term 'terminal residue' is seemingly hard to define. Recent results of metabolic studies, some of which have not yet been published, are presented for several selected groups of active ingredients. The compounds of each of these groups are interrelated by common structural features. Included are compounds in which the following substituents are esterified with (thio) phosphoric acids or (thio)phosphonic acids: aromatic thioethers, N-containing heterocycles (bound via a methylene group), halogenated phenols and nitrophenols, chains containing vinyl groups, several carboxylic acids and crotonic acids. Comparisons with metabolic pathways in animals or micro-organisms are not presented.

The title of my paper might suggest that I intend to give a complete review of the present level of research into this subject. This of course is impossible in the time allotted because it would mean that I would have only about 20 seconds for each active ingredient, and then only if I were to limit my comments to the 90 different organophosphates of commercial importance or experimental interest that were already listed three years ago in Spencer's *Guide to the Chemicals used in Crop Protection*[84] and Martin's *Pesticide Manual*[54]. Therefore, I wish to confine the scope of my paper to (1) a discussion of some general aspects that arise out of the existence of residues in foods of plant origin; (2) a presentation of several more recent results including some unpublished ones, which may help also towards explaining the general aspects. The compounds I shall mention have been chosen partly at random but this of course is unavoidable. It is only natural that interest always centres on the higher plant when one speaks of metabolism and of residues of pesticides because after all most pesticides are *plant* protection products. It is also not surprising that insecticidal, acaricidal and nematocidal organophosphates have always met with special interest. Many of them have a noteworthy level of mammalian toxicity, some of their physiological effects are easy to

---

* English translation by J. Edwards.

measure, and in the case of dithiophosphates and monothiophosphates primary transformation processes are not only easy to recognize but also have a direct effect on the toxicology of the residues. On the other hand, it is often just the more toxic organophosphates which, on account of their tendency to hydrolyse readily, present hardly any residue problems and more certainly pose no persistence problems. It is a known fact that the oxygen analogues, with some exceptions, hydrolyse with relatively greater ease than their parent thiophosphates. If, on the other hand, phosphates are compared with analogous phosphonates or, for example, diethyl phosphates are compared with homologous dimethyl phosphates, it is found that the relations are usually just the opposite:

Phosphate → Phosphonate
    more toxic
    acidic   hydrolyses *less readily*
    alkaline   hydrolyses more readily

Dimethyl → Diethyl phosphate
phosphate   *more toxic*
    acidic }
    alkaline}   hydrolyses *less readily*

When organophosphates hydrolyse, they lose their typical toxic effect and also their pesticidal effect. Nevertheless, a problem may still remain from the aspect of residue toxicology. This is the case when the so-called 'leaving group'* is still of some toxicological relevance. The probability of this is all the greater the more complex is the structure of the substituent, whereby consideration must perhaps be given chiefly to heterocycles.

The metabolism of chemicals in the plant is basically characterized by the far-reaching inability of the plant to excrete foreign substances. However, the plant has mechanisms for the degradation of almost every organic pesticide. The possession of a hydroxyl group enables phenols, for example, to unite with sugars to form glycosides. They are deposited in this form and are precluded from the plant metabolism, if only temporarily. In certain phases of plant growth, the glycosides may be cleaved again. Little is yet known about the further fate of aromatic aglycons. It is presumed that they are mainly deposited in correspondingly suitable parts of the plant organism or that they are further utilized in the biosynthetic metabolism. Some observations[13] support the findings of Miller[62] that apparently glycosides are not translocated from the tissues in which they are synthesized. It has also been suggested that uronic acids may serve as 'detoxication' agents in plants[85]. A still unsolved problem confronting the residue analyst lies in the question whether conjugated hydrolysis products of pesticides must be regarded as residues or not. Expressed otherwise, must a substance which, in free form, would have to be considered as a residue in accordance with the definition of the term, still have to be considered as 'residue' when it is in bound form?

---

    * Denotes anion of an XH-acidic compound according to the so-called 'Schrader rule' (see ref. 19); usually, this involves a phenol, an enol, an alcohol or a mercaptan. For the interpretation of the mechanisms of such 'phosphorylations' see e.g. refs. 27, 32, 79.

This problem becomes especially acute through the fact that—as we shall see—the amount of free phenols is, in general, relatively low as compared with the amount of conjugated phenols.

The animal excretes the greater part of an applied phosphoric ester, in changed or unchanged form, within a few hours or days; the plant tends to store chemicals and their metabolic products for longer periods. Whereas in animals, excretion and metabolism are parallel processes and excretion is often a direct consequence of metabolism, the plant must break down the active ingredient within its own organism and must convert or build up liberated cleavage products to physiological substances. For this reason, the term 'terminal residue' is problematic. The term 'residue' can be and has been defined[30], prime consideration being given to toxicological criteria.

But what does the word '*terminal*' really imply? If it is to be understood as relating to time, it will be necessary to define specifically the point of time which enters into consideration. It could, for example, be the time of harvest or the point of entry into trade channels to which tolerances usually apply. But it could also be the time of consumption, in other words when the residues enter the mouth of the consumer, which would be more to the point from the aspect of residue toxicology. A biochemist will not consider it essential to make such a distinction but a more practically-minded residue analyst knows that the metabolite pattern can undergo a change during the storage and processing of foods. In this point, our knowledge is still far from complete. The term 'terminal residue' could, however, also be understood as implying that the metabolism of a product has been studied down to the very final stages of chemical degradation. But this would be going far beyond the point necessary for residue toxicology and residue analysis. It should not be overlooked, either, that the majority of the known metabolic processes simply embrace '*initial*' residues. A definition of the term 'terminal residue' does not exist. While still upholding the definition of the term residue, it is my opinion that the expression terminal residue should relate simply to a definite point of time but not to the ultimate chemical fate of a pesticide molecule. In their very final stage of transformation, products can no longer be spoken of as residues but should be termed (bio)degradation products.

The metabolism of pesticides in plants cannot be viewed solely as an academic problem but rather it must be looked upon chiefly as a residue problem, in other words in close association with toxicology and residue analysis. Only by doing so can the complex findings of metabolism studies be translated to legislative measures, and thus contribute towards making foods 'safer', as well as placing the discussion of the subject on a more relevant basis. Thus residues in foods of plant origin are never 'terminal' because they still have to be consumed by human beings and metabolized in the human organism, which, in turn, may raise new, secondary metabolic problems.

The fortunate owner of a labelled active ingredient has hardly any difficulties in surprising the scientific community with the discovery of new radioactive spots on a chromatogram after he has once brought the compound into contact with the plant. We know the interpretation: spot No. 1 is the 'parent', spot No. 2 is the oxygen analogue, three other spots are unknowns A, B and C, the sixth spot was tentatively identified as the des-

11

methyl compound, etc. The residue analyst does not know, and the toxicologist cannot tell him, whether these metabolites are toxicologically significant, in other words whether he must co-analyse them as 'residue' because that would perhaps call for a special clean-up or even raise other technical difficulties. Whether it is worth concentrating the discovered metabolites, identifying them and perhaps synthesizing them for toxicological and analytical purposes will largely depend upon whether the same metabolites occur in the animal experiment. On this point, FAO and WHO have stated[31] that if the main metabolites present in the residues in the edible portions of farm animals, animal products or plants to which the pesticides were applied are identical with the main metabolites in experimental animals, then the ADI applies to both the pesticide and its metabolites; if the main metabolites are not identical, then the ADI applies only to the original pesticide, and separate studies on the main metabolites in the residues will be necessary for assessment of their toxicological properties.

I should now like to pass on to the discussion of the special problems. I shall, however, leave out of consideration those metabolic processes which take place simply as hydrolysis at the P atom (for details on such processes see, for example, the review in ref. 15). On the other hand, I do not propose in this discussion to distinguish pathways according to whether products found in or on plants arise from true metabolism or whether they stem from photodecomposition or other 'weathering' factors.

CONVERSIONS AT THE P-ATOM

Conversion from thionothiolo phosphates to thiolo phosphates or from thionophosphates to phosphates is a known phenomenon, as is likewise isomerization from the thiono form to the thiolo form. The acute toxicity can be very greatly altered as the result of such conversion. A simple example of this is provided by compounds of the parathion-methyl type (*Figure 1*).

$R = CH_3$ $\qquad R' = C_6H_4 \cdot NO_2(p)$

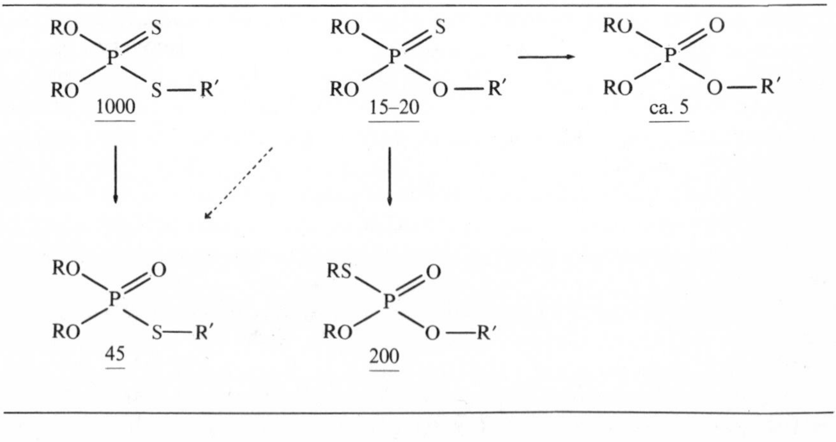

Figure 1. Oral LD_{50} for rats (mg/kg) of methyl-parathion type compounds.

12

The formation of S-alkyl isomers from thionophosphates due to exposure to heat is a phenomenon that is known for many compounds (e.g. malathion[61, 71], parathion[61], fenthion[60, 70], and fensulfothion[3]). With *phoxim* however, we observed, on cotton leaves as well as *in vitro*, a different kind of isomerization in which the oxyimino form is changed to the thioimino form[25]; see *Figure 2*. In this case the conversion is due to photosensitization

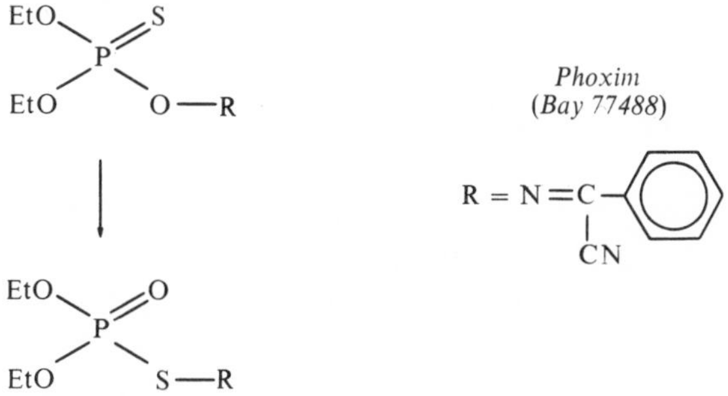

Phoxim
(Bay 77488)

$$ R = N = C - \bigcirc $$
$$ \overset{|}{C}N $$

Figure 2.

and not to heat exposure. After two days, the metabolite accounted for about 20 per cent of the applied amount of phoxim. However, it is broken down within a few days just like the metabolites tetraethyldiphosphate (TEPP) and tetraethylthiodiphosphate (monothio-TEPP) which likewise form, although in smaller amounts, during the course of the phoxim transformation. The structure of the metabolite was recognized by means of n.m.r. and mass spectra. The oral LD_{50} of phoxim for rats is 2000 mg/kg, and that of the photoisomeric form is seemingly lower. However, this substance could not yet be synthesized in pure form. The oxygen analogue did not occur in these experiments. The investigations were carried out with ^{32}P-labelled active ingredient.

THIOETHER (THIO)PHOSPHATES

Let us now turn to a number of compounds containing a methyl thiophenyl group. They undergo another typical reaction which Metcalf and his co-workers discovered on aliphatic thioether phosphates 20 years ago, namely oxidation to the sulphoxide and the sulphone. Owing to this reaction, the methylthio group is important in providing a delayed period of toxicity during and following absorption and translocation.

Some members of the group of aromatic thioether phosphates are shown in *Figure 3*. The arrows do not of course indicate metabolic pathways but merely represent lines of relationship in the sense of a 'family tree'.

The first report on the metabolism of one of the compounds included in this discussion concerned fensulfothion (Benjamini *et al.*, 1959[3]) but in the following years *fenthion* was studied more comprehensively. In 1961, Brady and Arthur[9] published results of investigations into the metabolism of fenthion in rats, as well as some results obtained in experiments on cotton. In 1962, results were published of investigations we carried out on beans[70],

13

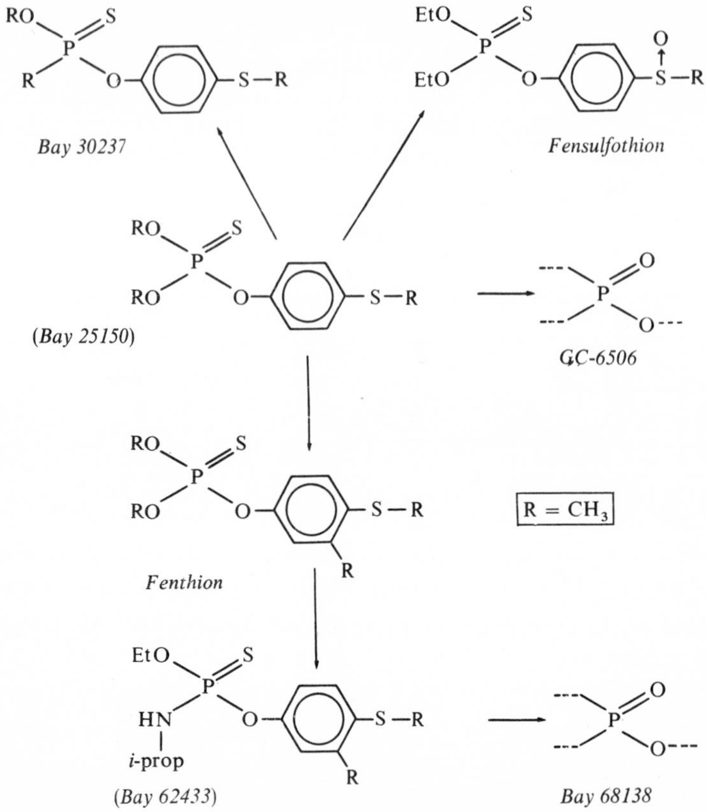

Figure 3.

and in the same year results of studies on rice, tea and cabbage were received from Japan[35,90]. In 1963, Metcalf et al. published corresponding qualitative data for cotton plants[60], and in 1966 Leuck and Bowman[48] reported on results obtained on maize plants, Bermuda grass and maize silage. The qualitative result of these studies which were supplemented by two additional recent papers[6,7], caused no surprise:—The sulphoxides and sulphones of the thionophosphate and of the phosphate are formed; when the S-methyl isomer is present as an impurity in the active ingredient, sulphoxide and sulphone are formed from it, too, but they are quickly broken down by hydrolysis[70]; photocatalytic oxidation takes place at the thioether group whilst enzymatic oxidation takes place at the phosphorus atom[70]. In corn silage, very small amounts of the oxygen analogue appear, which is indicative of transformation by reduction[48]. The Japanese experimenters found that the water-soluble metabolites present in rice plants included the O-desmethyl form of fenthion. The quantitative results available show far-reaching agreement for different plant species when the results are divided into three complexes: fenthion, fenthion–sulphoxide + fenthion–sulphone, oxygen analogue–sulphoxide + oxygen analogue–sulphone, as illustrated by four

14

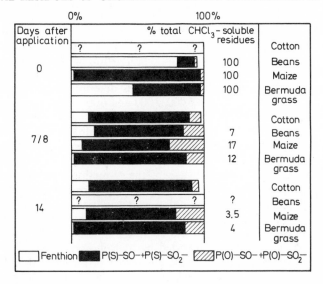

Figure 4. Percentage distribution of fenthion and its metabolites in plants.

examples (drawn from refs. 9, 48, 70) in *Figure 4*. Fenthion–sulphoxide and fenthion–sulphone account for the largest share of the chloroform-soluble metabolites as soon as the transformation processes become operative. The absolute amount of chloroform-soluble metabolites decreases within 14 days to a level equivalent to a few per cent of the initial amount.

It is not without interest to take a look at the physiological effect of such metabolites. In *Figure 5*, the principal metabolites are presented in the form of 'toxicity factors'[33], in other words the figures show by how many times the metabolites are more toxic or more effective than fenthion. It will be noted that the oxidation products are clearly more toxic to mammals whilst with respect to insecticidal activity they are no more than equally active at the best, being considerably less effective against mosquito larvae. In the case of flies, it is noted that in comparison with the topical application, the depression of cholinesterase activity is greatly increased, an effect that is

	Mosquito larvae (LC$_{50}$)			Housefly		Rat		Man
Compound	Aëdes	Anoph.*	Culex[a]	LD$_{50}$ topic.	ChE	LD$_{50}$ oral	ChE	ChE
Fenthion	1·0	1·0	1·0	1·0	1	1·0	1·0	<1
P(S)—SO—	0·005	0·2	0·16	0·96	500	1·8	44	11
P(S)—SO$_2$—	0·0005	0·06	0·08	0·64	90	1·8	5·1	1
P(O)—SO—	0·005	0·04	0·03	1·3	280	4·6	?	10
P(O)—SO$_2$—	0·025	0·03	0·03	1·3	2400	9·2	?	16

* resistant, [a] average of two investigators, ChE = cholinesterase depression.

Figure 5. Relative toxicity of fenthion and its main metabolites.

15

less marked in rats. For the residue analyst, such data are proof that residues of metabolite-forming pesticides cannot be determined quantitatively by means of bioassays.

The methylthiophenols, methylsulphinylphenols and methylsulphonylphenols liberated by hydrolysis from compounds of the fenthion type are practically non-toxic. The oral LD_{50} values determined in rats for these p-substituted phenols are above 6000, 3000 and 6000 mg/kg, respectively[68]. It is nonetheless of academic interest to follow their further fate in the plant. In this respect, interesting results were recently obtained in studies with GC-6506 which was labelled with both ^{32}P and S-methyl-^{14}C. Wendel and Bull[92] had found that in cotton plants GC-6506, its sulphoxide and sulphone were detoxified rapidly by cleavage of the O-methyl and P—O—phenyl linkages. Since the O-desmethyl derivatives were also shown to be unstable in the plant, which precludes accumulation, it was apparent that one ultimate end result of GC-6506 metabolism would be complete liberation of the substituted phenols into the plant system. From some of the metabolites, substituted phenols could be liberated by hydrolysis with β-glucosidase[13]. The predominant products were the glucosides of phenol–sulphoxide and phenol–sulphone. The glucosides, in turn, were changed slowly to an unidentified metabolite, possibly by alteration of the glucosyl moiety. When this metabolite was hydrolysed with β-glucosidase, the respective phenol was the only radioactive compound liberated. The authors speculate that the glycone portions of the conjugates are altered possibly by the formation of a β-gentiobiside comparable to those reported from studies of other phenols in plants. The quantitative relationships are shown in *Figure 6*; the sulphides have been combined with the sulphoxides and the sulphones also for the desmethyl compounds as well as the free phenols.

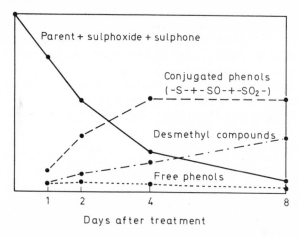

Figure 6. Relative concentrations in cotton leaves of GC-6506 and its metabolites.

The same phenols that are formed in the metabolism of GC-6506 are produced also in the metabolism of fensulfothion. A gas chromatographic method using a flame photometric detector operated in the sulphur mode was developed by Thornton for determining these phenols after acid hydrolysis and also for determining any conjugates that might be present (Chemagro 1968, unpublished[88]). A series of studies comprising 50 analyses was carried out by this method on maize and potatoes following treatment of the soil with fensulfothion[88]; the only notable residues of phenols were detected in corn fodder. In some cases, the phenols were of the same order as the residues of fensulfothion, in other cases they were present in considerably bigger amounts (e.g. approximately 6·5 p.p.m. after two months as against 0·1 p.p.m. of fensulfothion), and in yet another case the phenols were no longer detectable after 60 days whilst the fensulfothion residue then still amounted to 0·3 p.p.m.

The metabolism of fensulfothion was investigated in cotton, in 1959, by Benjamini and co-workers[3] who suggested that the sulphone, the S-ethyl–sulphoxide and the S-ethyl–sulphone were the major metabolites. Katague and Anderson[45], also working with cotton plants, were able to establish the absence of S-ethyl–isomers; the metabolites found were identified as the oxygen analogue and the sulphone of the parent compound. A small amount of the oxygen analogue sulphone was also detected. These results were confirmed by Everett and Gronberg (Chemagro 1967, unpublished[28]) in studies conducted not only on cotton but also on beans and corn. In corn, however, the oxygen analogue sulphone was found to account for up to 18 per cent of the total residue. A surprising result was also recorded, namely that the *sulphide* of fensulfothion (which is a sulphoxide) represented 10 to 20 per cent of the chloroform extractables in the bean plant. Lesser amounts, namely up to nine per cent were found in corn. According to these authors, the presence of this sulphide represents the first known case where a pesticidal sulphoxide was reduced by growing plants to the corresponding sulphide in substantial amounts.

In a study of the metabolism of *Bay 68 138* (®Nemacur P) in tomatoes, beans and groundnuts carried out by Waggoner (Chemagro 1969, unpublished[91]), further interesting observations were made. The compound was labelled in the ^{14}C-ethyl, ^{14}C-isopropyl and ^{3}H-methylthio positions. Two chloroform-extractable metabolites were detected in addition to the sulphoxide and the sulphone. The sulphoxide was predominating at all intervals studied. The parent compound disappeared completely at intervals of longer than 14 days. The sulphone was found in the least amounts of the three and was not present at the 14-day interval. One of the additional metabolites appeared very early, reached a very small concentration, and disappeared after three days. Although it could not be identified, all available evidence supported that it contained all substituents intact. The second additional metabolite accounted for 0·8 to 1·5 per cent of the total residue at 0 to 14 days and was not detected thereafter. It was tentatively identified as a ring hydroxylated derivative of the parent compound. This metabolite was about seven times more active than the parent compound with respect to horse serum cholinesterase inhibition. In tobacco plants, following soil treatment, neither of the two additional metabolites was detected (Chemagro 1971, unpublished[46]).

In connection with the compounds of the 'fenthion family', attention should be drawn also to a study by Neely and co-workers[67] who used multiple regression analysis to separate the contribution that the thiomethyl and sulphonylmethyl group as well as the P=O and P=S groups made on the insecticidal activity. The biological activity represented by the sulphonyl methyl and P=O group correlated well with the partition coefficient and the rate of alkaline hydrolysis. The analysis indicated: (a) that thiomethyl and the P=S group had to undergo transformation to a more reactive species; (b) that the thiomethyl phosphorothionate which is most stable to nucleophilic attack should be the most active as an insecticide.

In a more empirical approach, Reynolds and co-workers[77] investigated the systematic insecticidal action of 32 compounds of such type, including their methyl phosphonate and ethyl phosphonate analogues, as well as the compound *Bay 30 237* which was presented in *Figure 3* because it gave the best results in Reynolds's experiment.

I now wish to deal with some groups of compounds which each have certain structural features in common, and of which a few important members were studied recently. Due to the shortness of time available, I shall have to confine my comments to the more qualitative aspects.

DITHIOPHOSPHATES WITH A THIOMETHYLENE BRIDGE BETWEEN THE PHOSPHORUS AND DIFFERENT HETEROCYCLIC RINGS (*Figure 7*)

Studies with ^{14}C-carbonyl-labelled *R-1504* (®Imidan) on cotton showed a few years ago that in the case of this compound, hydrolysis predominates over oxidation[57]. The metabolism involves a hydrolytic step in the form of an amidase cleavage, and removal of the phosphorus-bearing N-substituent. The major product is phthalamic acid $[HO(O)C \cdot C_6H_4 \cdot C(O)NH_2]$ and/or phthalic acid $[C_6H_4 \cdot (COOH)_2]$. In addition, decarboxylation products were found (benzoic acid, hydroxybenzoic acid).

In the case of *phosalone*, a cleavage of the C—N bond was not observed; in addition to the oxon, the benzoxazolon ring system, conjugated at the N atom, occurred as glucoside[20, 24]. Both metabolites accounted for only a few per cent of the phosalone residue which can be determined either by gas chromatography or by colorimetry[23].

In the case of *GS-13 005* (®Supracide), a ring cleavage was not observed at first although the metabolism was studied very exhaustively with both ^{32}P-labelling as well as with ^{14}C-labelling in the carbonyl group and in the methoxy group[10, 16]. In cotton plants, the P—O—desmethyl compound is the dominant metabolic product and here, too, the oxon occurred only in very small concentrations. The authors concluded from the experimental findings that the oxidative mechanism responsible for biosynthesis of the oxon may have been inhibited by one or more of the compounds present. Studies on alfalfa[16] revealed that the desmethyl compound forms an unstable conjugate which is readily hydrolysed. Furthermore, fragmentation of the thiodiazole ring was suggested by a release of $^{14}CO_2$, irrespective of whether labelling was done in the carbonyl group or in the methoxy group. As the oxygen analogue is the only cholinesterase-inhibiting metabolite, determination of the residues is limited to the parent compound by gas chromatography

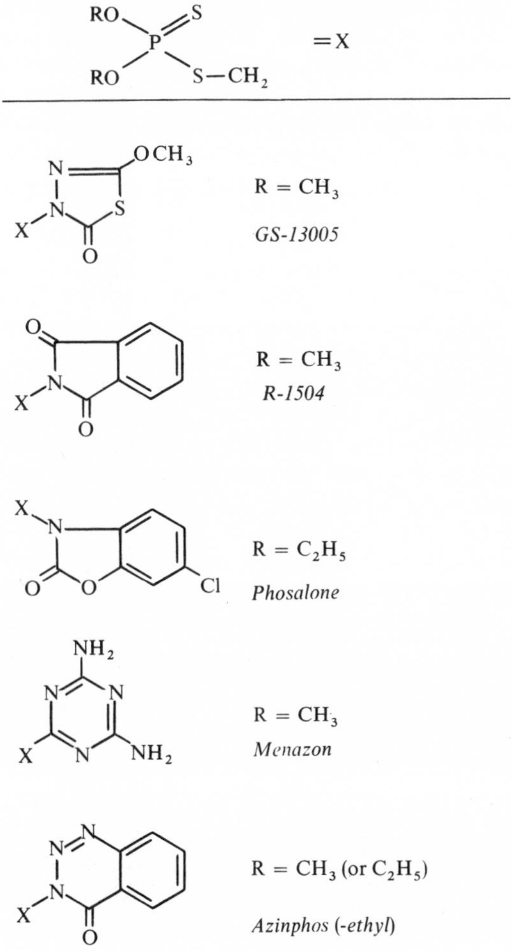

Figure 7.

and detection of the oxon by thin-layer chromatography[55]. However, it ought to be possible to determine both components by gas chromatography (see e.g. ref. 74).

Apart from hydrolysis experiments[14], no studies on plants seem to have been published for *menazon*.

Studies of *azinphos-methyl* on cotton made as long ago as 1957[89] showed that occurrence of the oxon as a metabolite is hardly to be expected. More recent studies (Chemagro 1966, unpublished[52]) with ^{14}C-carbonyl-labelled active ingredient were, therefore, undertaken with the object of determining the extent of formation of benzazimide metabolites following spray application to lettuce. The most remarkable observation made at first was that there was no apparent loss of radioactivity from the leaf. Most of the activity (80 to 95 per cent) remained on the surface through the entire fourteen-day observation period. Thin-layer chromatography showed that it was only in the 14-day benzene strip samples that there was any activity other than that corresponding to the parent compound; even in this sample, 95 per cent of the activity could be identified and shown to be azinphos–methyl. Two of the trace peaks observed had, in relation to azinphos, the same mobilities as the oxygen analogue and bis-*N*-methyl benzazimide sulphide; from its relative mobility, a third trace peak could not be identified either as mercapto methyl benzazimide or as hydroxymethyl benzazimide or as benzazimide. A fourth trace peak appeared at the starting point; it might have been identical with methyl benzazimide disulphide. Studies conducted by Crosby[21] showed that benzazimide is formed from azinphos in solution under the influence of ultra-violet light, together with very small amounts of anthranilic acid ($C_6H_4 \cdot NH_2 \cdot o\text{-}COOH$) and much cholinesterase-inhibiting polymer. In other words, azinphos appears to abstract hydrogen from its solvent in ultra-violet light.

In a field experiment, a study was made also of the possible primary metabolism of azinphos-ethyl in cotton and snap beans. Because of the greater chemical stability of azinphos-ethyl compared with the dimethyl compound, it was postulated that its oxygen analogue might be found to a greater extent. In actual fact, the oxon accounted for about ten per cent of the total residue after 14 days (Chemagro 1969, unpublished[72]).

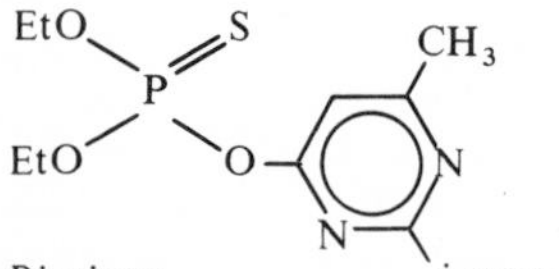

Diazinon

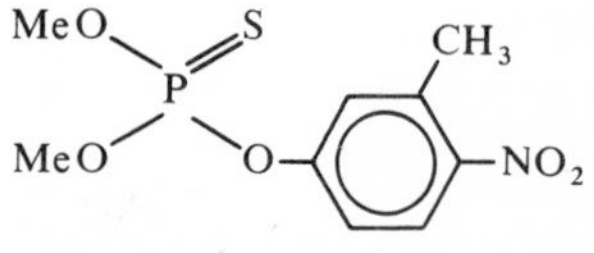

Fenitrothion

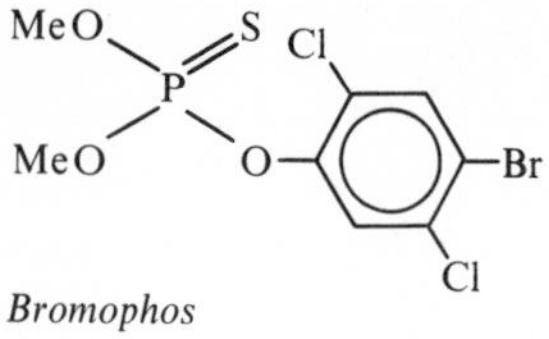

Bromophos

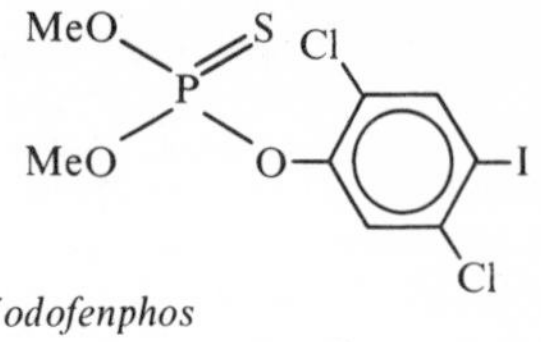

Iodofenphos

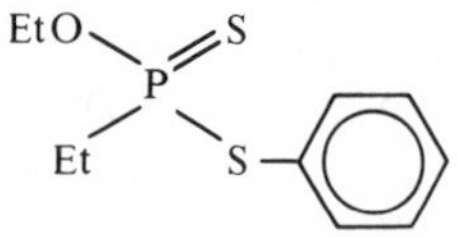

N-2790

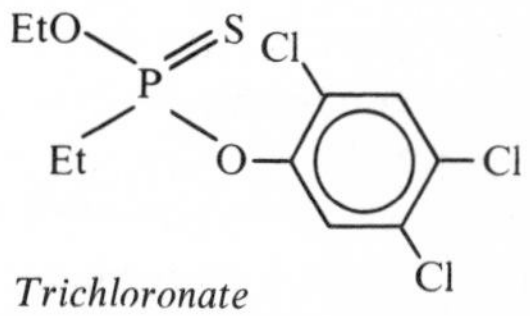

Trichloronate

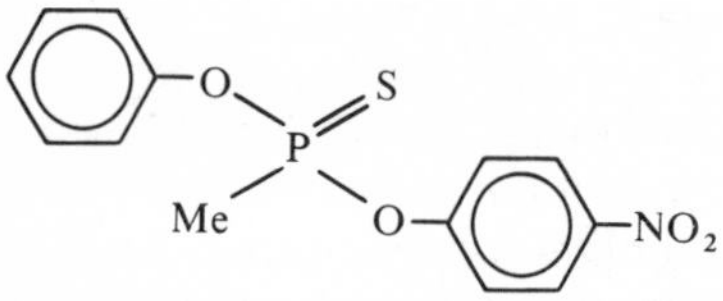

CP-40

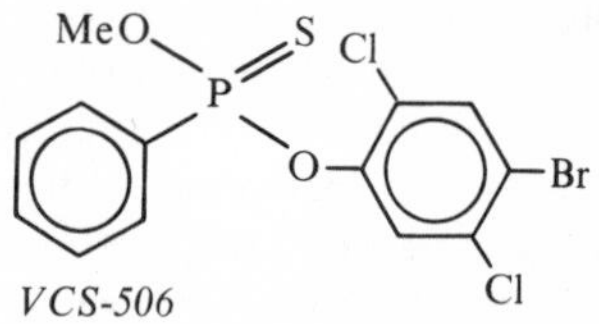

VCS-506

Figure 8.

COMPOUNDS IN WHICH AROMATIC HALOGEN-SUBSTITUTED, NITRO-SUBSTITUTED OR ALKYL-SUBSTITUTED OR UNSUBSTITUTED RINGS ARE THE SUBSTITUENTS OF THIOPHOSPHORIC AND THIOPHOSPHONIC ACIDS (*Figure 8*)

Diazinon uptake, translocation and metabolisms by plants and in the soil have been studied by many authors since 1957 (see summaries in refs 26 and 69); only little and partially contradictory information is available on biologically active metabolites formed from diazinon applied to food crops[26].

It appears that occurrence of diazinon metabolism largely depends on the plant species. The oxon either was not found at all or was detected only in very small amounts; this is confirmed also by results obtained in the last few years[26, 69]; however, Masuda and Fukuda[54a] found up to 40 per cent of the chloroform-solubles to be the oxygen analogue and detected two unknown metabolites in rice plants after application of diazinon on to the surface of paddy soil. One cholinesterase-inhibiting metabolite might possibly be the ethyl-*S* isomer[75]; if so, it would be one of the few cases of thiono-/thiol-rearrangement *in vivo*. In experiments with ring-labelled diazinon on tomatoes and beans, $^{14}CO_2$ was expired thus indicating cleavage of the pyrimidine ring which, however, was found also still intact as the 6-hydroxy form[44, 76]. Similar results were also obtained in studies of the degradation of diazinon in soil[36, 37, 80]. Nelson and Hamilton[69] made the interesting observation that diazinon is expired in intact form by alfalfa following uptake from the soil. Five of the known or possible transformation products can be detected by thin-layer chromatography[83]. A previously unreported alteration product of diazinon was recently isolated from field-sprayed kale and tentatively identified as diazinon, hydroxylated in the isopropyl group[73]. This compound can be determined by GLC. Interesting studies have also been published on the kinetics of *in vitro* hydrolysis of diazinon and diazoxon[40].

Compounds like *fenitrothion*, *bromophos* and *iodofenphos* are not expected to provide any surprises with respect to their metabolism. Therefore, I wish to mention only two studies by Bowman and co-workers on fenitrothion and iodofenphos (C-9491)[49, 8]. *Figure 9* shows that following degradation of fenitrothion, a very small amount of the *free* cresol is found in addition to slight amounts of the oxon (it should be noted that the residues are presented logarithmically). The results obtained with iodofenphos are completely similar (see also ref. 42a) to those recorded for fenitrothion. However, I should like to call to mind again the problem of free and bound phenols, which I referred to earlier in connection with the thioether phosphates. In studies to investigate the metabolism of bromophos in tomatoes, very small quantities of the oxon, the free phenols and *O*-desmethyl-bromophos were found but no desmethyloxon[86].

Let us now turn to the phosphonates*. Of the compounds shown in *Figure 8*, *CP-40* (®Colep) was studied as far back as 1964, using phenyl-^{14}C-labelling[53]. Acid and emulsin hydrolysis of benzene, chloroform and water extracts converted 75 to 80 per cent of the radioactivity to phenol, thus

---

* For a detailed treatise on metabolism of phosphonates, see paper by Menn, page 57.

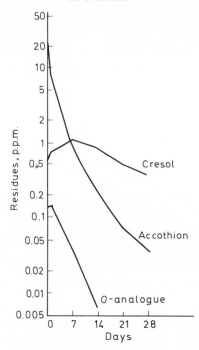

Figure 9. Residues of fenitrothion found in field corn after a spray application of ®Accothion* (2 lb a.i./acre). Reproduced by kind permission of the *Journal of Economic Entomology*[49] and the authors.

showing the association of the radioactivity with phenol-containing materials (among others, phenyl-β-glucoside, an α-glucoside, a phenyl-β-glycuronoside and a phenylsulphate); the oxon hardly occurred, and phenyl methyl phosphonate could not be traced with certainty. These studies are interesting because they shed light on various aspects of phenol conjugation from both methodical and biochemical angles. Analytical studies of *VCS-506* (®Phosvel) were confined to the oxon and the free phenol[50] which occur in known relations to each other. The same holds for *trichloronate*[66]. However, we have further investigated the fate of the phosphoric acid portion in the case of trichloronate[65]. The analyses on plants using the method developed by Möllhoff[64] are still in progress but I should nevertheless like to demonstrate the scope of these investigations by giving the results obtained from a degradation study in soil (*Figure 10*).

All the compounds presented in *Figure 10* can be extracted quantitatively from plants and soil and determined by gas chromatography[64]; only ethoxyethane phosphonic acid, ethane phosphonic acid and the phenol occur as non-bound ionic metabolites. Although these compounds have no toxicological relevance, their determination is not only of academic interest. They can, for example, be of significance for metabolite studies or also in cases where a certain compound cannot be determined even by gas chroma-

---

* Registered trademark of American Cyanamid Co.

R = (structure: benzene ring with three Cl substituents) — Cl

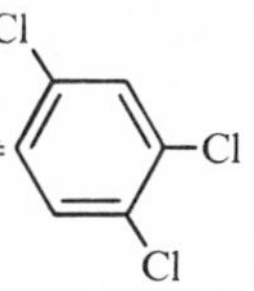

n.d. = none detectable

Days after applic.	EtO, Et, O—R (P=S)	EtO, Et, O—R (P=O)	HO, Et, O—R (P=S)	HO, Et, O—R (P=O)	HO—R
0	5500	n.d.	n.d.	n.d.	180
30	4860	n.d.	n.d.	n.d.	250
60	2340	trace	n.d.	n.d.	280
120	1120	n.d.	n.d.	n.d.	70

Days after applic.	EtO, Et, OH (P=S)	EtO, Et, OH (P=O)	HO, Et, OH (P=S)	HO, Et, OH (P=O)	Total P (%)
0	n.d.	60	n.d.	90	= 100
30	n.d.	80	n.d.	50	75
60	n.d.	80	n.d.	130	40
120	n.d.	< 10	n.d.	60	20

Figure 10. Residues of trichloronate and its metabolites in soil (p.p.b.).

tography, or if for screening purposes in the enforcement of food legislation it is required to establish whether insecticidal organophosphates are generally present or not. This development is apparently in progress in some laboratories[2, 42, 81, 82, 87]; for a more detailed discussion, see ref. 34. It will be noted from the results demonstrated here, that in the course of the experiment it was not possible to recover the total amount of the originally applied active ingredient in the form of parent compound and phosphorus-containing metabolites. Probably part of the phosphorus is present in the form of components which are bound by adsorption. Work is in progress to clarify this phenomenon.

Very interesting results concerning the metabolism of phosphonates were recently reported for *N-2790* (®Dyfonate)[56]. The studies were made on potatoes following treatment of the soil; the compound was labelled in the ethoxy group and in the ring. The metabolites found were the parent compound [15], the oxon [3], ethoxyethane phosphonic acid [2100] and ethoxyethane phosphonothioic acid [600] as well as their methyl esters, also methyl phenyl sulphoxide and methyl phenyl sulphone [1500]* as well as sulphates and glycoside conjugates of them, possibly partly in ring-hydroxylated form. Ethoxyethane phosphonic acid was the principal metabolite.

---

* The figures given in [ ] represent the acute oral toxicity values for rats expressed in mg/kg, and are rounded off.

ALIPHATIC PHOSPHONATES* AND VINYL PHOSPHATES
(*Figure 11*)

As expected, the unanimous result of the studies on aromatic phosphonates is that the P—C—bond of the phosphonates remains intact in the plant.

Following application of *trichlorfon* on cotton, dimethyl phosphate was found[12] but dichlorvos was also detected as a metabolite so that the

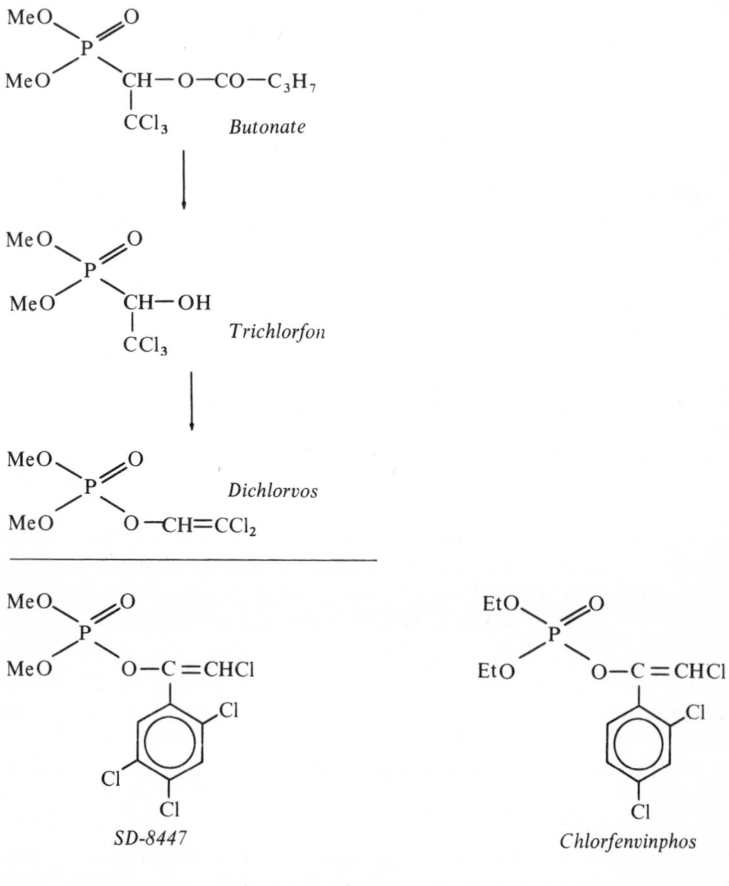

Figure 11.

question whether dimethyl phosphate is produced by direct hydrolysis of the P—C bond or by hydrolysis after the rearrangement of trichlorfon to dichlorvos was not resolved. These studies also did not clarify the structure of the principal metabolite cleavable with β-glucosidase. O-desmethyl-trichlorfon and O-desmethyl-dichlorvos also occurred. No O-desmethyl compounds were observed to be formed in the degradation of *butonate*[22].

---

* See footnote on page 21.

In contrast to its fate in dichlorvos, the chlorovinyl group does not remain intact in chlorfenvinphos which is closely related to SD-8477 (®Gardona). A major breakdown product was a sugar conjugate of the 1-dichlorophenyl-ethan-1-ol; a small amount of the corresponding acetophenone $[C_6H_3Cl_2 \cdot C(O)CH_3]$ as well as traces of the O-desmethyl compound were also formed[5]. There was also some evidence for conversion of the *trans* (β) to the *cis* (α) isomer. The breakdown is a detoxification process since the oral LD_{50} values for rats are 30 mg/kg (parent compound), more than 1 000 mg/kg (des-ethyl), and more than 800 mg/kg (..ethan-1-ol; ... aceto-phenone)[4]; all the mentioned transformation products and metabolites can be determined by gas chromatography[4]. In the case of *SD-8447* it was shown that weathered residues contained a large proportion of *trans* (low melting) to *cis* isomer than fresh residues[29].

CARBOXYLIC ACID DERIVATIVES OF DIMETHYL DITHIOPHOSPHORIC ACID (AS ESTERS OR AMIDES)
(*Figure 12*)

Koivistoinen and Aalto recently reported on the physical, chemical and biochemical behaviour of *malathion*[47]. In their report, they also referred to a research project which is being conducted at Helsinki University with the object of furnishing further information on the metabolism of malathion

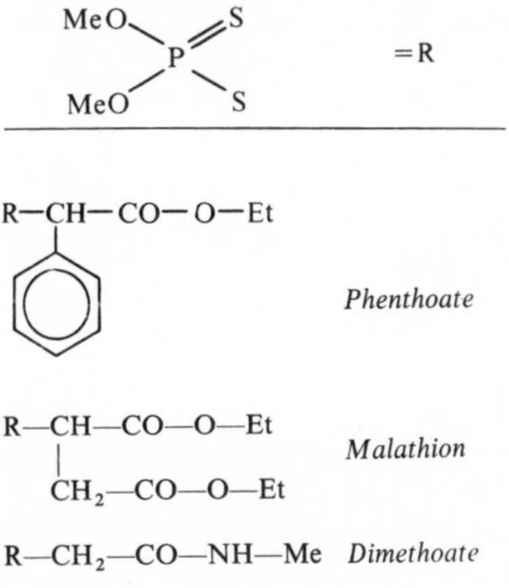

Figure 12.

because several metabolites have still not been identified. The results of these studies which are being carried out with P-, S-, C- and tritium-labelled active ingredient are being awaited with interest. Brief reference should also be made here to studies of theoretical interest undertaken by Dauter-man and co-workers[18, 41] who investigated the affinity and phosphorylation constants of the optical isomers of O,O-diethyl malathion and malaoxon. The biologically produced half-ester which is also termed malathion mono-

25

acid was identified as malathion α-monoacid, i.e. the 1-carboxy-2-carbethoxy-ethyl derivative[17]. Both the monocarboxylic and dicarboxylic acid can be determined by GLC[43].

The ester cleavage known for malathion was not observed with *phenthoate*[78].

Menzer and co-workers[51, 59] succeeded in identifying further metabolites of *dimethoate* from beans. Previously the oxon, *O*-desmethyl-dimethoate and the dimethoate and *O*-methoate carboxylic acids ('thiocarboxy' and 'oxycarboxy' compound) had been known but now the *N*-desmethyl and the *N*-hydroxymethyl compounds of dimethoate and *O*-methoate have also been found, plus another metabolite not yet identified. The *N*-desmethyl compounds are comparable with the corresponding *N*-methyl compounds with respect to intraperitoneal toxicity[51].

CROTONIC ACID DERIVATIVES OF DIMETHYLPHOSPHORIC ACID (*Figure 13*)

Mevinphos, like all members of this group, can occur in two isomeric forms. The *cis*- (α-) form is much more biologically active than the corresponding β-isomer (*trans*-crotonate). Winterlin and co-workers[93] published what is apparently the first GLC residue method capable of detecting the two isomers independently. A comparison with the cholinesterase inhibition that was used a lot earlier showed that, enzymatically, practically only the α-isomer is determined. On the other hand, the β-isomer appears to have a much longer residual effect. The studies on the optical isomers of malaoxon mentioned earlier also included the geometric isomers of mevinphos. The 20-fold difference in the inhibitory power of the *cis*-isomer was largely attributed to the difference in the phosphorylation rate[18].

As far as I know, no studies have been reported about the metabolism of *SD-4294* (®Ciodrin) in plants.

Just as with dimethoate, *N*-hydroxymethyl compounds of the amides *monocrotophos* and *dicrotophos* occur in the plant. In addition, dicrotophos is desmethylated to monocrotophos from which the unsubstituted amide is formed; only this amide is more toxic than the two parent compounds (intraperitoneal toxicity for female mice of 3 mg/kg as against 14 and 18 mg/kg for dicrotophos and monocrotophos, respectively[58, 59]). β-Glucose conjugates of the two *N*-hydroxymethyl compounds were also found[38]. All the metabolites I have mentioned can be determined by gas chromatography[38] or by thin-layer chromatography[39]. Unfortunately the reports on these studies contained no information on the quantitative interrelationships of the different metabolites in the plant.

Metabolites of *phosphamidon* found by Bull and co-workers were the *N*-hydroxyethyl form, the *N*-desethyl form and the *O*-desmethyl form[11]. The compounds were radiolabelled either with ^{14}C at the methylvinyl and carbonyl positions, or with ^{32}P, and the *cis*- and *trans*-isomers were compared. Although both isomers were converted to similar oxidative and hydrolytic metabolites, the rates of formation were somewhat different, the faster rate of oxidative *N*-desalkylation of *cis*-phosphamidon being

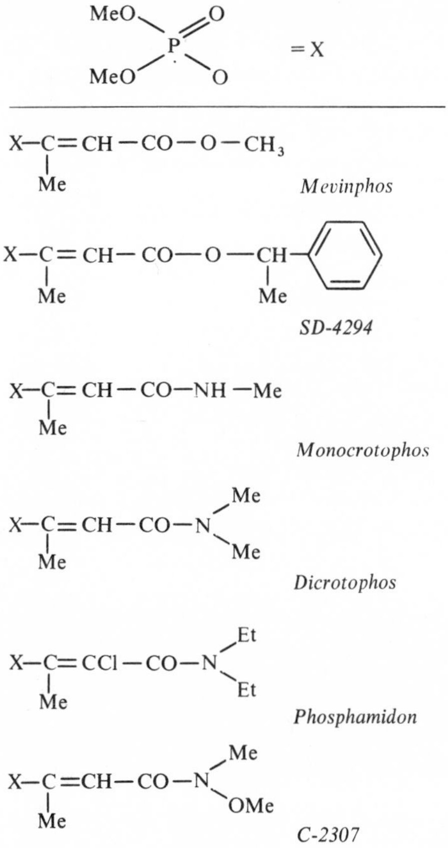

$$\begin{array}{c} MeO \\ \diagdown \\ P \\ \diagup \quad \diagdown \\ MeO \qquad O \end{array} \!\!\!\! = O \qquad = X$$

X—C=CH—CO—O—CH₃
|
Me
Mevinphos

X—C=CH—CO—O—CH—⟨phenyl⟩
| |
Me   Me
SD-4294

X—C=CH—CO—NH—Me
|
Me
Monocrotophos

X—C=CH—CO—N⟨Me, Me⟩
|
Me
Dicrotophos

X—C=CCl—CO—N⟨Et, Et⟩
|
Me
Phosphamidon

X—C=CH—CO—N⟨Me, OMe⟩
|
Me
C-2307

Figure 13.

particularly apparent. Five further metabolites were detected but not identified; some of them contained no phosphorus. In view of the results obtained with other crotonic amides, it is conceivable that these unknowns could quite well be accounted for by any of a number of transformation products already identified for the other crotonic amides. Menzer and Dauterman very recently published some further results[59] but it is not evident from their report whether the studies were made on animals, plants or soil*. The same holds for the metabolism of the newly developed Geigy compound *C-2307* which is closely related to dicrotophos[59].

There is no doubt that in the course of time these findings on the crotonic amide phosphates will complement each other to form a complete picture

---

* Dr Menzer has since kindly informed me that their new results were obtained from experiments with rats and liver microsomes. These findings have been submitted for publication in *J. Agr. Food Chem.*

common to all, and that some of them will then also touch upon the problems pertaining to the metabolism of other carboxylic amide phosphates. Results so far available indicate that as far as changes of the alkyl substituents at the nitrogen atom are concerned, crotonic amide phosphates already have something in common with insecticidal carbamates. And, as Menzer and Dauterman[59] pointed out, an understanding of the metabolism of compounds like C-2307 should enable us to understand the mechanism of oxidative desalkylation of other similar compounds, especially among the substituted phenylurea herbicides, as well as elucidating the actual mechanism of oxidative desalkylation.

Like all speakers who are compelled to cover a broad subject like this in such a short time, I do not doubt that in my review I have also touched upon points which seem trivial to some yet perhaps important to others. Therefore, I should like to close by making some comments which to me seem trivial and important at the same time.

The research work undertaken in the last few years has enormously broadened our knowledge of the behaviour of organophosphorus pesticides. From the scientific standpoint, this is most pleasing. But the pleasure does not remain unspoiled. In many instances, it will not be possible to regard the results of such investigations as being representative of the behaviour of the active ingredient. Sometimes transformation products are found which one would expect to be present also with a compound of similar structure, but which actually do not occur (e.g. the desmethyl compound of bromophos could be detected but not that of iodofenphos). There can be only one of two explanations for this: such compounds were not found due to methodical reasons, or the metabolism may differ very greatly from plant to plant. The first explanation seems to be the more probable one. An observation made in most investigations, however, is that the more toxic oxons occur only to a limited extent. This, in turn, is not surprising in view of their well-known instability on and in the plant; this phenomenon becomes especially obvious when, for comparison with the parent compound, oxons are applied to a plant in similar amounts and the degradation of both compounds is then studied. Desalkylation, on the other hand, which is repeatedly encountered also in plants, is usually accompanied by a many thousandfold reduction of the cholinesterase-inhibiting power[1].

Due to the never-ending development of new detector types, gas chromatography today enables us to find residues where previously there was 'none', and similarly isotope techniques enable us to find more and more metabolites where previously there was 'none'. Ultimately, we find ourselves confronted with the question what we are to do with the fruits of such eager research. It will soon be time for us to look back at what was once the starting point of it all, namely the endeavour to find efficient means of protecting crops and yet to keep our foods free from hazards. It is sometimes hard to see the real connection between the discovery of say a new oxy-carboxy compound and the realization of this after all humanitarian objective. I can do no more than draw attention, in all modesty, to the concern with which a residue analyst views this development.

APPENDIX

Tradenames of products are given in this paper only in cases where there is no generally known common name for the respective active ingredient. The given registered tradenames are as follows:

®Azodrin (Shell), ®Bidrin (Shell), ®Ciodrin (Shell), ®Colep (Monsanto), ®Dyfonate (Stauffer), ®Gardona (Shell), ®Imidan (Stauffer), ®Nemacur P (Bayer), ®Phosvel (Velsicol), ® Supracide (Geigy).

Chemical names of pesticides mentioned in text

azinphos-ethyl	S-(3,4-dihydro-4-oxobenzo[d]-[1,2,3]-triazin-3-ylmethyl) diethyl phosphorothiolothionate
azinphos-methyl	S-(3,4-dihydro-4-oxobenzo[d]-[1,2,3]-triazin-3-ylmethyl) dimethyl phosphorothiolothionate
Bay 30 237	methyl 4-methylthiophenyl methylphosphonothionate
Bay 68 138	ethyl 3-methyl-4-methylthiophenyl isopropylphosphoramidate
bromophos	4-bromo-2,5-dichlorophenyl dimethyl phosphorothionate
butonate	dimethyl 1-butyryloxy-2,2,2-trichloroethylphosphonate
C-2307	dimethyl cis-2-(N-methoxy-N-methylcarbamoyl)-1-methyl-vinyl phosphate
chlorfenvinphos	2-chloro-1-(2,4-dichlorophenyl)vinyl diethyl phosphate
CP-40	4-nitrophenyl phenyl methylphosphonothionate
diazinon	diethyl 2-isopropyl-6-methyl-4-pyrimidinyl phosphorothionate
dichlorvos	2,2-dichlorovinyl dimethyl phosphate
dicrotophos	dimethyl cis-2-dimethylcarbamoyl-1-methyl-vinyl phosphate
dimethoate	dimethyl S-(N-methylcarbamoylmethyl) phosphorothiolothionate
fenitrothion	dimethyl 3-methyl-4-nitrophenyl phosphorothionate
fensulfothion	diethyl 4-(methylsulphinyl)phenyl phosphorothionate
fenthion	dimethyl 3-methyl-4-methylthiophenyl phosphorothionate
GC-6506	dimethyl 4-methylthiophenyl phosphate
GS-13 005	S-(2,3-dihydro-5-methoxy-2-oxo-1,3,4-thiadiazol-3-ylmethyl) dimethyl phosphorothiolothionate
iodofenphos	2,5-dichloro-4-iodophenyl dimethyl phosphorothionate
malathion	S-[1,2-di(ethoxycarbonyl)ethyl] dimethyl phosphorothiolothionate
menazon	S-(4,6-diamino-1,3,5-triazin-2-ylmethyl) dimethylphosphorothiolothionate
mevinphos	2-methoxycarbonyl-1-methylvinyl dimethyl phosphate
monocrotophos	dimethyl cis-1-methyl-2-methylcarbamoyl-vinyl phosphate
N-2790	ethyl S-phenyl ethylphosphonothiolothionate
parathion	diethyl 4-nitrophenyl phosphorothionate
phenthoate	S-α-ethoxycarbonylbenzyl dimethyl phosphorothiolothionate

phosalone	*S*-(6-chloro-2-oxobenzoxazolin-3-yl)methyl diethyl phosphorothiolothionate
phosphamidon	2-chloro-2-diethylcarbamoyl-1-methyl-vinyl dimethyl phosphate
phoxim	α-(diethoxythiophosphoryloxyimino)-phenylacetonitrile
R-1504	dimethyl phthalimidomethyl phosphorothiolothionate
SD-4294	dimethyl *cis*-1-methyl-2-(1-phenyl-ethoxycarbonyl)-vinyl phosphate
SD-8447	2-chloro-1-(2,4,5-trichlorophenyl)vinyl dimethyl phosphate
TEPP	*bis*-*O,O*-diethylphosphoric anhydride
trichloronate	ethyl 2,4,5-trichlorophenyl ethylphosphonothionate
trichlorfon	dimethyl 2,2,2-trichloro-1-hydroxyethylphosphonate
VCS-506	4-bromo-2,5-dichlorophenyl methyl phenylphosphonothionate

REFERENCES

[1] A. H. Aharoni and R. D. O'Brien. *Biochemistry*, **7**, 1538 (1968).
[2] J. Askew, J. H. Ruzicka and B. B. Wheals, *J. Chromatogr.* **41**, 180 (1969).
[3] E. Benjamini, R. L. Metcalf and T. R. Fukuto, *J. Econ. Ent.* **52**, 94 and 99 (1959).
[4] K. I. Beynon, M. J. Edwards, K. Elgar and A. N. Wright, *J. Sci. Food Agr.* **19**, 302 (1968).
[5] K. I. Beynon and A. N. Wright, *J. Sci. Food Agr.* **19**, 146 (1968).
[6] M. C. Bowman, M. Beroza and D. B. Leuck, *J. Agr. Food Chem.* **16**, 796 (1968).
[7] M. C. Bowman, D. B. Leuck, J. C. Johnson Jr and F. E. Knox, *J. Econ. Ent.* **63**, 1523 (1970).
[8] M. C. Bowman and J. R. Young, *J. Econ. Ent.* **62**, 1468 (1969).
[9] U. E. Brady and B. W. Arthur, *J. Econ. Ent.* **54**, 1232 (1961).
[10] D. L. Bull, *J. Agr. Food Chem.* **16**, 610 (1968).
[11] D. L. Bull, D. A. Lindquist and R. R. Grabbe, *J. Econ. Ent.* **60**, 332 (1967).
[12] D. L. Bull and R. L. Ridgway, *J. Agr. Food Chem.* **17**, 837 (1969).
[13] D. L. Bull and R. A. Stokes, *J. Agr. Food Chem.* **18**, 1134 (1970).
[14] A. Calderbank, *J. Chem. Soc.* C, 56 (1966).
[15] J. E. Casida and L. Lykken, *Ann. Rev. Plant Physiol.* **20**, 607 (1969).
[16] J. E. Cassidy, D. P. Ryskiewich and R. T. Murphy, *J. Agr. Food Chem.* **17**, 558 (1969).
[17] P. R. Chen, W. P. Tucker and W. C. Dauterman, *J. Agr. Food Chem.* **17**, 86 (1969).
[18] Y. C. Chiu and W. C. Dauterman, *Biochem. Pharmacol.* **18**, 359 (1969).
[19] V. M. Clark, D. W. Hutchinson, A. J. Kirby and S. G. Warren, *Angew. Chem.* **76**, 704 (1964).
[20] D. L. Colinese and H. J. Terry, *Chem. Ind.* (*London*), 1507 (1968).
[21] D. G. Crosby, *Residue Rev.* **25**, 1 (1969).
[22] W. Dedek, *Z. Naturforsch.* **23b**, 504 (1968).
[23] J. Desmoras, F. Dubosq, M. Laurent, I. W. Bales and A. Guardigli, *Phytiat.-Phytopharm.* **4**, 277 (1968).
[24] J. Desmoras, M. Sauli and B. Terlain, *Phytiat.-Phytopharm.* **4**, 263 (1968).
[25] G. Dräger, 'Untersuchungen über den Metabolismus von Bay 77 488'. Leverkusen-Bayerwerk, 28 August 1969 (unpublished); 'Untersuchungen zum Metabolismus von Bay 77 488 (II)'. Leverkusen-Bayerwerk, 12 January 1970 (unpublished).
[26] D. O. Eberle and D. Novak, *J. Assoc. Offic. Analyt. Chem.*, **52**, 1067 (1969).
[27] M. Eto and H. Ohkawa, in: R. D. O'Brien and I. Yamamoto, *Biochemical Toxicology of Insecticides*, pp 93–104. Academic Press: New York and London (1970).
[28] L. J. Everett and R. R. Gronberg, Chemagro Corp., Research Dept., *Rep. No. 21513*, Kansas City, USA (November 1967).
[29] J. E. Fahey, P. E. Nelson and D. L. Ballee, *J. Agr. Food Chem.* **18**, 866 (1970).

[30] FAO/WHO *Pesticide Residues.* Report of the 1967 Joint Meeting of the FAO Working Party and the WHO Expert Committee. *Wld Hlth Org. Techn. Rep. Ser. No. 391,* 21 (1968).

[31] FAO/WHO *Wld Hlth Org. Techn. Rep. Ser. No. 417,* 7 (1969).

[32] Ch. Fest and K.-J. Schmidt, in: R. Wegler, *Chemie der Pflanzenschutz- und Schädlingsbekämpfungsmittel,* Vol. I, pp 246–453. Springer: Berlin, Heidelberg and New York (1970).

[33] H. Frehse, in: R. Wegler, *Chemie der Pflanzenschutz- und Schädlingsbekämpfungsmittel,* Vol. II, pp 433–515. Springer: Berlin, Heidelberg and New York (1970).

[34] H. Frehse, in *Methods in Residue Analysis,* edited by A. S. Tahori; pp 113–128. Gordon and Breach: New York, London, Paris (1971).

[35] H. Fukuda, T. Masuda, Y. Miyahara and C. Tomizawa, *Japan. J. Appl. Entomol. Zool.* **6,** 230 (1962).

[36] L. W. Getzin, *J. Econ. Ent.* **60,** 505 (1967).

[37] L. W. Getzin and I. Rosefield, *J. Econ. Ent.* **59,** 512 (1966).

[38] B. Y. Giang and H. F. Beckman, *J. Agr. Food Chem.* **16,** 899 (1968).

[39] B. Y. Giang and H. Beckman, *J. Agr. Food Chem.* **17,** 63 (1969).

[40] H. M. Gomaa, I. H. Suffet and S. D. Faust, *Residue Rev.* **29,** 171 (1969).

[41] A. Hassan and W. C. Dauterman, *Biochem. Pharmacol.* **17,** 1431 (1968).

[42] P. S. Jaglan, R. B. March, T. R. Fukuto and F. A. Gunther, *J. Agr. Food Chem.* **18,** 809 (1970).

[42a] F. R. Johannsen and C. O. Knowles, *J. Econ. Ent.* **63,** 693 (1970).

[43] A. M. Kadoum, *J. Agr. Food Chem.* **17,** 1178 (1969).

[44] A. S. H. Kansouh and T. L. Hopkins, *J. Agr. Food Chem.* **16,** 446 (1968).

[45] D. B. Katague and C. A. Anderson, *Bull. Environment. Contam. Toxicol.* **2,** 228 (1967).

[46] A. M. Khasawinah, Chemagro Corp., Research Dept, *Rep. No. 29142,* Kansas City, USA (January 1971).

[47] P. Koivistoinen and H. Aalto, in: *Nuclear Techniques for Studying Pesticide Residue Problems,* pp 11–21. International Atomic Energy Agency: Vienna (1970).

[48] D. B. Leuck and M. C. Bowman, *J. Econ. Ent.* **61,** 1594 (1968).

[49] D. B. Leuck and M. C. Bowman, *J. Econ. Ent.* **62,** 1282 (1969).

[50] D. B. Leuck, M. C. Bowman and J. M. McWilliams, *J. Econ. Ent.* **63,** 1346 (1970).

[51] G. W. Lucier and R. E. Menzer, *J. Agr. Food Chem.* **18,** 698 (1970).

[52] L. J. Magill and L. J. Everett, Chemagro Corp., Research Dept, *Rep. No. 18636,* Kansas City, USA (August 1966).

[53] G. J. Marco and E. G. Jaworski, *J. Agr. Food Chem.* **12,** 305 (1964).

[54] H. Martin, *Pesticide Manual.* British Crop Protection Council (1968).

[54a] T. Masuda and H. Fukuda, *Botyu-Kagaku,* **35,** 134 (1970).

[55] A. M. Mattson, R. A. Kahrs and R. T. Murphy, *J. Agr. Food Chem.* **17,** 565 (1969).

[56] J. B. McBain, L. J. Hoffman and J. J. Menn, *J. Agr. Food Chem.* **18,** 1139 (1970).

[57] J. J. Menn and J. B. McBain, *J. Agr. Food Chem.* **12,** 162 (1964).

[58] R. E. Menzer and J. E. Casida, *J. Agr. Food Chem.* **13,** 102 (1965).

[59] R. E. Menzer and W. C. Dauterman, *J. Agr. Food Chem.* **18,** 1031 (1970).

[60] R. L. Metcalf, T. R. Fukuto and M. Y. Winton, *Bull. Wld. Hlth Org.* **29,** 219 (1963).

[61] R. L. Metcalf and R. B. March, *J. Econ. Ent.* **46,** 288 (1953).

[62] L. P. Miller, *Contrib. Boyce Thompson Inst.* **11,** 271 (1940).

[63] E. Möllhoff, *Pflanzenschutz-Nachr. Bayer.* **21,** 331 (1968).

[64] E. Möllhoff, 'Methode zur Extraktion aus Pflanzen und Boden, zur Trennung und zum gaschromatographischen Nachweis von Organophosphorverbindungen und ihren Um- und Abbauprodukten'. *Vorläufiger Bericht,* Leverkusen-Bayerwerk (3 September 1970).

[65] E. Möllhoff, unpublished 1971a, cf. in ref. 34.

[66] E. Möllhoff, unpublished, 1971b.

[67] W. B. Neely, W. E. Allison, W. B. Crummett, K. Kauer and W. Reifschneider, *J. Agr. Food Chem.* **18,** 45 (1970).

[68] D. L. Nelson, Chemagro Corp., Research Dept, *Rep. No. 21488,* Kansas City, USA (December 1967).

[69] L. L. Nelson and E. W. Hamilton, *J. Econ. Ent.* **63,** 874 (1970).

[70] H. Niessen, H. Tietz and H. Frehse, *Pflanzenschutz-Nachr. Bayer.* **15,** 129 (1962).

[71] R. D. O'Brien, *J. Econ. Ent.* **49,** 484 (1956).

[72] T. J. Olson, Chemagro Corp., Research Dept, *Rep. No.25151,* Kansas City, USA (June 1969).

[73] J. R. Pardue, E. A. Hansen, R. P. Barron and J.-Y. T. Chen, *J. Agr. Food Chem.* **18,** 405 (1970).

[74] C. E. Polan, R. A. Sandy and J. T. Huber, *J. Dairy Sci.* **52,** 1296 (1969).

[75] J. W. Ralls and A. Cortes, *J. Econ. Ent.* **59**, 1296 (1966).
[76] J. W. Ralls, D. R. Gilmore and A. Cortes, *J. Agr. Food Chem.* **14**, 387 (1966).
[77] H. T. Reynolds, R. L. Metcalf and T. R. Fukuto, *J. Econ. Ent.* **59**, 293 (1966).
[78] R. Santi, M. Radice and P. Martinotti, *Chim. Ind. (Milano)*, **50**, 221 (1968).
[79] K.-J. Schmidt, *Pflanzenschutzberichte (Wien)*, **39**, 207 (1969).
[80] N. Sethunathan and T. Yoshida, *J. Agr. Food Chem.* **17**, 1192 (1969).
[81] M. T. Shafik, D. Bradway, F. J. Biros and H. F. Enos, *J. Agr. Food Chem.* **18**, 1174 (1970).
[82] M. T. Shafik and H. F. Enos, *J. Agr. Food Chem.* **17**, 1186 (1969).
[83] M. Siewierski and K. Helrich, *J. Assoc. Offic. Analyt. Chem.* **53**, 514 (1970).
[84] E. Y. Spencer, 'Guide to the chemicals used in crop protection'. Canada Department of Agriculture, *Publication No. 1093*, 5th ed., Queen's Printer: Ottawa (1968).
[85] C. M. Stewart, *Nature, London*, **186**, 374 (1960).
[86] M. Stiasni, W. Deckers, K. Schmidt and H. Simon, *J. Agr. Food Chem.* **17**, 1017 (1969).
[87] L. E. St John Jr and D. J. Lisk, *J. Agr. Food Chem.* **16**, 408 (1968).
[88] J. S. Thornton, Chemagro Corp., Research Dept, *Rep. No. 23316*, Kansas City, USA (September 1968).
[89] H. Tietz, R. L. Metcalf and T. R. Fukuto, *Höfchen-Briefe*, **10**, (Engl. Ed.) 279 (1957).
[90] C. Tomizawa, H. Fukuda, T. Masuda and Y. Miyahara, *Japan. J. Appl. Entomol. Zool.* **6**, 237 (1962).
[91] T. B. Waggoner, Chemagro Corp., Research Dept, *Rep. No. 25519*, Kansas City, USA (August 1969).
[92] L. E. Wendel and D. L. Bull, *J. Agr. Food Chem.* **18**, 420 (1970).
[93] W. Winterlin, C. Mourer and H. Beckman, *J. Agr. Food Chem.* **18**, 401 (1970).

TERMINAL RESIDUES OF ORGANOPHOSPHORUS INSECTICIDES IN ANIMALS

H. O. ESSER

Ciba-Geigy Ltd, Basle, Switzerland

ABSTRACT

The metabolic fate of the organophosphorus ester insecticides and the occurrence of their metabolites as final residues in animals is reviewed. In the first section reactions of toxicological relevance such as desulphuration, thio ether oxidation and N-dealkylation, are discussed. The second section summarizes the biochemical reactions by which animals get rid of these foreign chemicals. Reactions like cleavage of different phosphorus and carboxy ester or amide bonds and nitro group reduction are considered. Some links between physiological and pure chemical reactivity are outlined. In the third section the metabolism and the residue behaviour of groups of compounds, related by chemical structure or reactivity, are discussed on a comparative basis. The necessity for the adequate consideration of the mutual interdependence of metabolism, residue analysis and toxicology in the field of pesticide residues is stressed.

INTRODUCTION

It is intended in this Symposium to review the present knowledge of the terminal residues to which pesticides may give rise in our living environment. Taking into account the tremendous amount of information gathered up to now it is evident that such brief reviews of each of the important classes of pesticides must remain fragmentary. For even concentrating the lectures on single systems such as soil, plants and animals cannot prevent the imposition of strict limitations with respect to the number of representative compounds to be selected, and details of information to be given.

This holds true specially for the group of organic phosphorus acid esters, for Schrader's original finding of their insecticidal properties provided a concept of utmost variability for the chemist. Thus thousands of compounds have been synthesized in the past three decades and even those finally reaching the market represent an impressive number.

Despite this necessity for limitation full attention must be given to the mutual interdependence of metabolism, residue analysis and toxicology. It is evident that the conservative definition of the term 'residue', as that part of the parent compound present at a given time after application of the pesticide, no longer satisfies the requirements of today. Instead, the metabolic behaviour of the pesticide must be known, so that a qualitative and quantitative review of the pattern of parent and metabolites is at our disposal. This is valid for all types of compound, since it is not possible by looking even at a simple molecule or a fragment of it from a chemical viewpoint to predict the absence of a toxicological problem. If we recall that actually all residue work is done to guarantee the safety of our daily food it is obvious that we have to

C

have this knowledge of every foodstuff. Only then will we be in a position to evaluate a potential toxicological risk. An advantage of great practical value accompanying such a close association of metabolism and residue analysis is that it is possible to evaluate, quantitatively and qualitatively, all analytical procedures for their efficiency by means of the isotopically labelled parent and metabolites of the metabolism study.

Consequently, a synoptic compilation of quantitative residue data is dispensed with in this lecture in favour of a more qualitative consideration of the topic, referring to comparative aspects whenever possible. The term 'terminal residue' is understood as that part of a pesticide which is present in the form of parent or metabolites in any organ of an animal at the time of investigation. Residues eliminated with the excreta are also considered because they give valuable information on the metabolic processes taking place.

Generally, one has to realize that the statement 'terminal', for a residue in animals, is far less exactly defined than in plants or soil, since the presence of the said residue strongly depends on whether or not the excretion has already come to an end. This is valid especially for metabolites which may be stored more easily in plants, for example in the form of glucosides, than in animals where a potent excretory mechanism is available.

This problem can possibly be overcome by defining more standardized conditions for the animal experiments, as are already established for many analytical procedures. One can imagine that three types of standard experiments should be sufficient to satisfy our requirements, namely one each for oral and dermal application of the pesticide as well as one for prolonged feeding of pesticide-treated forage or silage. In this way a real comparison of different pesticides would be possible and, automatically, the basis for the definition of the term 'terminal' would be given. And, I can assure you, the work of later reviewers would be greatly facilitated.

Looking now at the objects of our discussion, the animals, we can distinguish between those being exposed directly or indirectly to phosphorus esters during routine agricultural practice and those being used as models in the laboratory. The first group primarily attracts our attention. Here we find the ruminants, the monogastric animals and the birds treated with phosphorus esters for the control of ecto- and endo-parasites or feeding on pasture or crops originally treated with this type of insecticide. Systemically acting phosphorus esters have to be mentioned here, too; for instance those fed to ruminants or birds to suppress larval development of flies in their manure. Finally, hygienic measures such as stall disinfection may give rise to insecticide residues in these animals.

These pesticide applications are intended and necessary. They increase and improve man's food production. Pesticide residues caused by incidental contamination of farm or wild animals will not be considered here. Some exceptions in the case of wild life will be mentioned for fish, because of their importance as a foodstuff.

The pesticides mentioned in this review have been selected without regard for their economic importance. Their selection was made simply because of the availability of results, suitable enough to serve as examples, for the comparative considerations intended.

Let us now look more closely at the reactivity of the phosphorus esters under physiological conditions and at some connecting links to pure chemical reactivity. Mechanistic considerations will not be included in this discussion. We will consider only some of the great variability to be observed among chemically related compounds or between the reaction products actually found as metabolites and those which are to be expected from a chemical point of view.

Relating our topic with toxicology we are confronted with two types of reactions. The first type leads to reaction products in which the toxicity of the parent compound is preserved or even increased. The second one represents a real detoxication, as the cholinesterase-inhibiting properties and, consequently, the acute toxicity of the parent molecule are completely lost.

REACTIONS OF PHOSPHORUS ESTERS RESULTING IN TOXICATION

The toxicating reactions are oxidative in character. The main representatives are shown in *Figure 1* in a schematic manner giving only starting and end products.

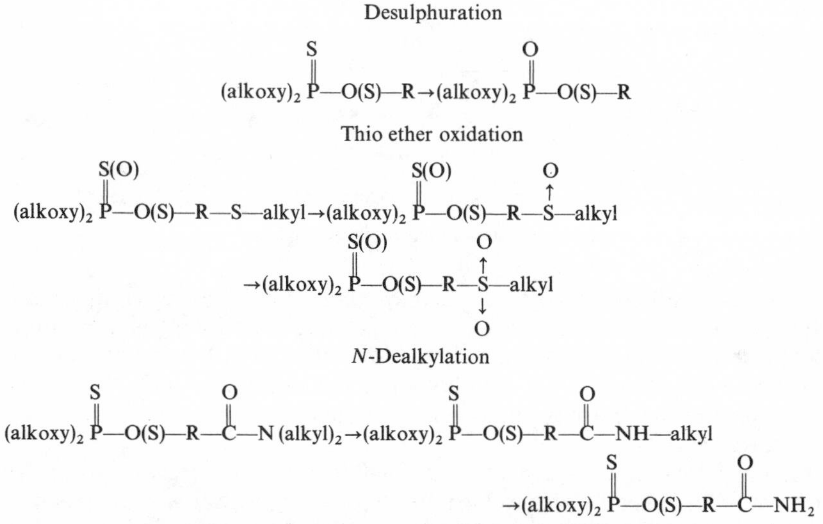

Desulphuration

$$(alkoxy)_2 \overset{S}{\underset{\|}{P}}-O(S)-R \rightarrow (alkoxy)_2 \overset{O}{\underset{\|}{P}}-O(S)-R$$

Thio ether oxidation

$$(alkoxy)_2 \overset{S(O)}{\underset{\|}{P}}-O(S)-R-S-alkyl \rightarrow (alkoxy)_2 \overset{S(O)}{\underset{\|}{P}}-O(S)-R-\overset{O}{\underset{}{S}}-alkyl$$

$$\rightarrow (alkoxy)_2 \overset{S(O)}{\underset{\|}{P}}-O(S)-R-\overset{O}{\underset{O}{S}}-alkyl$$

N-Dealkylation

$$(alkoxy)_2 \overset{S}{\underset{\|}{P}}-O(S)-R-\overset{O}{\underset{\|}{C}}-N(alkyl)_2 \rightarrow (alkoxy)_2 \overset{S}{\underset{\|}{P}}-O(S)-R-\overset{O}{\underset{\|}{C}}-NH-alkyl$$

$$\rightarrow (alkoxy)_2 \overset{S}{\underset{\|}{P}}-O(S)-R-\overset{O}{\underset{\|}{C}}-NH_2$$

Figure 1. Reactions of phosphorus esters resulting in toxication.

The first example represents the well-known desulphuration, a reaction all thionophosphates have to pass through in order to liberate their intrinsic toxicity. The term activation is widely used, pointing to the sharp increase in cholinesterase-inhibiting activity following this reaction. Increases by a factor of 10 000 and more have been observed. Simultaneously, the mammalian toxicity of the phosphate formed is enhanced, generally to a higher degree when phosphorodithioates have been activated than phosphorothioates.

Outlined next is a reaction not affecting phosphorus bonds, but the sulphur of thio ether groupings. The sulphoxides and sulphones formed under physiological conditions still represent intact phosphorus esters. But no uniform relationship is observable between the change in cholinesterase-inhibiting activity and mammalian toxicity. Successive thio ether oxidation to sulphoxide and sulphone increases cholinesterase inhibitory activity *in vitro* progressively (for Systox see ref. 1, for Di-Syston ref. 2, for Phorate ref. 3), whereas *in vivo* the situation is complicated by the simultaneous oxidation of thio ether and thionophosphates, although the two reactions often proceed at different rates. Nevertheless, metabolites both activated and sulphoxidized are the most toxic substances, thiolophosphates again being more toxic than orthophosphates.

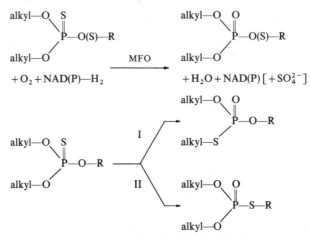

Figure 2. Activation of thionophosphates.

Whether another reaction at the thio ether group, namely sulphonium ion formation by alkylation, plays any role under physiological conditions is not known. Found as a chemical reaction with systox type compounds, it was shown to be the result of self-alkylation, increasing extremely the cholinesterase-inhibiting activity and, when applied intravenously, also mammalian toxicity[4, 5].

Finally a reaction sequence is outlined in which a series of oxidative carboxamide *N*-dealkylations lead to stepwise toxication of the reaction products without greatly changing their anticholinesterase activity. Other amides, for example phosphorus amides like Schradan, with which this activation in liver was originally found, or Dimefox, will not be considered because we are no longer confronted with them as agricultural chemicals.

Let us now revert to the phosphorothioate activation and discuss briefly what is known about the biochemical basis of desulphuration. This mechanism was first demonstrated in the early fifties[6] and later shown to take place in the microsomal fraction of the liver, requiring molecular oxygen and reduced NAD or NADP (nicotinamide–adenine dinucleotide or its phosphate) as outlined in the upper equation of *Figure 2*.

The enzyme catalysing the desulphuration is a mixed-function oxidase (MFO), an enzyme complex which is inducible, non-specifically, and capable of oxidizing an extreme variety of chemicals. It has been found in all species investigated so far[7, 8]. Although there are concrete ideas on the role of the cytochromes, flavoproteins and reduced nicotinamide–adenine nucleotides for the accomplishment of this cyclic process (for the present conception see ref. 9) we are far from understanding the activation of the molecular oxygen and the removal and further oxidation of the sulphur. All we know is that the sulphur is transiently bound to the microsomes and later excreted in the form of sulphate[10].

A reaction of great theoretical and practical importance, namely the action of synergists on this multi-enzyme complex and its consequences with respect to toxication or detoxication of phosphorus esters, will not be discussed. The interested are referred to the comprehensive review of this topic recently published[11].

Chemical isomerization must also be mentioned, because the same toxication is reached as in activation. Principally two end products can be formed, as shown schematically with the second example of *Figure 2*. Reaction I occurs preferably with compounds whose oxygen is connected with a benzene ring and requires a supply of energy in the form of heat or light to proceed to an appreciable degree within a reasonable time. Again, a pronounced increase of anticholinesterase activity follows, regardless of whether the thiono sulphur substitutes for the alkoxy oxygen or the oxygen connecting the leaving group. Whereas mammalian toxicity of the formed alkylthio derivatives may not be or may only moderately be enhanced, this increase, in the thiolo derivatives, is generally more pronounced. These isomerizations are of interest from our residue point of view when mixtures of isomers of a pesticide are applied. For the following degradation may leave either a sulphur or an oxygen atom with the leaving group thus possibly affecting a different further metabolism. The reader interested in details of these relationships is directed to the compilation of the properties of the members of the parathion and Systox (demeton) series[12, 13].

Examples for the activation *in vivo* of several thionophosphorus esters can be found in the following references: parathion[14, 15, 15a, 16], Sumithion[15, 15a], malathion[17, 18], Diazinon[14], acethion[14], dimethoate[14, 19–21], Guthion[7, 24, 26], Ronnel[26].

In the following references information is presented on comparative aspects of desulphuration with regard to chemical structure and animal species: mammalian[7, 14, 15a, 16, 22–24, 26], avian[7, 16, 24, 26], piscine[16, 24], ruminant[7] and human[25].

If we now look more closely at thio ether oxidation, we find a variety of aliphatic, mixed aliphatic–aromatic and aromatic examples of this reaction, a selection of which is listed in *Figure 3*.

As already mentioned, there is not a uniform correlation between cholinesterase inhibition and mammalian toxicity, as two examples show. The mammalian toxicity of phorate (LD_{50}, rat, subcutaneous application) increases evenly from parent to sulphoxide and sulphone, namely from 8–10 mg/kg body wt to 2–4 mg/kg and 1.8–2.0 mg/kg[27], as does the anticholinesterase activity (I_{50}) from 23×10^{-6} M to 3.7×10^{-6} M and 1.1×10^{-6} M [3]). The contrary is found for the thiono isomers of Systox and Metasystox. The mammalian toxity of their respective sulphoxides and

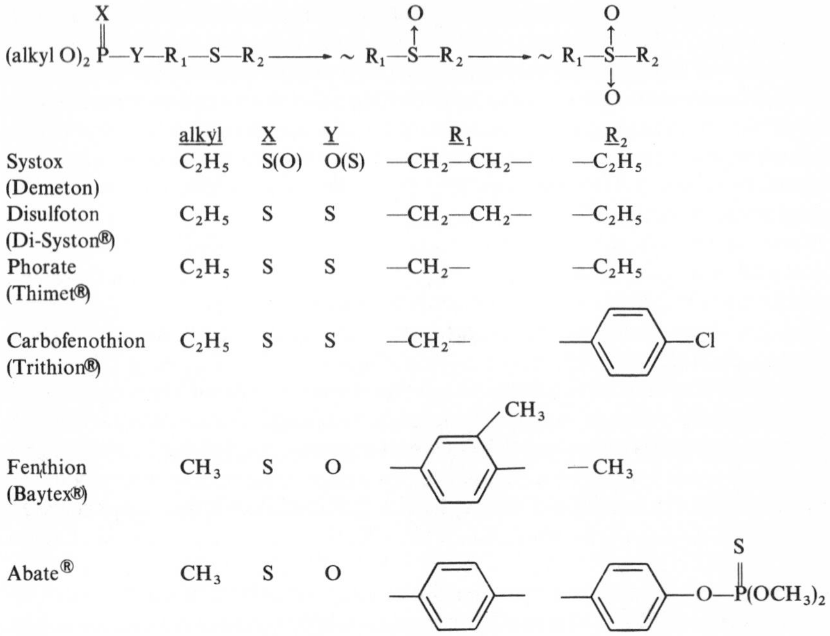

$$(\text{alkyl O})_2 \overset{X}{\underset{}{\overset{\|}{P}}}\text{—Y—R}_1\text{—S—R}_2 \longrightarrow \sim \text{R}_1\overset{O}{\underset{}{\overset{\uparrow}{\text{—S—}}}}\text{R}_2 \longrightarrow \sim \text{R}_1\overset{O}{\underset{\downarrow O}{\overset{\uparrow}{\text{—S—}}}}\text{R}_2$$

	alkyl	X	Y	R₁	R₂
Systox (Demeton)	C_2H_5	S(O)	O(S)	$-CH_2-CH_2-$	$-C_2H_5$
Disulfoton (Di-Syston®)	C_2H_5	S	S	$-CH_2-CH_2-$	$-C_2H_5$
Phorate (Thimet®)	C_2H_5	S	S	$-CH_2-$	$-C_2H_5$
Carbofenothion (Trithion®)	C_2H_5	S	S	$-CH_2-$	(benzene ring)—Cl
Fenthion (Baytex®)	CH_3	S	O	(benzene ring with CH_3)	$-CH_3$
Abate®	CH_3	S	O	(benzene ring)	(benzene ring)$-O-\overset{S}{\underset{}{\overset{\|}{P}}}(OCH_3)_2$

Figure 3. Thio ether oxidation in the phosphorus ester series.

sulphones was decreased by a factor of three, whereas their cholinesterase-inhibiting activity varied[28].

The increased stability towards hydrolysis of these oxidation products is of importance with respect to their final metabolic fate. Metasystox, with a half-life of 88 days in aqueous solution at pH 5 and 20°C, and its sulphoxide, with a half-life of 240 days, may serve as examples. This increase in stability was even more pronounced with Metasystox derivatives where the carbon atom, adjacent to the thiolo sulphur, was branched by a methyl group for example. This branching causes a sharp fall in hydrolytic stability from a half-life of 88 days to one of 1.8 days. This effect is not seen in the sulphoxide form, which has a half-life of 240 days[29].

Sulphoxide and sulphone of thiolo-Systox behave similarly in this respect, as long as a pH of six is not exceeded. Under neutral or alkaline conditions the sulphone is rapidly hydrolysed[30].

The sulphoxide and sulphone of Phorate also show a 100-fold increase in stability towards 0.1 M sodium carbonate over the parent compound. And even in the corresponding oxygen analogue this factor is still 40[27].

What had become important of these factors influencing the stability, if we look at the metabolites actually found after application of such insecticides? First it is astonishing that, despite a broad knowledge of the metabolic behaviour of these compounds in plants and even in insects, only limited information is at hand with respect to mammals. This is particularly true if one is interested in balance-type studies, which are a pre-requisite for a final evaluation of the importance of a single metabolite found.

Such information is available from studies with Systox in mice[31] and Di-Syston[32] and Phorate[27] in rats. Common to all studies is the poor recovery of the administered ^{32}P label (50–70 per cent in 24 h with both isomers of Systox, 28.6 per cent in 48 h with Di-Syston and 35 per cent in six days with Phorate). Only the ratio of the ionic degradation products, i.e. dimethyl phosphate, phosphorothioate and phosphorodithioate, was determined and found to be different for the three compounds. An attempt was made with Systox to determine urinary sulphoxides and sulphones. But only thiono sulphoxide was identified. No resolution or quantitation of metabolites was possible with the separation techniques available at that time. The pattern of oxidative metabolites of Phorate in the liver 30 or 120 min after dosage revealed 60 per cent to correspond to the thiolophosphate sulphone, 27 per cent to thiolophosphate sulphoxide and 13 per cent to parent sulphoxide.

Fenthion, an example of the mixed aryl alkyl thio ether type, was studied in the rat after a single oral dose or ten daily intraperitoneal injections[33] and in the cow after dermal or intramuscular application[34] with ^{32}P-labelled material. Only one to four per cent of the radioactivity, eliminated with the excreta of both species, consisted of sulphoxides and sulphones of the parent compound and oxygen analogue, whereas more than 95 per cent was found to be dimethyl phosphorothioate and phosphate. Analysis of the cow tissues showed, surprisingly, no parent or oxidation products to be present two weeks after dermal treatment. In contrast, three weeks after intramuscular application the organo-soluble radioactivity, representing 10 to 50 per cent of the total tissue residue (range; 0.03 p.p.m. steak, 0.76 p.p.m. liver, 76.5 p.p.m. injection site), consisted of up to 50 per cent (injection site) of mainly parent compound and small amounts of sulphoxides and sulphones of parent and oxygen analogue.

The oxidative metabolism of Bayer 9017, which differs from Fenthion only in an additional methyl group in the 5-position, was investigated in calves with thio ether ^{35}S-labelled compound[35]. The analysis of the tissues performed 24 h after dermal or oral treatment showed small amounts of sulphoxide and sulphone to be present in addition to the parent compound, which was the main constituent of the organo-soluble radioactivity. The oxygen analogue was the main oxidation product and, in this series, thio ether oxidation was more prominent. Sulphoxides and sulphones of the free xylenols have also been found in tissues and, in conjugated form, in the urine.

Information on structure–toxicity relationships within this series can be found in ref. 36.

Abate[37], a symmetrical diphenyl thio ether derivative, is rapidly excreted in rats dosed with ^{3}H-labelled insecticide (75 per cent in 24 h, > 95 per cent total recovery). Appreciable levels of radioactivity were found only in the gastrointestinal tract and fatty tissue (range 1.25 p.p.m. after 48 h to 1.75 p.p.m. after 72 h) and consisted of mainly parent compound and minor amounts of its sulphoxide (ratio 7:1). Sulphuric acid esters of the phenolic hydrolysis products, i.e. 4,4′-thio-, 4,4′-sulphinyl and 4,4′-sulphonyl diphenol were the principal metabolites in the urine.

Some examples for carboxamide N-dealkylations, the third reaction with a toxicating effect (for examples see refs 36, 38) are shown in Figure 4.

Again, the mixed-function oxidase of the liver is responsible for the catalysis

39

of this reaction. Discussions on the nature of the primary oxidation products lasted for years. The first idea, that N-oxides should be the intermediates[39, 40], was revised[41, 42] and replaced by the N-methylol derivatives as first oxidation products. This reaction is now well established not only in the carboxamide group of phosphorus esters, but also in the carbamate and phenylurea series. Intermediary N-oxides have been found in the course of the oxidation of aryl dialkyl amines[43]. In a study of this reaction in the alkylated amine series with ^{18}O, molecular oxygen was shown to be incorporated into the leaving aldehyde[44].

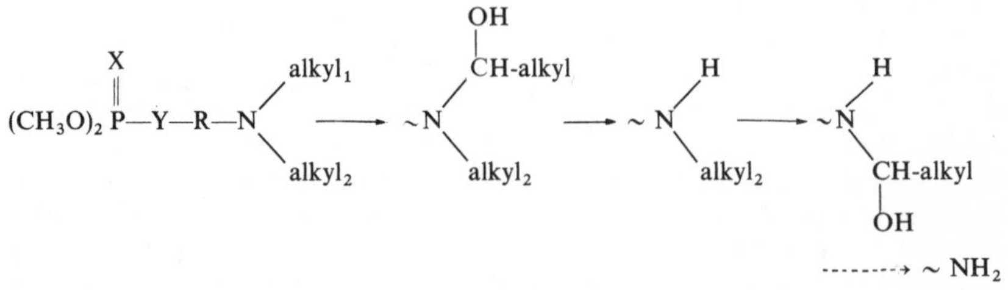

$$(CH_3O)_2\ \overset{\overset{X}{\parallel}}{P}-Y-R-N\overset{alkyl_1}{\underset{alkyl_2}{\diagdown}} \longrightarrow \ \sim N\overset{CH\text{-alkyl (OH)}}{\underset{alkyl_2}{\diagdown}} \longrightarrow \ \sim N\overset{H}{\underset{alkyl_2}{\diagdown}} \longrightarrow \ \sim N\overset{H}{\underset{CH\text{-alkyl (OH)}}{\diagdown}}$$

$$\cdots\cdots\rightarrow\ \sim NH_2$$

	X	Y	R	alkyl$_1$	alkyl$_2$
Dicrotophos (Bidrin®)	O	O	$-\underset{\underset{CH_3}{\vert}}{C}=CH-\underset{\underset{O}{\parallel}}{C}-$	CH$_3$	CH$_3$
Monocrotophos (Azodrin®)	O	O	$-\underset{\underset{CH_3}{\vert}}{C}=CH-\underset{\underset{O}{\parallel}}{C}-$	H	CH$_3$
Phosphamidon (Dimecron®)	O	O	$-\underset{\underset{H_3C}{\vert}}{C}=\underset{\underset{Cl}{\vert}}{C}-\underset{\underset{O}{\parallel}}{C}-$	C$_2$H$_5$	C$_2$H$_5$
Dimethoate (Rogor®)	S	S	$-CH_2-\underset{\underset{O}{\parallel}}{C}-$	H	CH$_3$
Famphur (Warbex®)	S	O	⬡$-SO_2-$	CH$_3$	CH$_3$

Figure 4. Carboxamide N-dealkylation in the phosphorus ester series.

After a first report on the occurrence of N-hydroxymethyl derivatives of Bidrin and Azodrin in urine of rats dosed with ^{32}P-labelled insecticides[45], a thorough study of these compounds with the aid of O- and N-$^{14}CH_3$- and ^{32}P-labelled materials has been performed. It showed that all possible single dealkylating steps had been passed through in the rat, mouse, rabbit, dog and goat[38]. These compounds represented from 5 to 25 per cent of the meta-bolites in the urine, but the mono-demethylation product, i.e. Azodrin, constituted in all cases the most important metabolite. Traces of some of the oxidative products, mainly in the form of Azodrin, occurred transiently in the milk of the goat.

Degradation of Bidrin in egg yolk, following essentially the same sequence of reactions, has also been reported[46].

The metabolic behaviour of phosphamidon has been extensively studied. A review of the results obtained so far is to be published[47]. These results, of studies in the rat[48] and in the rat and goat[47, 49], demonstrate that oxidative N-de-ethylation also takes place with this substance. Mono- and bis-de-ethylated derivatives have been identified in the urine and as transitory metabolites in the milk. In addition dechlorination and, to a minor extent, O-demethylation have also been observed. The occurrence of hydroxy vinyl metabolites, as a consequence of hydrolytic dechlorination, was strongly indicated in these studies[50]. In summary, the oxidative degradation of phosphamidon accounts for a small fraction of the total metabolism, since more than 90 per cent of the urinary radioactivity consisted of non-organo-soluble compounds.

As the numerous publications on the metabolic fate of the systematic insecticide dimethoate have just been competently reviewed[21], we can concentrate on the essential results of the oxidative metabolism of this compound. In addition to potent desulphuration, N-demethylation of the parent compound, and especially of its oxygen analogue, to the respective carboxamides via the N-methylol intermediates was observed in the rat. As with other alkyl carboxamides the oxidative part of the degradation of this compound represents only a limited fraction of the total metabolism. To date, we have no conclusive evidence that N-dealkylations have to occur before cleavage by amidases can take place.

On the other hand, the oxidation of the N-methyl group, as determined by the liberation of $^{14}CO_2$, is very rapid (more than 90 per cent within 6 h after dosage, totalling 15 to 18 per cent of the dose applied), as demonstrated in rat balance studies with O- and N-$^{14}CH_3$-labelled dimethoate[51].

An interesting N-demethylation of a sulphonamide was observed with famphur to occur in insects[52] and in sheep and calves[53], but not in practice in mice[52].

REACTIONS OF PHOSPHORUS ESTERS RESULTING IN DETOXICATION

The reactions of *Figure 5*, to be discussed now, generally result in the cleavage of ester or amide bonds, the nitro group reduction of parathion and its analogues being an exception.

They represent by far the most important reactions if one considers the overall metabolism of a given phosphorus ester. Common to them all is the complete loss of cholinesterase-inhibiting activity and a sharp reduction in mammalian toxicity of the formed phosphorus di- and tri-esters. This effect depends on the formation of an anionic centre either in the direct neighbourhood of the phosphorus atom or in the form of a carboxyl group which is capable of exerting a field effect.

Comparative determinations of the esterase-inhibiting activity between parent insecticides and their O-dealkyl derivatives revealed 6 000-(Ronnel) to 665 000-(dimethoate, —P=O) fold losses of activity in the course of demethylation or de-ethylation[54]. Similar relationships hold for amino-parathion, which no longer inhibits cholinesterase and is more than 100-fold less toxic than the parent parathion[55].

Since it is outside the scope of this presentation to consider structure–reactivity relationships (which can be referred to, for example. in ref. 56),

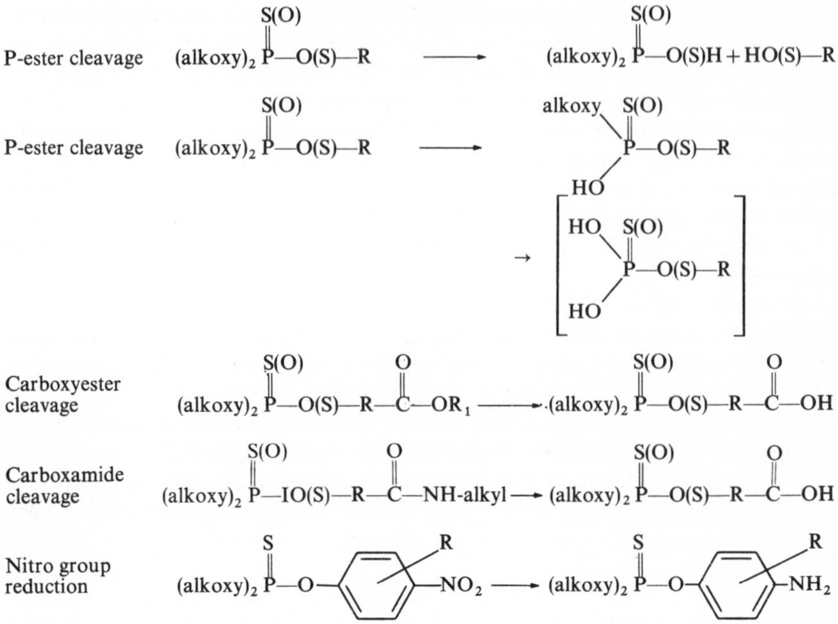

Figure 5. Reactions of phosphorus esters resulting in detoxication.

we will briefly look only at the chemical stability of the phosphorus bond. In *Figure 6* the various starting and end products participating in the ester cleavage are outlined.

Generally the ease of hydrolytic cleavage of the ester bond increases in the series dithiophosphates, thionophosphates, orthophosphates and thiolophosphates, although exceptions exist. The increased susceptibility of phosphates and thiolophosphates essentially facilitates the metabolic attack of an organism enabling it to prevail over the cholinergic toxicant. Furthermore, thiolophosphorus esters are hydrolysed under alkaline conditions about 1 000 times faster, with cleavage of their P—S bond, than the respective phosphorus esters[57, 58], but exceptions to this rule are known (see thiolo-Systox and the corresponding orthophosphate, as well as the sulphoxides of both compounds, as examples[1]).

The dialkyl phosphates (I) to (IV) of *Figure 6*, although considerably less susceptible to hydrolysis than the triesters[59] and the monoesters (methyl phosphate is about 100 times more reactive than dimethyl phosphate at pH 4 to 5; for detailed information see refs 60, 61), will not be further considered.

Finally I would like to point out the ready susceptibility of phosphorus ester bonds to catalytic hydrolysis (for review see ref. 62), which may greatly influence the rate and possibly type of cleavage under physiological conditions.

Looking from the residue point of view, the problem is greatly simplified because we only have to know whether or not the sulphur atom of dithio- or

42

thiolo-phosphates accompanies the leaving group. We are especially interested in this leaving group, because as far as possible we should know its metabolic fate in addition to that of the toxic activation products.

Various types of phosphorus ester cleavage are known to occur in animal metabolism, according to the tri-, di- or mono-phosphates found as metabolites. In addition it was observed that these reactions may take place in different subcellular fractions of different organs and, finally, that they evidently follow different types of chemical reactions.

If we differentiate according to chemical reactions, we can distinguish between an oxidative and a hydrolytic type, both affecting three groups of starting materials via routes B, namely activated esters already present or previously formed via route A, and thiono- and dithio-phosphorus esters. Whereas until recently the cleavage of phosphorus ester bonds was assumed to be simply a hydrolytic reaction, evidence has accumulated demonstrating that at least a part of the thiono- and, probably, dithio-phosphates found as metabolites are the result of an oxidative process. This process was originally found with parathion when it was proved that both activation to paraoxon and cleavage to diethyl phosphorothioate required NADPH and molecular oxygen[10, 63, 64]. The liver microsomal system of a variety of animals was found capable of performing this cleavage. The study was then extended to

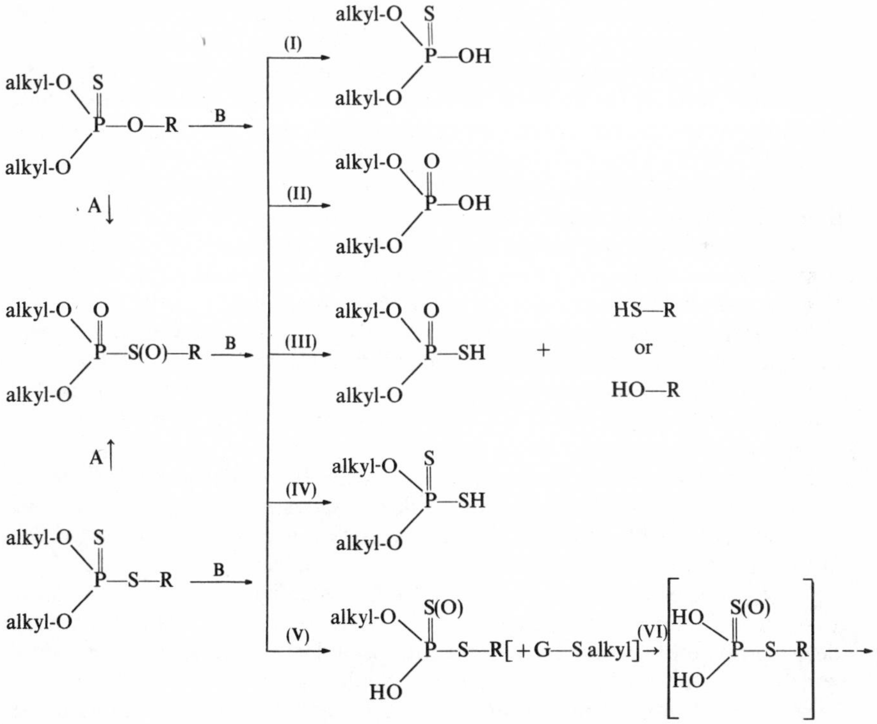

Figure 6. Cleavage of phosphorus ester bonds.

a series of parathion analogues[15a], to Diazinon[65,66] and malathion[65], demonstrating also the quantitative importance of this reaction within the overall degradation.

Esteratic cleavage of various phosphorus esters in different organs, especially in serum and liver, is well known (for the influence of animal species, i.e. mammalian, avian and piscine, on this cleavage of activated phosphorus esters see refs. 7, 24). It was shown with Diazinon[67] and parathion[10] that a minor part of such an esteratic cleavage also occurs in the supernatant fraction of rat liver, with reduced glutathione as a cofactor. On the other hand, the existence of esteratic enzymes, which cleave Diazinon with Ca^{2+} for activation, has also been demonstrated in microsomes[67]. Activation of esterases by Ca^{2+} (mitochondria) and Mn^{2+} (supernatant) has been shown in DDVP hydrolysis by rats and rabbits[68].

The same activation by Ca^{2+} has been found to occur with three different paraoxon-hydrolysing enzymes, which have been located in the microsomal, mitochondrial and supernatant fractions of rat liver[68a].

However, the reduced glutathione-dependent fission of phosphorus esters evidently has its significance in the O-dealkylation reaction (pathway V of *Figure 6*). Even in the first studies, the favoured cleavage of dimethyl over diethyl esters and the increase of this demethylation with increasing dosages of the investigated insecticides were noted (Ronnel[69], dicapthon, Chlorthion, methyl parathion[70] and DDVP[68]). In experiments *in vitro* with methyl parathion[71,72] the properties of the enzyme and its dependence on reduced glutathione were stated. These relationships have been confirmed and found to occur in a variety of phosphorus esters (Sumithion[15,73]; *cis*-Phosdrin[74,75]; methyl paraoxon and alkyl analogues[76]; Guthion and Ronnel[26]; bromophos[76a,77]). Finally, the products of this reaction have been identified as the corresponding demethyl derivatives and methylated glutathione[74–76,78].

Bromophos[77] seems to be an exception to this reaction, because no mono-demethylation, but bis-demethylation to form 4-bromo-2,5-dichlorophenyl phosphorothionic acid, has been reported (see route VI of *Figure 6*). An even more striking exception of dealkylation is available in the form of Dursban, the bis- de-ethyl derivative of which was found in rats[77a].

This is an interesting variation of the O-dealkylation reaction as it is well documented that mono-demethyl phosphorus esters (route V of *Figure 6*) are readily hydrolysed to mono-alkyl phosphates in contrast to dialkyl phosphates (e.g. II of *Figure 6*), which are excreted unchanged, even when applied directly to rats[68,79].

Let us now revert to the remaining examples of detoxication of *Figure 5*, namely cleavage of carboxy ester or amide linkages and nitro group reduction. The metabolism of phosphorus esters carrying a carboxy ester or amide group, as for example malathion, acethion and dimethoate, has intensively been studied, especially with regard to the selectivity of these insecticides. But it is unnecessary to repeat the results of these studies, because they have been competently summarized and interpreted[80,81]. Thus I will only add some new results, which make some of the well-known facts more precise. New types of metabolites, in addition to malathion mono- and di-acid or demethyl malathion, have not been demonstrated. But it was not until 1969, when the structure of the main metabolite of various animals, malathion mono-acid, was reported to be definitely in the α-form[82].

Phosphorus ester cleavage with malathion, both sulphur atoms of which were labelled with ^{35}S, is probably also of the oxidative type requiring NADPH and molecular oxygen[65].

So far, no indication is available for the biological formation of free or esterified maleic acid. Such substances could be expected as chemically, under alkaline conditions, the carboxy group in the β-position directs not to P—S cleavage but to a β-elimination liberating an olefin, in this case maleic acid diethyl ester[83]. Minor amounts of $^{14}CO_2$ (2.8 per cent of the dose applied) have been liberated in rats dosed with malathion, ^{14}C-labelled at C-2 and C-3, but, of course, no deductions can be made with regard to the mechanisms involved[84].

The optical isomers of malathion have been found to have different toxicities to mice, the D-form being more than twice as toxic as the L-form (LD_{50}, per os: L-form 2357 mg/kg, D-form 1014 mg/kg). This was related to the better inhibition of the carboxyl esterase by the formed D-malaoxon[85]. Whether or not these properties are the expression of a different metabolism of each isomer is not known.

With regard to dimethoate, only some newer references are cited. In a balance study in the rat, with ^{32}P- and O- and N-$^{14}CH_3$-labelled materials, very rapid liberation of $^{14}CO_2$ from the N-$^{14}CH_3$ group (15 to 18 per cent of the dose applied) has been observed in addition to the excretion of small amounts of $[^{14}C]$formate in the urine. Dimethoate carboxylic acid was the main metabolite, in addition to dimethyl phosphate and phosphorothioate[51]. Detoxication of dimethoate by the action of amidases of human liver, ranging from 20 to 100 per cent of the total degradation (corresponding to 0.23 to 0.37 $\mu g/g$ of liver per 30 min) has been reported[86].

Details on the reductive and oxidative metabolism of Parathion and some of its analogues will be presented in the next section.

COMPARATIVE METABOLISM OF PHOSPHORUS ESTERS

In this section the metabolic fate of a number of phosphorus esters closely related by chemical structure or reactivity is discussed on a comparative basis. On this basis not only the common reactions come to light, but also the extreme variations in metabolic behaviour. Again, it must be stressed that the metabolic fate of the leaving group of many phosphorus esters is not yet known, so that only a limited selection of examples can be given in the following figures.

The examples of *Figure 7*, with the exception of menazon, can be assumed to be derived from cyclic carboxamide N-methylol compounds. The metabolites of Supracide shown have been identified in the rat, demonstrating methylation and sulphoxidation of the intermediate mercaptomethyl derivative. By means of ^{14}C labelling in the methylene, carbonyl and ring-methoxy groups, the cleavage of most of the molecule, not excreted as the sulphinyl or sulphonyl metabolites, and the final oxidation of the formed C-1 fragments to $^{14}CO_2$ have been demonstrated[87-89]. The efficient oxidation of the different C-1 fragments to carbon dioxide has been confirmed

45

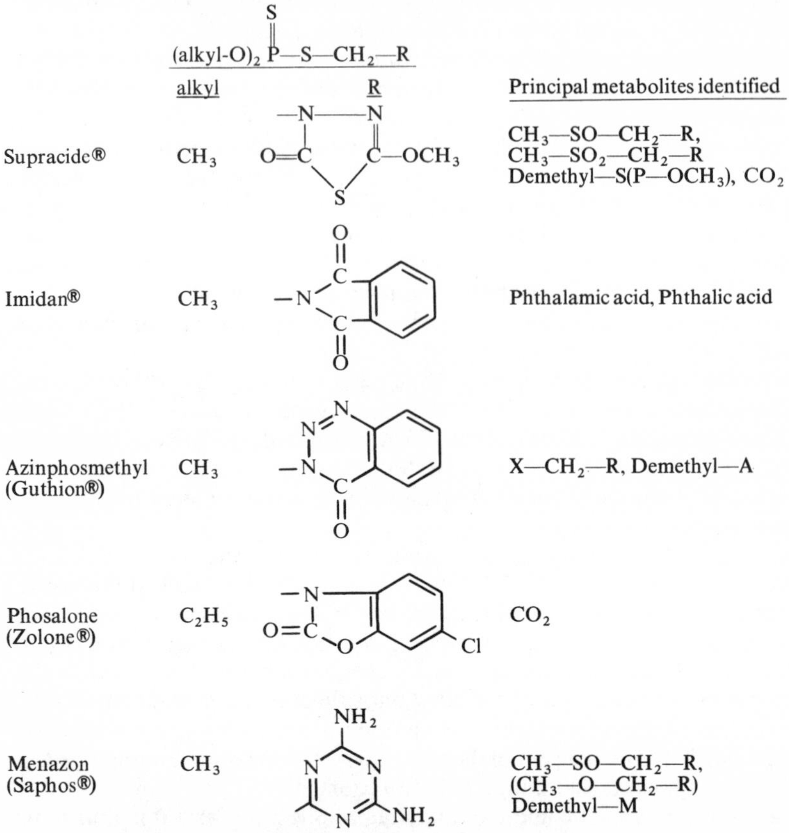

$$(\text{alkyl-O})_2 \overset{\overset{\text{S}}{\|}}{\text{P}}\text{—S—CH}_2\text{—R}$$

	alkyl	R	Principal metabolites identified

Supracide® CH$_3$ —N——N , O=C, C—OCH$_3$, S (ring)
CH$_3$—SO—CH$_2$—R,
CH$_3$—SO$_2$—CH$_2$—R
Demethyl—S(P—OCH$_3$), CO$_2$

Imidan® CH$_3$ —N (phthalimide ring, C=O, C=O)   Phthalamic acid, Phthalic acid

Azinphosmethyl (Guthion®) CH$_3$ —N, N=N, C=O (benzotriazinone ring)   X—CH$_2$—R, Demethyl—A

Phosalone (Zolone®) C$_2$H$_5$ —N, O=C, O (benzoxazolone ring), Cl   CO$_2$

Menazon (Saphos®) CH$_3$ triazine ring with NH$_2$, NH$_2$ CH$_3$—SO—CH$_2$—R, (CH$_3$—O—CH$_2$—R) Demethyl—M

Figure 7. Comparative metabolism of heterocyclic dithiophosphorus esters.

and, in addition, the excretion of demethyl-Supracide has also been demonstrated[90]. The methyl group of the sulphoxide metabolite was shown to be donated by methionine. Whether or not these oxidized thio ether metabolites have to be passed through for final oxidation of the molecule to carbon dioxide cannot be decided, although both sulphoxide and sulphone liberate large portions of their *carbonyl*-^{14}C label as $^{14}CO_2$ when they are applied orally and intravenously to rats[91].

Results on the tissue residue behaviour of Supracide in the rat[87], in a lactating cow after treatment for five days[92] or after chronic feeding to ruminating bull calves for ten weeks[93] show rapid elimination of the parent and its metabolites.

Imidan shows a completely different behaviour in the rat. The ester, ^{14}C-labelled at both carbonyl groups, has been shown to be split, and the resulting phthalimide ring to be opened hydrolytically to form phthalamic acid, which, in part, is further cleaved by amidase action to phthalic acid. Both substances were excreted in the free form, even when applied directly to the rat[94,95]. Similar findings have been made in a steer dermally treated with the ^{14}C-labelled insecticide[96].

46

The residue behaviour of Imidan has been investigated in cattle after spraying[97] and in dairy cows after feeding with Imidan-treated silage[98].

The fate of the heterocyclic moiety of Guthion is not completely understood. In addition to desulphuration and hydrolysis of the formed oxygen analogue, which have been repeatedly reported[7, 24, 26], reduced glutathione-dependent demethylation has been demonstrated[26]. The ^{14}C-labelled methylene group was found to be partly incorporated into milk sugars of cows feeding on Guthion-treated forage. Simultaneously metabolites have been found still containing the ^{14}C-labelled methylene group and the benztriazine ring[99, 100]. The question of their exact nature, and of their possible similarity

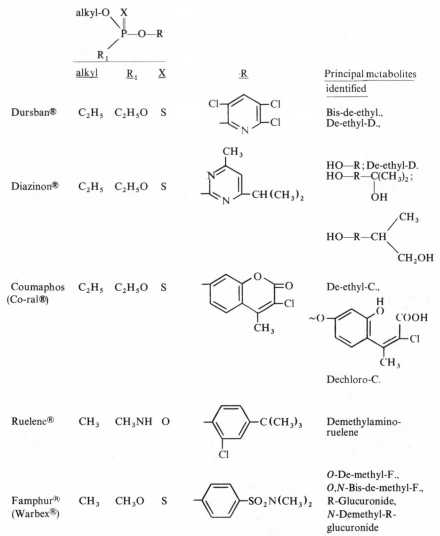

Figure 8. Comparative metabolism of enolic and phenolic phosphorus esters.

to the sulphoxide type metabolites of Supracide, cannot yet be answered. For information on the residue behaviour of Coumaphos see refs 101, 102.

The rapid and complete excretion of phosalone in the rat has been reported[103]. In this study two thirds of the *carbonyl-*[14]C label was recovered in the form of [14]CO_2, demonstrating the efficient cleavage of the benzoxazoline ring. The nature and the fate of the remaining part of the molecule has not been reported on so far.

Menazon is the second example of *Figure 7* which gives rise to a methylated sulphoxide metabolite. In addition to the oxygen analogue and minor amounts of, probably, methoxy methyl derivative, this metabolite was found to be the main excretion product in the urine of rats dosed with *ring-2-*[14]C- and ^{35}S-labelled insecticide[104, 105].

Dursban, the first representative of the class of phosphorus esters with enolizable heterocycles, has been investigated by means of [14]C- (C–2 and C–6 of the ring) and [36]Cl-(3,5-chloro) labels in the rat[77a], in a lactating cow[106] and in fish[107]. Bis-de-ethylated parent compound has been found as the main metabolite in the urine of the rat in addition to appreciable amounts of the leaving chlorinated pyridinol. The heterocyclic moiety of Dursban was also found to be the main metabolite of fish, which excrete this compound into the surrounding water. Intermediate de-ethylation is probable, as mono-ethyl phosphate and phosphorothioate have been found.

Information is available on the tissue residues of Dursban and its oxygen analogue in cattle, dipped or sprayed with the insecticide[108], and in turkeys held on Dursban-treated soil[109–111].

The metabolism of Diazinon has been studied intensively in the rat both *in vitro*[14, 65–67] and *in vivo*[112]. The leaving pyrimidinol R—OH has been determined both in the studies *in vitro*, as a result of oxidative or esteratic cleavage, and in the studies *in vivo*, as a urinary and, to a lesser extent, as a faecal metabolite. In addition, side-chain oxidation has been observed *in vivo* yielding mainly the tertiary alcohol of the pyrimidine isopropyl group. Primary alcohol formation at this group has been found to a lesser extent (by a factor of three to four)[112].

The pyrimidinol R—OH, when fed to rats, is partly excreted unchanged, partly in the form of the tertiary and primary alcohols showing the same ratio as after Diazinon dosage. In contrast, the tertiary alcohol derivative is excreted unchanged in the urine[112].

Of the great number of references available on the residue behaviour of Diazinon some newer examples will be given: sheep[113], cows fed[114] or cattle dermally treated[102, 115, 116] with the insecticide, pheasants and pigeons[117], dogs[118] and guinea-pigs[119].

Although extensive information exists on the excretion and the general residue behaviour in different animals treated with coumaphos (examples: cattle dermally treated[120, 121, 121a], poultry drenched[122], cows fed for the control of house fly larvae in their manure[123], metabolism *in vitro* by tissues of different species[124]), only limited knowledge on the fate of the benzpyrone ring is available. In addition to the relatively efficient de-ethylation, indications have been obtained for the presence, in the urine of a goat and a cow, of parent compound and/or oxygen analogue, the pyrone ring of which was partly opened, as can occur with alkaline treatment[125].

Small amounts of dechloro-coumaphos have been observed in the faeces of cows orally tested with the insecticide for the control of house fly larvae in their manure[123].

Interestingly, phosphorus deamination has been reported to be more efficient than O-demethylation, in sheep orally treated with Ruelene, since a metabolite, without the methylamino group, has been found in the urine[126].

Both O- and N-demethylation determine the metabolic behaviour of famphur after its intravenous and intramuscular injection into sheep and cattle[53]. Thus O-demethyl and O,N-bis-demethyl derivatives of the parent compound have been found in blood plasma and urine, in addition to the corresponding glucuronides of the parent phenol and of its N-demethyl derivative. p-Hydroxybenzenesulphonic acid, the most extensively degraded metabolite found, was present in the urine only in very small amounts.

The fate of famphur and its oxygen analogue has been determined in bovine milk and edible tissues[127].

Some selective insecticides, which have an enolized vinyl group as a common feature, are shown in Figure 9.

Intensive metabolism of dichlorvos, the oldest representative of this group, has been found to occur in the rat, goat and cow[79]. In addition to mono- and di-methyl phosphate as the main excretion products containing the ^{32}P

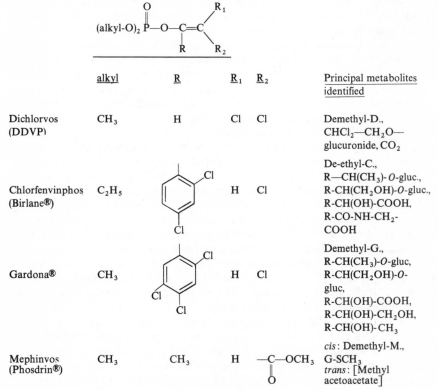

$$(alkyl\text{-}O)_2 \overset{O}{\underset{}{\overset{\|}{P}}} - O - \underset{R}{\overset{}{C}} = \underset{R_2}{\overset{R_1}{C}}$$

	alkyl	R	R₁	R₂	Principal metabolites identified
Dichlorvos (DDVP)	CH₃	H	Cl	Cl	Demethyl-D., CHCl₂—CH₂O— glucuronide, CO₂
Chlorfenvinphos (Birlane®)	C₂H₅	(2,4-dichlorophenyl)	H	Cl	De-ethyl-C., R—CH(CH₃)-O-gluc., R-CH(CH₂OH)-O-gluc., R-CH(OH)-COOH, R-CO-NH-CH₂-COOH
Gardona®	CH₃	(2,4,5-trichlorophenyl)	H	Cl	Demethyl-G., R-CH(CH₃)-O-gluc, R-CH(CH₂OH)-O-gluc, R-CH(OH)-COOH, R-CH(OH)-CH₂OH, R-CH(OH)-CH₃
Mephinvos (Phosdrin®)	CH₃	CH₃	H	—C(=O)—OCH₃	cis: Demethyl-M., G-SCH₃ trans: [Methyl acetoacetate]

Figure 9. Comparative metabolism of vinyl phosphorus esters.

49

label, mono-demethyl dichlorvos has been identified as a metabolite in each species. By use of a ^{14}C label in the C-1 position of dichlorvos, the leaving group was shown to undergo mainly conjugation after ester hydrolysis, as more than 90 per cent of the urinary radioactivity has been found to consist of the glucuronide of dichloroethanol. The entrance of the C-2 fragment of the leaving group into the intermediary metabolism of the rat has been demonstrated by the liberation of part of the ^{14}C label in the form of $^{14}CO_2$, and by the fact that appreciable amounts of the ^{14}C label had not yet been excreted seven days after the application of the insecticide. The reduction by NADH of dichloroacetaldehyde, the product of direct dichlorvos hydrolysis to form dichloroethanol, has been proved to occur in studies *in vitro*[68]. Glutathione-dependent demethylation of dichlorvos has been demonstrated in experiments *in vitro* investigating the influence of different alkyl groups on the rate of the *O*-dealkylation reaction[76].

The rapid detoxication of dichlorvos by the liver has been confirmed in studies demonstrating that, after oral application, the insecticide primarily enters the hepatic portal vein system of the rat before reaching the systemic circulation[127a].

Chlorfenvinphos and the closely related Gardona undergo similar de-alkylation, but an interesting difference has come to light. De-ethylation of chlorfenvinphos was established to be an oxidative process that is performed by liver microsomes requiring oxygen and reduced NADP. By means of a ^{14}C label at C–1 of the ethyl groups it has been shown that acetaldehyde is the product of spontaneous cleavage of the intermediate *O*-alkylol derivative. A pronounced difference in the efficiency with which different animal species perform this reaction has been observed (dog:rabbit:rat, 88:24:1)[128]. In contrast, in the demethylation of Gardona, which can also be performed by liver microsomes, the highest activity has been located in the supernatant fraction and requires reduced glutathione as described for other demethylations. Methylated glutathione has in this case also been identified as the primary reaction product[78].

The leaving groups of both chlorfenvinphos[129] and Gardona[130] have been found to give rise to the same pattern of metabolites, but remarkable differences have been observed between rat and dog metabolism. Whereas in the dog *O*-dealkylation dominated (70 per cent of the dose applied with chlorfenvinphos and 46 per cent with Gardona occurred as dealkylated derivatives in the urine), esteratic cleavage and conjugation have been found to be the main pathways used by the rat. Both reductive and hydrolytic dechlorination had taken place as di- and tri-chlorophenyl ethan-1-ol and the corresponding ethanediol have been identified, mostly in the form of their β-D-glucuronides (for example R—CH(CH$_3$)—O—gluc: 41 per cent in the rat, 4 per cent in the dog for chlorfenvinphos, 35 per cent in the rat, 0 per cent in the dog for Gardona, have been found as metabolites in urine).

The remarkable difference between dog and rat metabolism has also been observed with toxicity (LD$_{50}$, per os, for chlorfenvinphos:dog > 5000 mg/kg, rat 10–15 mg/kg). Obviously the concerted interaction in absorption, metabolism, availability in blood, rate of brain uptake and sensitivity of brain cholinesterase, is sufficient to explain the difference, as these factors accounted for a 900–1350-fold difference in the two species[131].

Data on the residue behaviour of ^{32}P-labelled chlorfenvinphos in cattle after various application techniques[132], on the general metabolism of ^{32}P-labelled Gardona[133] and on its residue behaviour in cattle[134], poultry[135, 136] and bovine milk and excreta[121a, 137] are available.

Mephinvos and some of its analogues can be used as examples to discuss the differences observed between the metabolism of *cis* and *trans* isomers of vinyl esters. It has been found in studies *in vitro* that the *cis* isomer is detoxified by an enzyme system of mouse liver supernatant fraction, requiring reduced glutathione, to yield demethyl mephinvos and methyl glutathione. The *trans* isomer, in contrast, is split by esterase action of the same cell fraction to dimethyl phosphate and, probably, methyl acetoacetate as primary products.

These relationships have not been found with closely related Bomyl, where group R of mephinvos is substituted by a methoxy carbonyl methyl group. Both geometric isomers of Bomyl have been found to be degraded by esterases of both microsomal and supernatant fractions[74, 75].

Selective activation of the *cis* isomer of the thiono analogue of Phosdrin, in contrast to that of the *trans* isomer, has also been observed in mouse liver microsomes[138]. These differences have been discussed with respect to steric hindrance of the metabolic reactions involved.

Esteratic cleavage of the phosphorus ester bond was supposed to be the exclusive route in cattle as only dimethyl phosphate was found as the ^{32}P-labelled metabolite in urine and in studies *in vitro* in plasma[139].

The examples of phenolic phosphorus esters presented in *Figure 10* are closely related, but, nevertheless, pronounced differences in their metabolic and toxicological behaviour in animals can be observed.

Parathion and its analogues have regained attention recently when the mechanisms involved in ester bond cleavage had begun to be studied in detail. The basis of these reactions has been discussed in the last section. Here, we will restrict ourselves to a comparative consideration of the first three compounds on the one hand and the final ones on the other.

From the pattern of metabolites in urine of rats dosed with [32]P- and ^{35}S-labelled parathion, it is evident that activation to paraoxon and oxidative cleavage to dimethyl phosphorothioate had occurred to the same degree. This was indicated by the ratios found of both inorganic sulphate to dimethyl phosphorothioate and orthophosphates to dimethyl phosphorothioate. With increasing dosages increasing amounts of de-ethyl paraoxon were excreted. Non-oxidative cleavage of the aryl moiety by soluble enzymes requiring glutathione was small[10].

Hydrolysis of the paraoxon, formed by activation, has been shown to occur in several tissues. The liver again showed the highest activity, plasma being the next important tissue in this respect[140]. In addition to three different Ca^{2+}-activated liver enzymes, a fourth soluble enzyme has been isolated capable of cleaving paraoxon to de-ethyl paraoxon[68a]. The properties of this enzyme have not yet been explored, so that a comparison with the oxidative mechanism found with the de-ethylation of chlorfenvinphos is not yet possible.

Many investigations on the cleavage of dimethyl phosphorus esters have been performed in order to search for an explanation of the striking increase

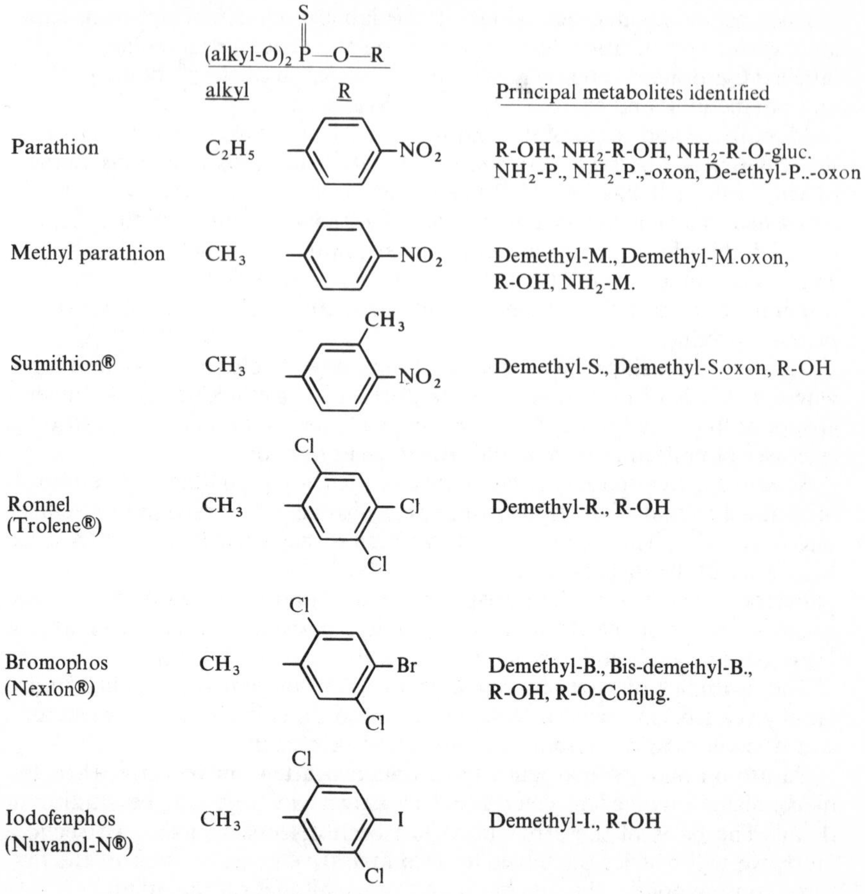

$$(\text{alkyl-O})_2 \overset{\displaystyle S}{\underset{\displaystyle \|}{P}}\text{—O—R}$$

	alkyl	R	Principal metabolites identified
Parathion	C_2H_5	⟨benzene⟩–NO_2	R-OH, NH_2-R-OH, NH_2-R-O-gluc. NH_2-P., NH_2-P.,-oxon, De-ethyl-P..-oxon
Methyl parathion	CH_3	⟨benzene⟩–NO_2	Demethyl-M., Demethyl-M.oxon, R-OH, NH_2-M.
Sumithion®	CH_3	⟨benzene, CH_3⟩–NO_2	Demethyl-S., Demethyl-S.oxon, R-OH
Ronnel (Trolene®)	CH_3	⟨benzene, Cl, Cl⟩–Cl	Demethyl-R., R-OH
Bromophos (Nexion®)	CH_3	⟨benzene, Cl, Cl⟩–Br	Demethyl-B., Bis-demethyl-B., R-OH, R-O-Conjug.
Iodofenphos (Nuvanol-N®)	CH_3	⟨benzene, Cl, Cl⟩–I	Demethyl-I., R-OH

Figure 10. Comparative metabolism of phenolic phosphorus esters.

in selectivity of Sumithion caused by the introduction of a simple methyl group into methyl parathion. However, in studies *in vivo* with guinea pigs and rats no difference has been found great enough to account for the lower mammalian toxicity of Sumithion[73]. With both compounds, in contrast to the diethyl analogue, O-dealkylation has been found to compete with aryl bond cleavage. On the other hand, when equitoxic amounts (200 mg of Sumithion/kg corresponded to 3 mg of methyl parathion/kg) of both compounds had been fed to mice, O-demethylation of Sumithion, to mainly demethyl parent compound and demethyl oxygen analogue, prevailed over aryl bond cleavage when higher dosages had been applied (e.g. at the 200 mg/kg dosage, 51 per cent of demethyl Sumithion and 25 per cent of demethyl Sumioxon had been excreted in 24 h[15]).

Other factors than metabolism have been related to Sumithion's selectivity, such as differences in inhibition of the target enzymes in mammals and insects due to variations in the distance between anionic and esteratic sites[141].

The fate of methyl paraoxon *in vivo* and the mechanisms involved in its dealkylation and in that of some of its O-alkyl analogues have been thoroughly studied[76]. It has been found that, at normal levels of liver glutathione, aryl bond cleavage contributes to two thirds, demethylation to one third of the total degradation occurring in the supernatant fraction of mouse liver. A similar ratio has been observed in vivo, which shifted at higher dosages of the applied methyl parathion in favour of demethylation. Methyl gluta-thione, isolated and identified in the experiments in vitro, was not excreted in the urine, probably owing to its rapid degradation.

Detoxication of the nitrophenyl esters by a reductive mechanism should be mentioned. It was first observed with parathion when, in studies both in vitro[55, 142] and in vivo[55], amino-parathion was identified in rumen fluid and in the cow as a major metabolite. In addition dimethyl phosphorothioate and small amounts of dimethyl phosphate were also found. This reaction was also shown to occur with other parathion analogues, such as methyl parathion and a number of chlorinated nitrophenyl esters. The recoveries of the corresponding amino derivatives were in the range 25 per cent (parathion) to 80 per cent (2-chloro-4-nitrophenyl dimethyl phosphate) after an incuba-tion period of 160 min[55]. The aminophenols formed in the studies in vivo were excreted, depending on the species, in free or conjugated forms.

Although this enzymatic reduction has been shown to occur in various tissues of a variety of mammals, birds and fish[143], no reports have been found of the occurrence of metabolites containing aminophenol groups in these species.

As the last three phosphorus esters of Figure 10 differ only in the halogen atom of the 4-position, a similar metabolism can be expected to take place. Actually, all compounds are subject to intense demethylation, owing to the fact that their favourable mammalian toxicity allows higher dosages to be applied (see for Ronnel in the rat and cow[69]; bromophos in the rat[76a] and in hog and mouse liver[77]; iodofenphos in hens[144]). With the exception of bromophos, where bis-demethylation has been reported to occur[77], only mono-demethylated original compounds have been identified. The leaving phenolic groups have been found partially in conjugated form.

The question whether the different halogen atoms at the 4-position give rise to a different metabolism of these phenols, especially whether or not the bromo and iodo atoms are selectively split off, cannot yet be answered. So far, there is good evidence that the phenolic moieties are rapidly excreted. This has been shown for bromophos, the ^{3}H-labelled moiety of which had been applied subcutaneously to rats. More than 95 per cent of the ^{3}H label was recovered within 48 h in the excreta, mainly in the urine[76a]. An interesting example of further degradation of mono-demethyl phosphorothioates has been reported to occur with demethyl Ronnel, which, after being fed to rats, was excreted in the urine almost exclusively as the corresponding P=O analogue[69].

Finally, some information is presented on the residue behaviour of the individual members of the last group: on residues of Ronnel, applied by different techniques, in bovine tissues and milk[69, 121a, 145–147] and in sheep[148]; of closely related OO-diethyl-O-(2,4-dichlorophenyl)phosphorothioate in cattle, goats and sheep[149]; of bromophos in the rat[76a] and in dipped sheep[150]; of iodofenphos in the rat[151] and in hens[144].

REFERENCES

[1] T. R. Fukuto, R. L. Metcalf, R. B. March and M. G. Maxon, *J. Econ. Ent.* **48**, 347 (1955).
[2] R. L. Metcalf, T. R. Fukuto and R. B. March, *J. Econ. Ent.* **50**, 338 (1957).
[3] J. J. Menn, and W. M. Hoskins, *J. Econ. Ent.* **55**, 90 (1962).
[4] D. F. Heath and M. Vandekar, *Biochem. J.* **67**, 187 (1957).
[5] H. Niessen, H. Tietz, G. Hecht and G. Kimmerle, *Archiv für Toxikologie*, **20**, 44 (1963).
[6] R. D. O'Brien. In *Toxic Phosphorus Esters*. p. 133. Academic Press: New York (1960).
[7] R. E. Johnsen and P. A. Dahm, *J. Econ. Ent.* **59**, 1437 (1966).
[8] J. E. Casida. In *Microsomes and Drug Oxidation*, pp 517–30. Ed. by J. R. Gillette, A. H. Conney, G. J. Cosmides, R. W. Estabrook, J. R. Fouts and G. J. Mannering. Academic Press: New York (1969).
[9] R. W. Estabrook and B. Cohen. In *Microsomes and Drug Oxidation*. Ed. by Gillette *et al*. p. 95–105. Academic Press: New York (1969).
[10] T. Nakatsugawa, N. M. Tolman and P. A. Dahm, *Biochem. Pharmacol.* **18**, 1103 (1969).
[11] J. E. Casida, *J. Agr. Food Chem.* **18**, 753 (1970).
[12] T. R. Fukuto and R. L. Metcalf, *J. Am. Chem. Soc.* **76**, 5103 (1954).
[13] G. Schrader, *Die Entwicklung neuer insektizider Phosphorsäurester*. Verlag Chemie: Weinheim/Bergstr. (1963).
[14] H. R. Krueger, R. D. O'Brien and W. C. Dauterman, *J. Econ. Ent.* **53**, 25 (1960).
[15] R. M. Hollingworth, R. L. Metcalf and T. R. Fukuto, *J. Agr. Food Chem.* **15**, 242 (1967).
[15a] T. Nakatsugawa, N. M. Tolman and P. A. Dahm, *Biochem. Pharmacol.* **17**, 1517 (1968).
[16] J. L. Potter, and R. D. O'Brien, *Science*, **144**, 55 (1964).
[17] R. B. March, T. R. Fukuto, R. L. Metcalf and M. G. Maxon, *J. Econ. Ent.* **49**, 185 (1956).
[18] R. D. O'Brien, *J. Econ. Ent.* **50**, 159 (1957).
[19] D. L. Bull, D. A. Lindquist and J. Hocskaylo. *J. Econ. Ent.* **56**, 129 (1963).
[20] U. E. Brady and B. W. Arthur, *J. Econ. Ent.* **56**, 477 (1963).
[21] G. W. Lucier and R. E. Menzer. *J. Agr. Food Chem.* **18**, 698 (1970).
[22] P. A. Dahm, B. E. Kopecky and C. B. Walker, *Toxicol. Appl. Pharmacol.* **4**, 683 (1962).
[23] R. A. Neal, and K. P. DuBois, *J. Pharm. Exp. Ther.* **148**, 185 (1965).
[24] S. D. Murphy, *Proc. Soc. Exp. Biol. Med.* **123**, 392 (1966).
[25] F. Matsumura and C. T. Ward, *Arch. Environ. Health*, **13**, 257 (1966).
[26] S. L. N. Rao and W. P. McKinley, *Canad. J. Biochem.* **47**, 1155 (1969).
[27] J. S. Bowman and J. E. Casida, *J. Econ. Ent.* **51**, 838 (1958).
[28] W. Wirth, *Naunyn-Schmiedebergs Arch. Exp. Pathol. Pharmacol.* **234**, 352 (1958).
[29] G. Schrader, *Angew. Chem.* **69**, 86 (1957).
[30] R. Mühlmann and G. Schrader, *Z. Naturforsch.* **12b**, 196 (1957).
[31] R. B. March, R. L. Metcalf, T. R. Fukuto and M. G. Maxon, *J Econ. Ent.* **48**, 355 (1955).
[32] D. L. Bull, *J. Econ. Ent.* **58**, 249 (1965).
[33] U. E. Brady and B. W. Arthur, *J. Econ. Ent.* **54**, 1232 (1961).
[34] C. O. Knowles and B. W. Arthur, *J. Econ. Ent.* **59**, 1346 (1966).
[35] S. Y. Young and R. S. Berger, *J. Econ. Ent.* **62**, 929 (1969).
[36] W. Lorenz and K. Sasse, *Pflanzenschutz-Nachrichten Bayer.* **21**, 5 (1968).
[37] R. C. Blinn, *J. Agr. Food Chem.* **17**, 118 (1969).
[38] R. E. Menzer and J. E. Casida, *J. Agr. Food Chem.* **13**, 102 (1965).
[39] G. S. Hartley, *15th Int. Congr. Pure Appl. Chem., New York: section 13, Pesticides* (1951).
[40] J. E. Casida, T. C. Allen and M. A. Stahman, *J. Biol. Chem.* **210**, 607 (1954).
[41] D. F. Heath, D. W. J. Lane and P. O. Park, *Phil. Trans. Roy. Soc.* **239B**, 191 (1955).
[42] E. Y. Spencer, R. D. O'Brien and R. W. White, *J. Agr. Food Chem.* **5**, 123 (1957).
[43] D. M. Ziegler and F. H. Pettit, *Biochemistry*, **5**, 2932 (1966).
[44] R. E. McMahon, H. W. Culp and J. C. Occolowitz, *J. Am. Chem. Soc.* **91**, 3389 (1969).
[45] D. L. Bull and D. A. Lindquist, *J. Agr. Food Chem.* **12**, 310 (1964).
[46] J. C. Roger, D. G. Upshall and J. E. Casida, *Biochem. Pharmacol.* **18**, 373 (1969).
[47] H. Geissbühler, G. Voss and R. Anlicker, *Res. Revs.* (In press).
[48] D. L. Bull, D. A. Lindquist and R. R. Grabbe, *J. Econ. Ent.* **60**, 332 (1967).
[49] G. P. Clemons and R. E. Menzer. *J. Agr. Food Chem.* **16**, 312 (1968).
[50] R. E. Menzer and W. C. Dauterman, *J. Agr. Food Chem.* **18**, 1031 (1970).
[51] A. Hassan, S. M. A. D. Zayed and M. R. E. Bahig, *Biochem. Pharmacol.* **18**, 2429 (1969).
[52] R. D. O'Brien, E. C. Kimmel and P. R. Sferra. *J. Agr. Food Chem.* **13**, 366 (1965).
[53] P. E. Gatterdam, L. A. Wozniak, M. W. Bullock, G. L. Parks and J. E. Boyd, *J. Agr. Food Chem.* **15**, 845 (1967).

[54] A. H. Ahorni and R. D. O'Brien, Biochemistry, 7, 1538 (1968).

[55] M. K. Ahmed, J. E. Casida and R. E. Nichols, J. Agr. Food Chem. 6, 740 (1958).

[56] R. D. O'Brien. In Toxic Phosphorus Esters, Ch. 2. Academic Press: New York and London (1960).

[57] R. F. Hudson and L. Keay, J. Chem. Soc. p. 3269 (1956).

[58] D. F. Heath, J. Chem. Soc. p. 3796, p. 3804 (1956).

[59] J. Kumamoto and F. H. Westheimer, J. Am. Chem. Soc. 77, 2515 (1955).

[60] P. W. Barnard, C. A. Bunton, D. R. Llewellyn, C. A. Vernon and V. A. Welch, J. Chem. Soc. p. 2670 (1961).

[61] C. A. Bunton, M. M. Mhala, K. G. Oldham and C. A. Vernon, J. Chem. Soc. p. 3293 (1960).

[62] R. D. O'Brien. In Toxic Phosphorus Esters, p 43. Academic Press: New York (1960).

[63] T. Nagatsugawa and P. A. Dahm, Biochem. Pharmacol. 16, 25 (1967).

[64] R. A. Neal, Biochem. J. 103, 183 (1967).

[65] T. Nakatsugawa, N. M. Tolman and P. A. Dahm, Biochem. Pharmacol. 18, 685 (1969).

[66] R. S. H. Yang, W. C. Dauterman and E. Hodgson, Life Sci. 8, 667 (1969).

[67] K. Fukunage, T. Shishido and J. Fukami, 6th Intern. Congr. Plant Protection, Vienna, Abstr. p. 202 (1967).

[68] E. Hodgson and J. E. Casida, J. Agr. Food Chem. 10, 208 (1962).

[68a] K. Kojima and R. D. O'Brien, J. Agr. Food Chem. 16, 574 (1968).

[69] F. W. Plapp and J. E. Casida, J. Agr. Food Chem. 6, 662 (1958).

[70] F. W. Plapp and J. E. Casida, J. Econ. Ent. 51, 800 (1958).

[71] J. Fukami and T. Shishido, Botyu-Kagaku, 28, 77 (1963).

[72] J. Fukami and T. Shishido, J. Econ. Ent. 59, 1338 (1966).

[73] J. Miyamoto Agr. Biol. Chem., Japan, 28, 411 (1964).

[74] A. Morello, A. Vardanis and E. Y. Spencer, Biochem. Biophys. Res. Commun. 29, 241 (1967).

[75] A. Morello, A. Vardanis and E. Y. Spencer, Canad. J. Biochem. 46, 885 (1968).

[76] R. M. Hollingworth, J. Agr. Food Chem. 17, 987 (1969).

[76a] M. Stiasni, D. Rehbinder and W. Decker, J. Agr. Food Chem. 15, 474 (1967).

[77] J. Stenersen, J. Econ. Ent. 62, 1043 (1969).

[77a] G. N. Smith, B. S. Watson and F. S. Fischer, J. Agr. Food Chem. 15, 132 (1967).

[78] D. H. Hutson, B. A. Pickering and C. Donninger, Biochem. J. 106, 20 P (1968).

[79] J. E. Casida, L. McBride and R. P. Niedermeier, J. Agr. Food Chem. 10, 370 (1962).

[80] R. D. O'Brien. In Toxic Phosphorus Esters, p 320. Academic Press: New York (1960).

[81] R. D. O'Brien. In Insecticides, Action and Metabolism, p 262. Academic Press: NY (1967).

[82] P. R. Chen, W. P. Tucker and W. C. Dauterman, J. Agr. Food Chem. 17, 86 (1969).

[83] J. A. A. Ketelaar and H. R. Gersmann, Rec. Trav. Chim. Pays-Bas, 77, 973 (1958).

[84] J. B. Bourke, E. J. Broderick, L. R. Hackler and P. C. Lippold, J. Agr. Food Chem. 16, 585 (1968).

[85] H. Hassan and W. C. Dauterman, Biochem. Pharmacol. 17, 1431 (1968).

[86] T. Uchida and R. D. O'Brien, Toxicol. Appl. Pharmacol. 10, 89 (1967).

[87] H. O. Esser and P. W. Müller, Experientia, 22, 36 (1966).

[88] H. O. Esser, G. Dupuis, W. Muecke and P. W. Müller, 6th Intern. Congr. Plant Protection, Vienna, Abstr. p. 199 (1967).

[89] W. Muecke, K. O. Alt and H. O. Esser, Helv. Chim. Acta, 51, 513 (1968).

[90] D. L. Bull, J. Agr. Food Chem. 16, 610 (1968).

[91] G. Dupuis, W. Muecke and H. O. Esser, J. Econ. Ent. 64, 588 (1971).

[92] J. E. Cassidy, R. T. Murphy, A. M. Mattson and R. A. Kahrs, J. Agr. Food Chem. 17, 571 (1969).

[93] C. E. Polan, J. T. Huber, R. W. Young and J. C. Osborn, J. Agr. Food Chem. 17, 857 (1969).

[94] J. M. Ford, J. J. Menn and G. D. Meyding, J. Agr. Food Chem. 14, 83 (1966).

[95] J. B. McBain, J. J. Menn and J. E. Casida, J. Agr. Food Chem. 16, 813 (1968).

[96] W. F. Chamberlain, J. Econ. Ent. 58, 51 (1965).

[97] W. M. Rogoff, G. Brody, A. R. Roth, G. H. Batchelder, G. D. Meyding, W. S. Bigley, G. H. Gretz and R. Orchard, J. Econ. Ent. 60, 640 (1967).

[98] J. C. Johnson and M. C. Bowman, J. Dairy Sci. 51, 1225 (1968),

[99] W. W. Loeffler, G. W. Trimberger, F. H. Fox, R. L. Ridgeway, D. J. Lisk and G. G. Gyrisco. J. Agr. Food Chem. 14, 46 (1966).

[100] L. J. Everett, C. A. Anderson and D. MacDougall, J. Agr. Food Chem. 14, 46 (1966).

[101] G. Schrader, see ref. 13, p 195.

[102] J. G. Matthysse and D. J. Lisk, J. Econ. Ent. 61, 1394 (1968).

103 R. M. Ings. Unpublished, cited by D. L. Colinese and H. J. Terry, *Chem. & Ind.* 1507 (1968).
104 J. C. Gage, *Food Cosmet. Toxicol.* **5**, 349 (1967).
105 M. A. Stevens and G. H. Walker, *J. Heterocyclic Chem.* **4**, 268 (1967).
106 W. H. Gutenmann, L. E. St. John and D. J. Lisk, *J. Agr. Food Chem.* **16**, 45 (1968).
107 G. N. Smith, B. S. Watson and F. S. Fischer, *J. Econ. Ent.* **59**, 1464 (1966).
108 H. V. Claborn, R. A. Hoffman, H. D. Mann and D. D. Oehler, *J. Econ. Ent.* **61**, 983 (1968).
109 L. M. Hunt, B. N. Gilbert and J. C. Schlinke, *J. Agr. Food Chem.* **17**, 1166 (1969).
110 H. J. Dishburger, J. R. Rice, W. S. McGregor and J. Pennington, *J. Econ. Ent.* **62**, 181 (1969).
111 H. V. Claborn, S. E. Kunz and H. D. Mann, *J. Econ. Ent.* **63**, 422 (1970).
112 W. Muecke, K. O. Alt and H. O. Esser, *J. Agr. Food Chem.* **18**, 208 (1970).
113 J. G. Matthysse, W. H. Gutenmann and R. Gigger, *J. Econ. Ent.* **61**, 207 (1968).
114 J. C. Derbyshire and R. T. Murphy, *J. Agr. Food Chem.* **10**, 384 (1962).
115 H. V. Claborn, H. D. Mann, R. L. Younger and R. D. Radeleff, *J. Econ. Ent.* **56**, 858 (1963).
116 J. R. Bourne and B. W. Arthur, *J. Econ. Ent.* **60**, 402 (1967).
117 P. J. Bunyan, D. M. Jennings and A. Taylor, *J. Agr. Food Chem.* **17**, 1027 (1969).
118 K. R. Millar, *N.Z. Vet. J.* **11**, 141 (1963).
119 J. N. Kaplanis, S. J. Louloudes and C. C. Roan, *Trans. Kansas Acad. Sci.* **65**, 70 (1962).
120 W. E. Robbins, T. L. Hopkins, D. I. Darrow and G. W. Eddy, *J. Econ. Ent.* **52**, 214 (1959).
121 T. R. Adkins, D. H. Kropf and S. G. Woods, *J. Econ. Ent.* **56**, 759 (1963).
121a D. D. Oehler, J. L. Eschle, J. A. Miller, H. V. Claborn and M. C. Ivey, *J. Econ. Ent.* **62**, 1481 (1969).
122 F. R. Shaw, C. T. Smith, D. L. Anderson, W. J. Fischang, W. H. Ziener and J. Hurny, *J. Econ. Ent.* **57**, 516 (1964).
123 R. W. Miller, C. H. Gordon, N. O. Morgan, M. C. Bowman and M. Beroza, *J. Econ. Ent.* **63**, 853 (1970).
124 R. D. O'Brien and L. S. Wolfe, *J.Econ. Ent.* **52**, 692 (1959).
125 H. R. Krueger, J. E. Casida and R. P. Niedermeier, *J. Agr. Food Chem.* **7**, 182 (1959).
126 W. R. Bauriedel, and M. G. Swank, *J. Agr. Food Chem.* **10**, 150 (1962).
127 N. R. Pasarela, R. E. Tondreau, W. R. Bohn and G. O. Gale, *J. Agr. Food Chem.* **15**, 920 (1967).
127a E. R. Laws, *Toxicol. Appl. Pharmacol.* **8**, 193 (1966).
128 C. Donninger, D. H. Hutson and B. A. Pickering, *Biochem. J.* **102**, 26 P (1967).
129 D. H. Hutson, D. A. A. Akintonwa and D. E. Hathway, *Biochem. J.* **102**, 133 (1967).
130 D. A. A. Akintonwa and D. H. Hutson, *J. Agr. Food Chem.* **15**, 632 (1967).
131 D. H. Hutson and D. E. Hathway, *Biochem. Pharmacol.* **16**, 949 (1967).
132 M. C. Ivey, H. V. Claborn, R. A. Hoffman, O. H. Graham, J. S. Palmer and R. D. Radeleff, *J. Econ. Ent.* **59**, 379 (1966).
133 R. R. Whetstone, D. D. Philips, Y. P. Sun, L. F. Ward and T. E. Shellenberger, *J. Agr. Food Chem.* **14**, 352 (1966).
134 M. C. Ivey, R. A. Hoffman and H. V. Claborn, *J. Econ. Ent.* **61**, 1647 (1968).
135 M. C. Ivey, R. A. Hoffman, H. V. Claborn and B. F. Hogan, *J. Econ. Ent.* **62**, 1003 (1969).
136 C. P. Yadava and F. R. Shaw, *J. Econ. Ent.* **63**, 1097 (1970).
137 R. W. Miller, C. H. Gordon, M. C. Bowman, M. Beroza and N. O. Morgan. *J. Econ. Ent.* **63**, 1420 (1970).
138 A. Morello, A. Vardanis and E. Y. Spencer, *Biochem. Pharmacol.* **17**, 1795 (1968).
139 J. E. Casida, P. E. Gatterdam, J. B. Knaak, R. D. Lance and R. P. Niedermeier, *J. Agr. Food Chem.* **6**, 658 (1958).
140 R. L. Lauwerys and S. D. Murphy, *Biochem. Pharmacol.* **18**, 789 (1969).
141 R. M. Hollingworth, T. R. Fukuto and R. L. Metcalf, *J. Agr. Food Chem.* **15**, 235 (1967).
142 J. W. Cook, *J. Agr. Food Chem.* **5**, 859 (1957).
143 M. Hitchcock and S. D. Murphy, *Biochem. Pharmacol.* **16**, 1801 (1967).
144 J. A. Rose, *Internal Report*, Ciba-Geigy Ltd, Agricultural Chemicals Research Department.
145 C. O. Knowles and B. W. Arthur, *J. Econ. Ent.* **59**, 752 (1966).
146 M. C. Ivey, J. E. Eschle, H. V. Claborn and O. M. Graham, *J. Econ. Ent.* **60**, 712 (1967).
147 H. V. Claborn, H. D. Mann, J. L. Berry and R. A. Hoffman, *J. Econ. Ent.* **58**, 922 (1965).
148 H. R. Crookshank and H. E. Smalley, *J. Agr. Food Chem.* **18**, 326 (1970).
149 M. C. Ivey, H. V. Claborn and R. L. Younger, *J. Econ. Ent.* **57**, 8 (1964).
150 D. E. Clark, R. L. Younger and C. H. Ayala, *J. Agr. Food Chem.* **14**, 608 (1966).
151 F. R. Johannsen and C. O. Knowles, *J. Econ. Ent.* **63**, 693 (1970).

TERMINAL RESIDUES OF PHOSPHONATE INSECTICIDES

J. J. MENN

Stauffer Chemical Company, Agricultural Research Center, Mountain View, California 94040, USA

ABSTRACT

Although the chemical properties of phosphonates (compounds with a P—C bond) have been known for almost a century, their excellent insecticidal properties have been discovered only recently. Metabolic studies with several phosphonothioate and phosphonodithioate insecticides showed that in most respects they resemble the phosphate ester insecticides. Neither in plants nor in animals is there evidence for P—C bond cleavage, with the exception of trichlorfon. Terminal residues consist of alkyl or aryl phosphonothioic and phosphonic acids. These acids are essentially non-toxic and readily excreted primarily in the urine. It might be possible in the future to include analytical tests for these terminal metabolites in crops and soils to serve as ancillary indicators in determining the dissipation rates of parent phosphonate insecticides.

INTRODUCTION

Organophosphorus (OP) insecticides comprise a large proportion of all available insecticides. They are coming into even more prominence today owing to the greater emphasis which our society places on preserving environmental quality by means of utilization of less persistent insecticides. As far back as 1959 it was estimated that 50 000 OP insecticides had been made[1]. Currently, it has been estimated that approximately 80 000 new pesticidal compounds are synthesized annually by US companies, and possibly as many as one-half are OP esters. Only a handful of these comprise phosphonate esters that are commercially available.

Generalized structural formulae of phosphonate ester insecticides are given in *Figure 1*, where R and R′ are usually similar or dissimilar, straight or branched alkyl chains ranging from one to five carbon atoms, and R can also consist of chloroalkyl, cyclic or aromatic moieties. The 'leaving group' (R″) is susceptible to displacement by a nucleophilic reagent such as a water molecule or an OH⁻ ion.

The first definite OP compound with a P—C bond, diethyl ester of methane phosphonic acid, was synthesized by A. V. Hofmann in 1873[2]. Hofmann also established the extreme chemical stability of the P—C bond. These studies eventually gave rise in 1938[3] to the synthesis of the powerful cholinesterase inhibitor, Sarin (I) (*Figure 2*), a forerunner of the phosphonate insecticides.

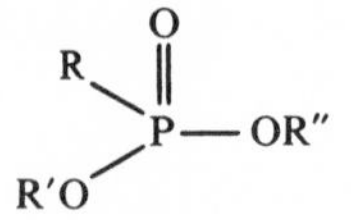

Phosphonate

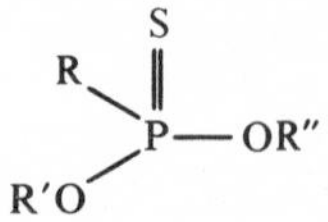

Phosphonothioate

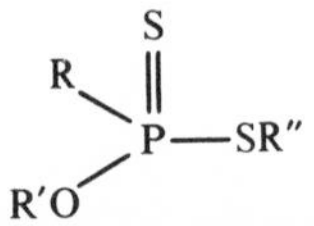

Phosphonodithioate

R,R' = lower alkyl
chloroalkyl,
or phenyl
R'' = leaving group.

Figure 1. Generalized structures of phosphonate esters.

A search through several references[4, 5, 1, 6] revealed a number of phosphonic acid ester insecticides. The compounds are illustrated in *Figure 2*, where they are grouped into phosphonates, phosphonothioates and phosphonodithioates.

Since, in many instances, phosphonates display excellent insecticidal activity in comparison to their phosphate analogues[7–10], it is surprising that so few have reached commercial status. One possible explanation is that phosphonates require more complicated synthetic procedures than those commonly in use for OP esters[7] and, consequently, they are more expensive.

This paper reviews the metabolism and degradation of phosphonate insecticides, with special attention to the biotransformation steps and products formed in animals and plants.

Since the parent phosphonates and, in some instances, one or more of their metabolites or degradation products are toxic to living organisms, it is important to determine their nature, the amounts in which they are formed and their ultimate disposition.

This knowledge is also needed to provide a better understanding of the mode of action of these materials, and ultimately to generate the basic information necessary for development of meaningful residue analysis methods and to

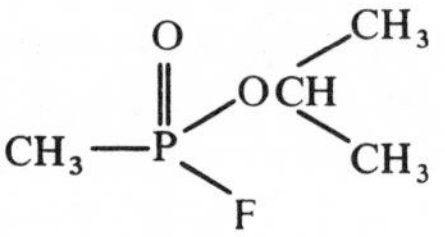

(I) Sarin

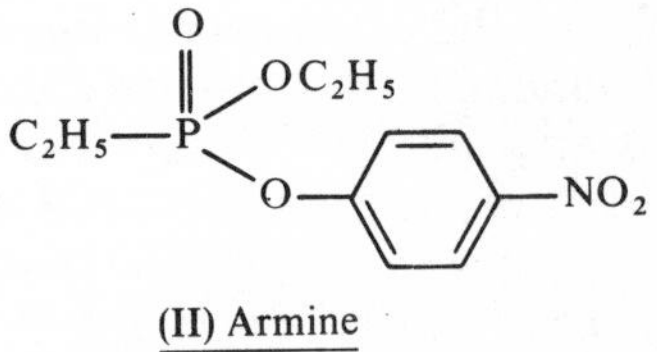

(II) Armine

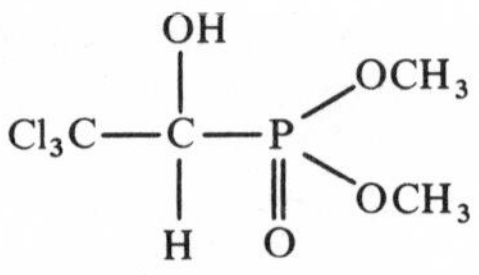

(III) Trichlorfon

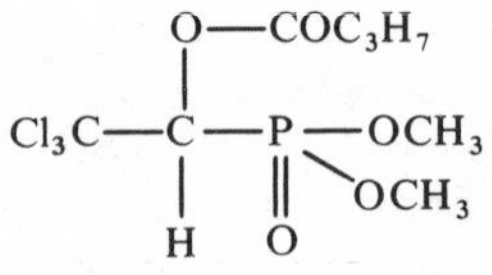

(IIIa) Butonate

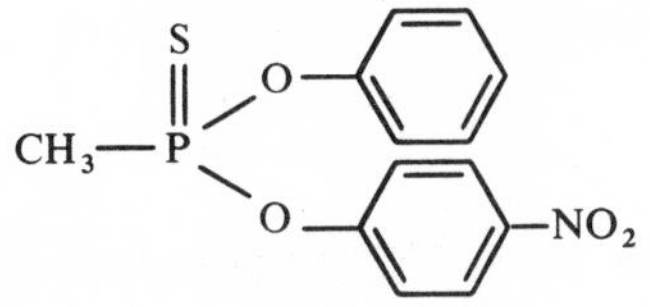

(IV) Colep

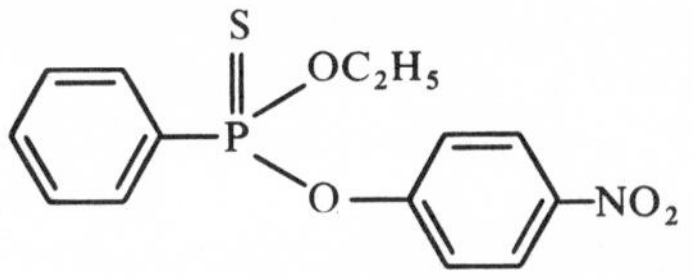

(V) EPN

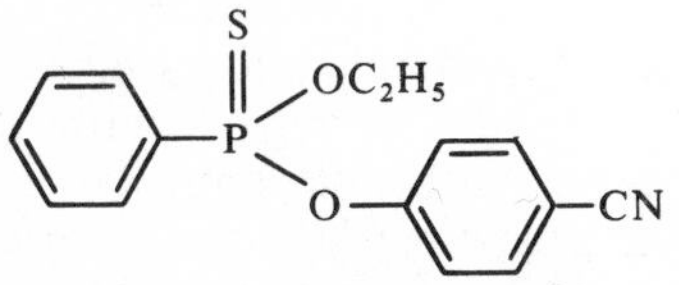

(VI) Surecide

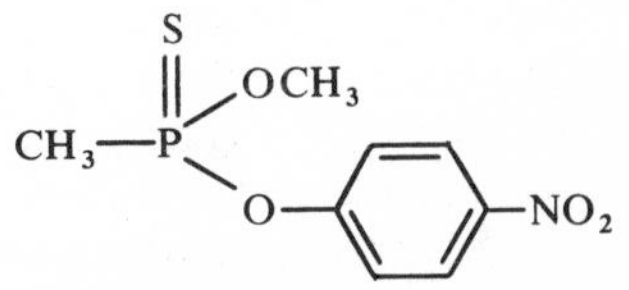

(VII) Methyl paraphonothion

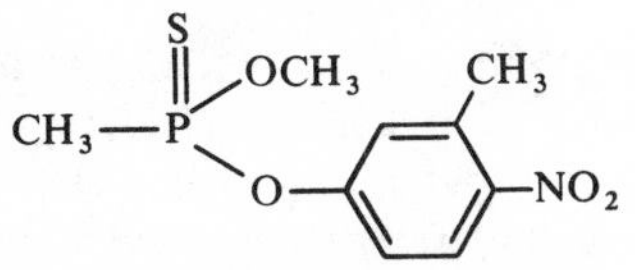

(VIII) Sumiphonothion

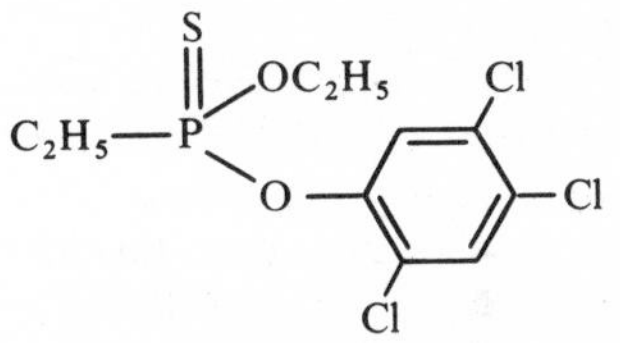

(IX) Agritox

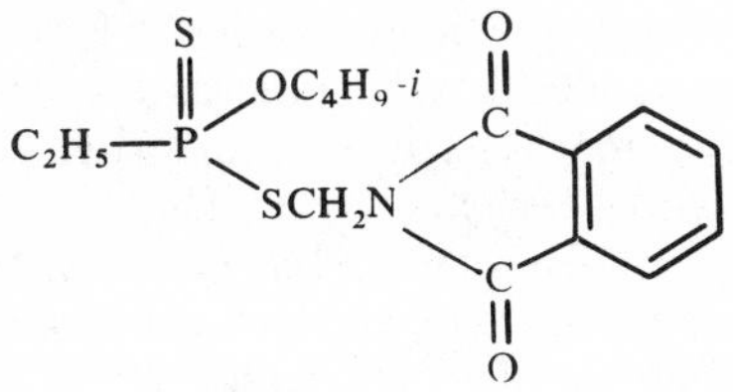

(X) N-4543

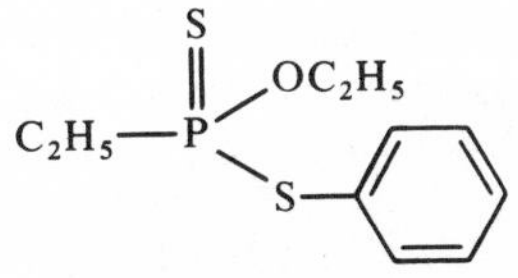

(XI) Dyfonate

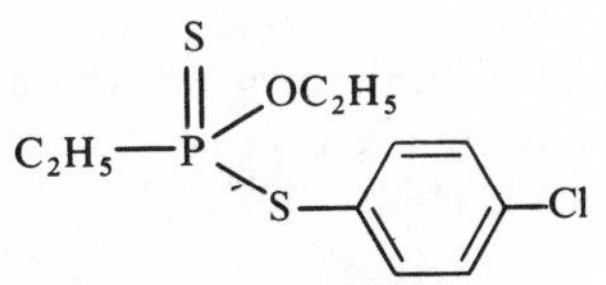

(XII) N-2596

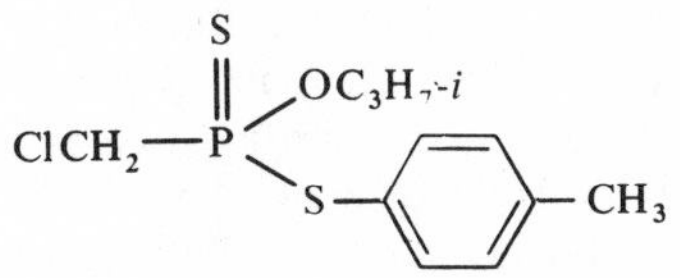

(XIII) B-10119

Figure 2. Structures of selected phosphonate (I, II, III, IIIa), phosphonothioate (IV to IX inclusive) and phosphonodithioate (X to XIII) insecticides.

provide a comprehensive basis for establishment of tolerances for permissible, negligible or finite residues.

TRICHLORFON

Four phosphonate esters are shown in *Figure 2*: Sarin (I), a model compound in many pharmacological studies; Armine (II), a phosphonate analogue of paraoxon used for glaucoma therapy in the USSR; trichlorfon (III); Butonate (IIIa).

Trichlorfon [dimethyl(2,2,2-trichloro-1-hydroxyethyl)phosphonate] is, perhaps, the best-known phosphonate insecticide. However, in a sense it is an anomalous phosphonate if considered in terms of the generalized phosphonate structures shown in *Figure 1*; the P—C bond of trichlorfon involves the 'leaving group' rather than an alkyl group. Furthermore, whether trichlorfon exerts its toxic action in the phosphonate form or by arrangement to dichlorvos (2,2-dichlorovinyl dimethyl phosphate) is still disputed[7, 1]. *In vitro*, the rearrangement, coupled with a loss of hydrogen chloride, occurs spontaneously at pH 6 or higher[7, 11].

However, metabolism in animals and plants may not involve primarily this pathway. Metabolic studies in the dog with [32P]trichlorfon (III) injected intraveneously at a dose of 150 mg/kg[12] showed rapid and extensive cleavage of the P—C bond, as evidenced by recovery in 48 h of 67 per cent of the injected dose in urine as trichloroethyl glucuronide (TEG), which was identified by chemical tests. Trichlorfon levels fell rapidly in blood and urine. The apparent half-life of the parent insecticide in blood was less than 30 min, based on water-solvent partitioning experiments.

Only one per cent of the dose was recovered as unchanged trichlorfon in urine, from zero to two days post-treatment. The remaining 32P-labelled materials were described as hydrolysis products. No evidence was obtained for dehydrochlorination *in vivo* and rearrangement to the more toxic dichlorvos.

In pea plants, [32P]trichlorfon hydrolyses rapidly[12]. The metabolic products of [32P]trichlorfon in the plant were identified as dimethyl phosphoric acid (DMP), methyl phosphoric acid (MP) and inorganic phosphate[13].

Robbins *et al.*[14] studied the metabolic fate of [32P]trichlorfon after oral administration of 25 mg/kg to a lactating cow. Excretion of metabolic products in urine was very rapid; 66 per cent of the administered does was recovered during the first 12 h after dosing. Only 0.17 per cent of the administered does was unchanged trichlorfon; 16.8 per cent consisted of what was considered to be DMP and 76 per cent of an unknown phosphorus-containing metabolite. Milk contained less than 0·2 per cent of the radioactive dose, of which less than 0.02 per cent was trichlorfon. No dichlorvos was found in blood, milk or urine. The authors concluded from their work that trichlorfon is metabolized, leaving the P—C bond largely intact. However, it is difficult to reconcile this conclusion with other available data.

Labelling the α-carbon atom of the hydroxyethyl moiety of trichlorfon with 14C would provide more direct biochemical evidence for the biotransformation *in vivo* of this phosphonate insecticide.

Application of [32P]trichlorfon to lactating cows by dipping, intravenous or intramuscular injection resulted in excretion of dichlorvos, DMP and demethyltrichlorfon (DTCP) in the aqueous phase of milk[15]. Subcutaneous

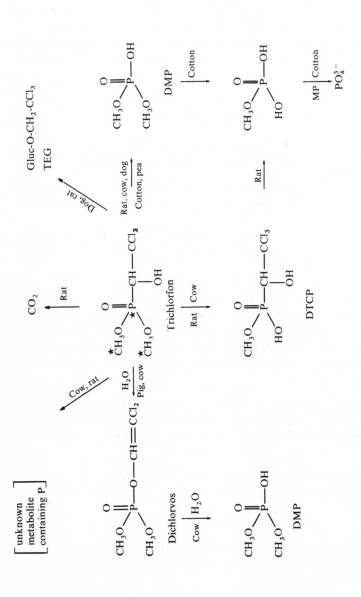

Figure 3. Proposed metabolic pathway for trichlorfon (see refs. 11, 12, 17). DMP, dimethylphosphoric acid; MP, methylphosphoric acid; DTCP, demethyl-trichlorfon: TEG trichlorethyl glucuronide.

61

injection of [³²P]trichlorfon into piglets also resulted in appearance of dichlorvos in the blood and intestines up to 3.5 h after injection[16].

Intraperitoneal injection of [²³P]trichlorfon into rats at a dose of 100 mg/kg resulted in the recovery of 75 to 85 per cent of the administered dose in urine within 48 h after injection. Of that recovered, methyl phosphate (MP) accounted for 20 to 30 per cent, DMP for 60 to 70 per cent and an unidentified metabolite for about 10 per cent[17].

The proposed metabolic pathway for trichlorfon in mammals and plants is presented in *Figure 3*. It is readily seen that the compound is metabolized: by de-alkylation to DTCP and MP; by hydrolytic cleavage to TEG, DMP and MP; by rearrangement to dichlorvos.

Although it has been stated[18] that trichlorfon is metabolized largely by cleavage of the P—C bond, the only direct evidence for this pathway is the isolation of TEG[12].

Thus it appears that further metabolic studies are needed to determine clearly the sequence of biochemical steps involved in the biotransformation of trichlorfon.

It is apparent from the foregoing studies that, regardless of the mechanism involved, the P—C bond of trichlorfon is broken, giving rise to terminal residues derived from phosphoric acid.

BUTONATE

The selective insecticide Butonate (IIIa) (*O,O*-dimethyl 2,2,2-trichloro-1-butyryloxyethyl phosphonate), an acyloxy ethyl derivative of trichlorfon, was synthesized by Arthur and Casida[19]. In most respects it resembles trichlorfon and yields similar metabolic products in plants[20] and rats[19].

Butonate is equitoxic to trichlorfon in houseflies but two- to three-fold less toxic to rats. The differential toxicity has been attributed to esteratic cleavage of the acyl group yielding trichlorfon in insects, whereas in mammals demethylation and cleavage of the phosphonate moiety predominate.

In fruit and grain crops Butonate is rapidly converted into trichlorfon[20] and further degraded to water-soluble metabolites.

Consequently, with the addition of the de-esterification step, Butonate undergoes the same biotransformation reactions in plants and animals as shown for trichlorfon in *Figure 3*.

COLEP

The experimental insecticide Colep [*O*-phenyl (*O*-4-nitrophenyl)methyl-phosphonothioate] (IV) is an interesting methyl phosphonate analogue of parathion. The metabolic fate of Colep was studied by Marco and Jaworski[21] in the rat, apple and cotton plants.

Phenyl-¹⁴C-labelled Colep was orally administered to rats at two doses: 0.45 mg/kg and 1.19 mg/kg, one rat per dose. Plant foliage was topically treated at the rate of 52 µg/leaf.

Radioactive samples were prepared for analyses by means of selective solvent extraction, ion-exchange column chromatography, thin-layer chromatography (TLC) and chromatographically separated metabolites were quantified by liquid scintillation counting (LSC).

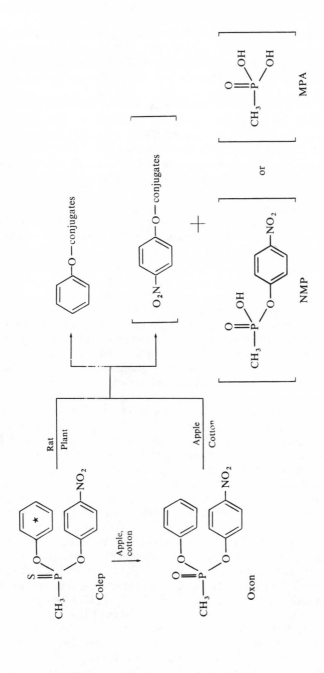

Figure 4. Suggested metabolic pathway for Colep in plants and animals (see ref. 21). Phenol conjugates: α- and β-glycoside in plant, glucuronide in rat. Oxon, O-phenyl O-(4-nitrophenyl)methylphosphonate; NMP, O-(4-nitrophenyl)methylphosphonic acid; MPA, methylphosphonic acid.

The suggested metabolic pathway for Colep is presented in *Figure 4*.

Limited desulphuration of Colep to the oxon was indicated in plants. The major radioactive plant metabolites and metabolites in rat urine appeared to be conjugates of the cleaved phenol. By means of column elution patterns, acid hydrolysis and emulsin (β-glucosidase) cleavage experiments it appeared that the phenol moiety was conjugated in plants as β- or α-glucoside and as the glucuronide in the rat. This detoxication mechanism implies that O-(4-nitrophenyl)methyl phosphonic (NMP) and phosphono-thioic acids were also formed as metabolites. Furthermore, cleavage of the nitrophenyl moiety is also likely since it is a better leaving group than phenol. Cleavage of both phenolic groups would give rise to methyl phosphonic acid (MPA) as the terminal metabolite. However, it was not possible to determine this since only one labelling position was employed in the foregoing studies.

The methyl phosphonate portion is the unusual moiety in Colep. A *methyl*-^{14}C label would provide a very useful metabolic handle to determine the nature of the metabolites arising from the methyl phosphonic acid moiety.

EPN

Although the arylphosphonothioate insecticide and acaricide EPN (V) (O-ethyl O-p-nitrophenyl phenyl phosphonothioate) was commercially introduced 22 years ago, only fragmentary published information is available on its metabolism in animals, and none exists for plants. The few available published reports deal with metabolic degradation of EPN in isolated biological systems, and on this basis an attempt is made to construct a reasonable degradative pathway for this arylphosphonothioate insecticide.

Ahmed et al.[22] incubated EPN and EPNO (O-ethyl O-p-nitrophenyl phenyl phosphonate) at 300 p.p.m. each in one litre of cow rumen juice at 28°C. After 3 h, they recovered five per cent of the EPN as amino-EPN and 50 per cent of the EPNO as amino-EPNO. The remaining material from each starting product was accounted for as hydrolysis products. The formation of the reduction products was confirmed by derived coloured products, column chromatography and infra-red spectra. The better recovery of the amino phosphonate was due to the greater hydrolysis rate of the phosphono-thioate than the phosphonate by rumen juice. The reduction reaction is a clear-cut example of detoxication in mammals and insects; toxicity was reduced by a factor greater than 100 and 10000 respectively, based on comparison of LD_{50} values for parathion, paraoxon and the respective amino products. By analogy, the respective detoxication mechanism would apply to the biochemical reduction of EPN and EPNO to their respective amino products. Reduction in vitro of EPN to amino EPN was also demonstrated with liver homogenates from mammalian and avian species in the presence of $NADPH_2$ and FAD cofactors[23]. The aminated parathion and paraoxon were rapidly eliminated from a cow after feeding of parathion. Only trace amounts were recovered from milk and fat and then only after the first 24 h after treatment. The aminated products readily cleaved in vivo to hydrolysis products which were excreted largely in urine[22]. Again, and in a

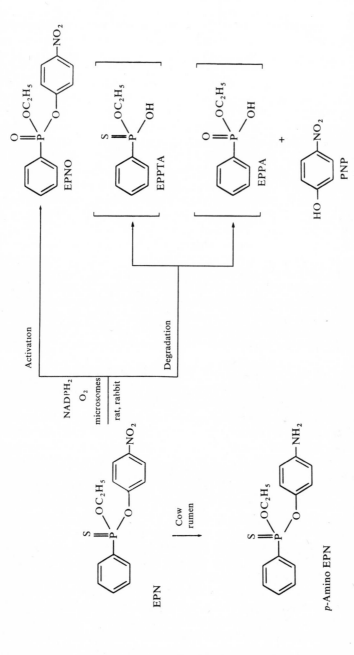

Figure 5. Proposed metabolic pathway for EPN in animals (see refs 22, 24). EPNO, *O*-ethyl *O-p*-nitrophenyl phenyl phosphonate; EPPTA, *O*-ethyl phenyl phosphonothioic acid; EPPA, *O*-ethyl phenyl phosphonic acid; PNP, *p*-nitrophenol.

65

speculative manner, it is reasonable to assume that EPN would undergo similar degradative events in the cow.

Nakatsugawa et al.[24] examined the microsomal degradation of EPN using rabbit liver microsomal pellets in the presence of $NADPH_2$. EPN and EPNO were extracted from the incubation mixtures and estimated by electron-capture gas chromatography (GLC). Production of p-nitrophenol (PNP) was measured colorimetically at 400 nm. Further identification of metabolites was carried out with TLC, and co-chromatography with authentic reference standards. Metabolic products consisted of PNP, EPNO and O-ethyl phenyl phosphonothioic acid (EPPTA) and, very likely, O-ethyl phenyl phosphonic acid (EPPA). Hydrolysis of EPNO was not enhanced by $NADPH_2$, indicating that hydrolytic, rather than oxidative, reactions were primarily involved in cleaving EPNO.

The metabolic pathway for EPN, proposed in *Figure 5*, is based largely on information derived from the foregoing studies. By analogy with other organophosphorus esters, it appears that EPNO is the only toxic metabolite of EPN which is of biological significance in terms of residues of this insecticide. Amino-EPN, PNP and the implied metabolites, EPPTA and EPPA, represent detoxication products.

Since the phenyl phosphonate moiety is biologically novel, it would be of interest to study the metabolism *in vivo* of EPN in animals and plants with EPN labelled with ^{14}C in the phenyl ring. Such studies would supplement and complement the limited, currently available, metabolic data on the biotransformation *in vivo* of EPN. Such studies would also be applicable to elucidate the metabolic fate of the more recently introduced phenyl phosphonothioate insecticide, Surecide (VI).

METHYL PARAPHONOTHION

The studies reviewed so far shed little light on the fate of the phosphonic acid moiety liberated as a result of metabolism of phosphonate esters *in vivo*.

Hollingworth et al.[25] studied the metabolism in mice of the phosphonothioate analogue of methyl parathion, which they named methyl paraphonothion (VII). In comparison with other phosphonate–phosphate pairs, here, too, methyl paraphonothion proved to be an excellent insecticide, superior to methyl parathion against susceptible and phosphate-resistant house flies[26]. However, (VII) proved to be also substantially more toxic orally to mice than methyl parathion.

Male Swiss mice were orally dosed with ^{32}P-labelled methyl paraphonothion at the rate of 2.5 mg/kg and maintained in Roth metabolism cages, enabling separate collection of urine and faeces, up to 72 h after dosing.

Metabolites in urine were separated by gradient elution ion-exchange column chromatography. Metabolites were quantified by planchet counting in a gas flow counter. Identity of metabolites was established by column and paper chromatography with known reference metabolites. Of the 60 per cent of the administered radioactivity recovered in urine through 72 h, 97·8 per cent was distributed among six metabolites in the amounts (percentages) shown in *Figure 6*. The remaining 2.2 per cent was distributed between two minor unknown metabolites.

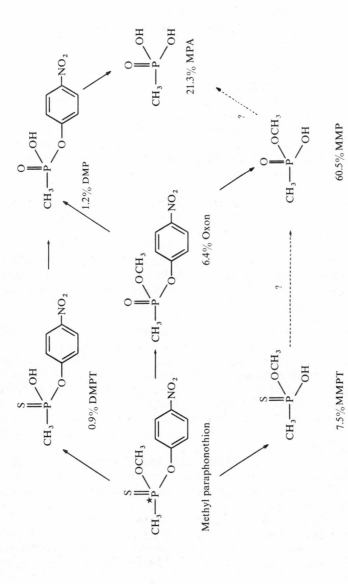

Figure 6. Proposed metabolic pathway for methyl paraphonothion in mice (see ref. 25). Oxon, *O*-methyl *O-p*-nitrophenyl methane phosphonate; DMPT, *O-p*-nitrophenyl methane phosphonothioic acid: DMP, *O-p*-nitrophenyl methane phosphonic acid: MPA, methylphosphonic acid; MMPT, *O*-methyl methane phosphonothioic acid; MMP, *O*-methyl methane phosphonic acid.

It is significant that, in all the biotransformation steps, the P—C bond remains intact. Furthermore, unlike the metabolism of methyl parathion[25], where demethylation played a key role in detoxication, demethylphosphono-thioate (DMPT) and demethylphosphonate (DMP) are only minor metabolic products. Consequently, detoxication appears to involve primarily cleavage of the *P-O*-aryl bond. The proposed sequence of reactions shown in *Figure 6* is drawn largely by analogy with the pathway proposed by Hollingworth *et al.*[26] for methyl parathion and Sumithion. No evidence is available on the precise sequence of metabolite formation, and whether P═O metabolites are formed primarily before or after hydrolysis.

However, it appears that all the metabolites, with the exception of the oxon, are readily excreted, non-toxic terminal residues. The same studies were conducted also with Sumiphonothion (VIII) and provided similar metabolic findings.[32]P-labelled residues were not quantified in faeces and tissue in the foregoing studies. Consequently it is not possible to determine from this work whether all phosphonate residues were readily eliminated from the organism.

The biological stability of alkyl phosphonic acids was first demonstrated by Hoskin[27]. He injected intraperitoneally into rats ^{32}P-labelled methyl phosphonic acid and isopropyl methyl phosphonic acid, the metabolic product of Sarin (I) in rats. Both acids were recovered unchanged in urine. Furthermore, rat muscle phosphorylase was unable to catalyse the synthesis of hexose phosphonate esters from these phosphonic acids under conditions where hexose phosphates are readily synthesized from phosphoric acid.

N-4543

The previously reviewed studies have demonstrated the metabolic stability of the P—C bond in phosphonate terminal residues consisting of methyl and phenyl phosphonic acid derivatives. The experimental insecticide N-4543 (*S*-phthalimidomethyl *O*-isobutyl ethylphosphonodithioate) is a phosphonate insecticide where the alkyl moiety of the phosphonic acid portion of the molecule is an ethane group.

The chemistry and biological properties of this heterocyclic phosphono-dithioate insecticide and acaricide were described by Szabo and Menn[10], and van den Brink *et al.*[28].

It appeared likely that N-4543 would undergo hydrolytic cleavage in a manner analogous with the related phosphorodithioate insecticide Imidan®[29], giving rise to phthalate and phosphonate moieties. Consequently, two labelled preparations, namely, *i*-BuO-1-^{14}C and carbonyl-^{14}C, were studied to elucidate the metabolic fate of N-4543 in rats[30].

Rats were orally dosed with each labelled preparation at a dosage of 4.5 mg/kg and placed individually in metabolism cages, enabling separate collection of urine, faeces and exhaled air, according to the method described by Ford *et al.*[31].

The absorption, distribution and excretion pattern of ^{14}C from both preparations was similar and paralleled results obtained with other OP compounds. Within 96 h after dosing with N-4543-*i*-BuO-1-^{14}C, the radio-activity recovered as a percentage of the administered dose was distributed as follows: 62 per cent in urine, 34 per cent in faeces and 0.6 per cent in expired air. The carbonyl-^{14}C labelled residues yielded 69 per cent ^{14}C in urine and 19 per cent in faeces within 24 h after dosing. In neither case was there any accumulation of ^{14}C in tissues.

No common metabolites were detected in the urine of rats receiving either labelled preparation of N-4543, thus indicating that the carbonyl and isobutyl moieties were no longer linked together. Since only a trace amount of ^{14}CO$_2$ was recovered in the expired air of rats dosed with N-4543-i-BuO-1-^{14}C, it is apparent that the P-O-isobutyl bond remained intact. Had such cleavage occurred it would have resulted in liberation of isobutanol, which is mainly converted into ^{14}CO$_2$ in $vivo$[32].

Metabolites in urine were separated by TLC, co-chromatographed with reference metabolites and detected by radioautography.

The proposed metabolic pathway of N-4543 in the rat is shown in $Figure$ 7.

The phthaloyl portion of N-4543 is excreted in urine in a similar fashion to Imidan[29], with phthalamic acid (PAA) and phthalic acid (PA) constituting the major metabolites in urine, and acid hydrolysis converting six remaining metabolites in urine into PA. Four metabolites in urine from rats treated with N-4543-i-BuO-1-^{14}C were detected by TLC. It appears that i-butoxy ethane phosphonic acid (BEP) ($Figure$ 7) is the major terminal metabolite in urine. Enzymatic and hydrolysis cleavage experiments suggest that a portion of BEP is excreted in urine as a conjugate other than a sulphate or glucuronide. Incubation with β-glucuronidase or arylsulphatase + β-glucuronidase mixture did not release BEP, but acid hydrolysis of urine yielded one radioactive product which co-chromatographs with BEP.

DYFONATE®

The soil insecticide Dyfonate, O-ethyl S-phenylethylphosphonodithioate (XI), labelled in the α-ethoxy carbon of the phosphonothioate moiety (E-^{14}C), in the ring of the thiophenyl moiety (R-^{14}C) and the sulphur of thiophenyl moiety (T-^{35}S), was used to facilitate studies useful in characterizing and identifying metabolites arising from both the thiophenyl and thiophosphonic acid moieties of Dyfonate in animals and plants. These studies may serve as a more complete model for studying the metabolic fate of phosphonate insecticides.

$Table$ 1 summarizes the radioactivity recovered from two groups of four rats, each dosed orally with Dyfonate-(T-^{35}S) and -(E-^{14}C) according to the procedure described by Ford et $al.$[31].

Table 1. Average radioactivity recovered from rats 96 h after receiving single oral doses* of Dyfonate-(E-^{14}C) and -(T-^{35}S)

Source	Administered radioactive dose (%)	
	E-^{14}C	T-^{35}S
Urine	94.5	63.8
Faeces	5.0	33.1
Tissues	0.0	3.0
Expired air	0.5	<0.1

* 0.08 mg of Dyfonate -(F-^{14}C)/kg;
  2.0 mg of Dyfonate -(T-^{35}S)/kg.

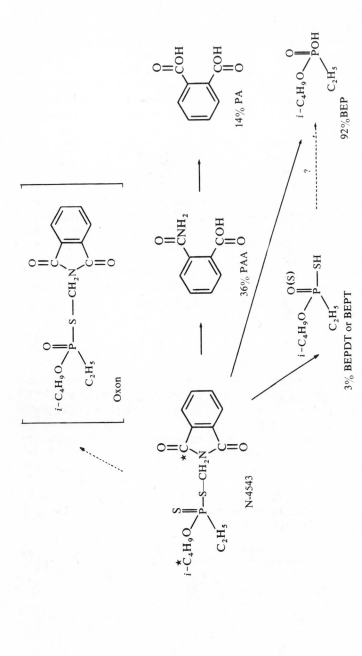

Figure 7. Proposed metabolic pathway of N-4543 in rats (see ref. 30). Oxon; [S-phthalimidomethyl O-isobutyl ethyl phosphonothioate]; PAA, phthalamic acid, PA, phthalic acid; PAA, phthalamic acid; BEPDT, i-butoxy ethane phosphonodithioic acid; BEPT, i-butoxy ethane phosphonothiolic acid; BEP i-butoxy ethane phosphonic acid.

It is evident that Dyfonate residues in the animal are eliminated primarily in the urine, as is the case with all other phosphate insecticides[1] and the phosphonates discussed so far in this paper. The dissimilarity in faecal radioactivity from both labels also suggests that Dyfonate metabolites may also be excreted in the bile as a secondary route of residue elimination. Recent studies have indicated that the E-^{14}C faecal residue is largely unchanged Dyfonate[33]. Only a trace amount of E-^{14}C activity was recovered as [14]CO$_2$, indicating that de-ethylation is at best only a minor detoxication pathway for this compound. Had cleavage occurred at the α-ethoxy carbon, large amounts of [14]CO$_2$ would have been expected as a result of ethanol metabolism[34]. Animal balance studies of short duration (24 to 96 h), usually indicate small radioactive residues in tissues. With OP insecticides, these are almost always uniformly distributed without evidence of selective accumulation in storage organs or tissues. Biological half-life experiments conducted with Dyfonate-(T-^{35}S) have shown rapid removal of essentially all ^{35}S residues from rats within 16 days after dosing[35].

Irish potatoes were selected as a representative root crop for determining the metabolism of Dyfonate-(E-^{14}C) and -(R-^{14}C) in plants. Sprouting potato pieces were planted in soil containing uniformly incorporated radioactive Dyfonate at the rate of 2.64 p.p.m. (approximating actual field rates). Plant material was analysed through 87 days after planting. Details of the plant study were reported by McBain et al.[36].

The proposed metabolic pathway of Dyfonate in plants and animals is presented in *Figure 8*. This is based on metabolites which were identified by thin-layer chromatography, radio-gas–liquid chromatography, hydrolysis, enzymatic cleavage, derivation of metabolites and mass spectrometry. In the rat, the biotransformation pathway for the thiophenol (PSH) moiety was also established from separate metabolism studies with ^{35}S-labelled PSH, methylphenyl[^{35}S]sulphide (MPS) and methylphenyl[^{35}S]sulphone (MPSO$_2$)[37]. These studies indicated that the same products are formed from PSH, MPS and MPSO$_2$, and so each product must ultimately be derived from MPSO$_2$.

MPSO$_2$ is further biotransformed to more polar products in the animal and plant. Acid hydrolysis yields 3-(hydroxyphenyl)methylsulphone (3-OH-MPSO$_2$) and 4-(hydroxyphenyl)methylsulphone (4-OH-MPSO$_2$) as the major water-soluble metabolites in urine[33].

Although the polar, thiophenyl-derived plant metabolites have not been conclusively identified, enzyme cleavage and acid hydrolysis studies indicate that very likely MPSO$_2$ is hydroxylated and further metabolized via glycoside and, to a lesser extent, sulphate conjugation.

Cleavage of Dyfonate at the P—S junction converts the phosphonate moiety primarily into O-ethyl ethane phosphonothioic acid (ETP) and to O-ethyl ethane phosphonic acid (EOP) in the animal and plant.

Quantitation of the Dyfonate metabolites found in foliage of 60-days-old potato plants and rat urine collected from 0 to 48 h is shown in *Figure 9*. Of the total plant ^{14}C, 41.4 per cent represents, in descending order: EOP, MPSO$_2$, oxon, ETP, MPSO and Dyfonate. An additional 15 per cent of the ^{14}C in plants, arising primarily from the phosphonate moiety, has been incorporated into plant constituents. The remainder primarily represents

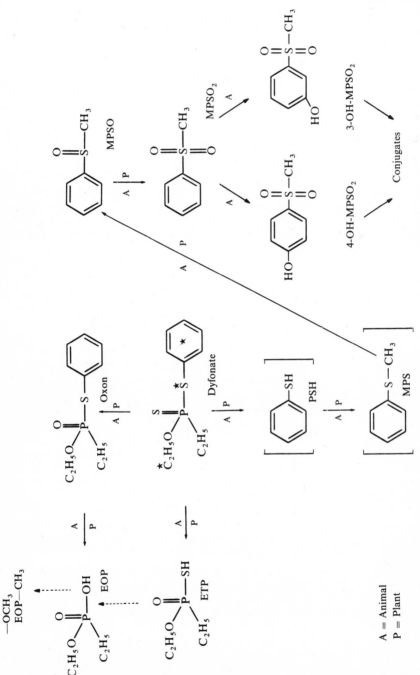

Figure 8. Proposed metabolic pathway of Dyfonate in the rat and the potato plant: metabolites and routes (see refs 33, 35, 36). Oxon, *O*-ethyl *S*-phenyl ethyl-phosphonothiolate; ETP, *O*-ethyl ethane phosphonothioic acid; EOP, *O*-ethyl ethane phosphonothioic acid; PSH, thiophenol; MPS, methylphenylsulphide; MPSO, methylphenylsulphoxide; MPSO$_2$, methylphenylsulphone; 4-OH-MPSO$_2$, 4-(hydroxyphenyl)methylsulphone; 3-OH-MPSO$_2$, 3-(hydroxyphenyl)methyl-sulphone; EOP-CH$_3$, *O*-ethyl ethyl phosphonate; ETP-CH$_3$, *O*-ethyl *O*-methyl ethyl phosphonothioate.

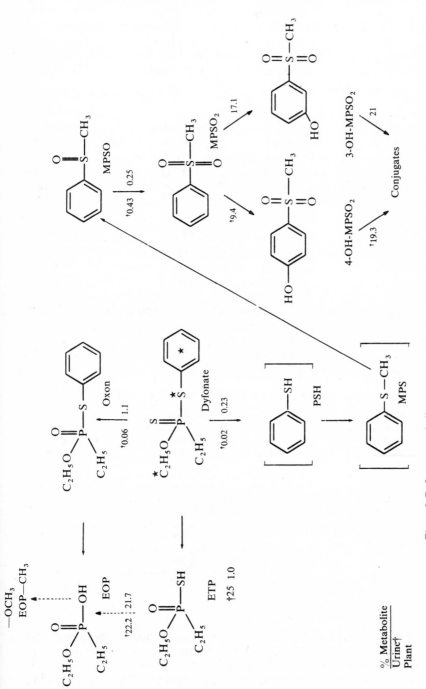

Figure 9. Dyfonate metabolites (percentages) recovered from potato foliage and rat urine.

73

two polar derivatives of $MPSO_2$ (35.1 per cent). In urine, 97 per cent of the ^{14}C represents, in descending order: ETP, EOP, 3-OH-$MPSO_2$, 4-OH-$MPSO_2$, $MPSO_2$, MPSO and traces of the oxon and Dyfonate.

Each biotransformation step in the metabolism of Dyfonate, with the exception of oxon formation, is associated with detoxication. The acute toxicities of Dyfonate metabolites to the rat, orally, and the house fly, by topical application, are shown in *Figure 10*.

PSH is toxic to rats, but *S*-methylation and sulphoxidation are highly effective detoxication steps, as shown by the rat LD_{50} values for MPS and $MPSO_2$. *S*-Methylation is apparently non-reversible in animals, based on our findings and those of Bull[38], who reported the sulphoxidation of intact dimethyl *p*-(methylthio-^{14}C)phenyl phosphate (GC-6506) in the cotton plant, and subsequent cleavage to derivatives of MPSO and $MPSO_2$. The phosphonic acid terminal residues, ETP and EOP, are only slightly toxic to rats and the house fly, and both are readily and completely excreted by the rat.

CONCLUSION

This paper provides information which demonstrates that phosphonate insecticides undergo activation and detoxication reactions in plants and animals similar to those so abundantly described for the phosphate insecticides.

The major metabolic difference between the two groups is confined to the stability of the P—C bond of the phosphonate insecticides in plants and animals.

The identity and occurrence of terminal phosphonic acid-derived residues in plants and animals are summarized in *Table 2*.

Table 2. Terminal phosphonate residues in animals and plants

Parent phosphonate	Metabolite (s)	Occurrence
Sarin (I)	*i*-Propyl methyl phosphonic acid	Rat
Colep (IV)	Methyl phosphonic acid	Rat, apple cotton
EPN (V)	*O*-Ethyl phenyl phosphonothioic acid	Rat, rabbit
	O-Ethyl phenyl phosphonic acid	Rat, rabbit
Methyl paraphonothion (VII)	*O*-Methyl methane phosphonothioic acid	Mouse
	O-Methyl methane phosphonic acid	Mouse
Sumiphonothion (VIII)	*O*-Methyl methane phosphonothioic acid	Mouse
	O-Methyl methane phosphonic acid	Mouse
N-4543 (X)	*i*-Butoxy ethane phosphonothioic acid	Rat
	i-Butoxy ethane phosphonic acid	Rat
Dyfonate (XI)	*O*-Ethyl ethane phosphonothioic acid	Rat, potato
	O-Ethyl ethane phosphonic acid	Rat, potato

Data presented in this paper show that where the alkyl moiety comprising the P—C bond of the phosphonic acid consists of methyl and ethyl groups, these terminal residues are readily voided from animals, primarily in urine. This was demonstrated with the following compounds: methyl paraphonothion (VII), Sumiphonothion (VIII), Dyfonate (XI), Sarin (I) and N-4543 (X).

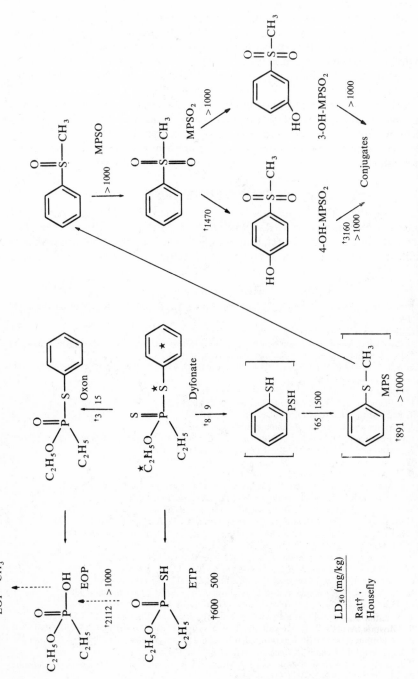

Figure 10. Comparative acute toxicity of Dyfonate metabolites to the rat (oral) and housefly (topical) in mg/kg.

75

It is also likely that ethyl ethane phosphonothioic and phosphonic acids are the terminal residues of the soil insecticides Agritox (IX) and N-2596 (XII). Data for the remaining phosphonates *in vivo* are either lacking or inconclusive owing to the inadequate selection of a labelling position in the insecticide molecule. It would be especially interesting to determine the fate of the phenyl phosphonic acid moiety of EPN (V) *in vivo*. Nothing is known of the metabolic fate of chloroalkyl phosphonates, such as B-10119 (XIII), in animals and plants.

Both methyl and ethyl phosphonic acids are essentially nontoxic to rats and insects and presumably to other animals and man. By virtue of non-accumulation and ready removal from animals, they appear to be innocuous terminal residues whose impact on the environment would seem to be minimal.

ACKNOWLEDGEMENT

I thank the following persons for their critical review of this paper and constructive comments: J. R. DeBaun, L. J. Hoffman and J. B. Miaullis, Agricultural Research Center, Stauffer Chemical Company, Mountain View, California; and L. Lykken, University of California, Berkeley, California.

REFERENCES

[1] R. D. O'Brien. In *Insecticides, Action and Metabolism*, Academic Press: New York and London (1967).

[2] G. Schrader. *Pflanzenschutz Berichte.* **36**, 29 (1967).

[3] G. Schrader. *Die Entwicklung neuer Insektizider Phosphorsäure-Ester* (*Monograph No. 62*, 3rd ed.), Verlag Chemie GmbH, Weinheim/Bergstr. (1963).

[4] G. Schrader. *Die Entwicklung neurer Insektizider Phosphorsäure-Ester.* Verlag Chemie GmbH. Weinheim/Bergstr. (1963).

[5] G. Schrader. *World Rev. Pest Cont.* **4**, 140 (1965).

[6] E. E. Kenaga and W. E. Allison. *Bull. Ent. Soc. Am.* **15**, 85 (1969).

[7] T. R. Fukuto. *Ann. Rev. Entomol.* **6**, 313 (1961).

[8] J. J. Menn and K. Szabo. *J. Econ. Ent.* **58**, 734 (1965).

[9] R. B. Fearing, E. N. Walsh, J. J. Menn and A. H. Freiberg. *J. Agr. Food Chem.* **17**, 1261 (1969).

[10] K. Szabo and J. J. Menn. *J. Agr. Food Chem.* **17**, 863 (1969).

[11] W. Dedek and H. Schwarz. *Atompraxis*, **12**, 603 (1966).

[12] B. W. Arthur and J. E. Casida. *J. Agr. Food Chem.* **5**, 186 (1957).

[13] I. Y. Mostafa, A. Hassan and S. M. A. D. Zayed. *Z. Naturforsch.* (B), **20**, 67 (1965).

[14] W. E. Robbins, T. L. Hopkins and G. W. Eddy. *J. Econ. Ent.* **49**, 801 (1956).

[15] W. Dedek and H. Schwarz. *Arch. Exp. Veterinaermed.* **20**, 849 (1966).

[16] H. Schwarz and W. Dedek. *Zentr. Veterinaermed., Reihe B.* **12**, 653 (1965).

[17] A. Hassan, S. M. A. D. Zayed and S. Hashish. *Biochem. Pharmacol.* **14**, 1692 (1965).

[18] L. Lykken and J. E. Casida. *Canad. Med. Assoc. J.* **100**, 145 (1969).

[19] B. W. Arthur and J. E. Casida. *J. Agr. Food Chem.* **6**, 360 (1958).

[20] W. Dedek. *Z. Naturforsch. B*, **23**, 504 (1968).

[21] G. J. Marco and E. G. Jaworski. *J. Agr. Food Chem.* **12**, 305 (1964).

[22] M. K. Ahmed, J. E. Casida and R. E. Nichols. *J. Agr. Food Chem.* **6**, 740 (1958).

[23] M. Hitchcock and S. C. Murphy. *Biochem. Pharmacol.* **16**, 1801 (1967).

[24] T. Nakatsugawa, N. M. Tolman and P. A. Dahm. *Biochem. Pharmacol.* **17**, 1517 (1968).

[25] R. M. Hollingworth, R. L. Metcalf and T. R. Fukuto. *J. Agr. Food Chem.* **15**, 242 (1967).

[26] R. M. Hollingworth, T. R. Fukuto and R. L. Metcalf. *J. Agr. Food Chem.* **15**, 235 (1967).

[27] F. C. G. Hoskin. *Canad. J. Biochem. Physiol.* **34**, 743 (1956).

[28] B. J. van den Brink, J. Antognini and J. J. Menn. *Proceedings of the 4th British Insecticide and Fungicide Conference* **1**, 406 (1967).

[29] J. B. McBain, J. J. Menn and J. E. Casida. *J. Agr. Food Chem.* **16**, 813 (1968).

[30] H. Lee and J. J. Menn. *Metabolism of S-Phthalimidomethyl O-isobutyl Ethylphosphonodi-thioate (N-4543) in the Rat.* Tech. Report ARC-B-20. Stauffer Chemical Co., Agric. Res. Cent., Mountain View, Calif. 94040. (1968).

[31] I. M. Ford, J. J. Menn and G. D. Meyding. *J. Agr. Food Chem.* **14**, 83 (1966).

[32] H. Lee and J. J. Menn. *Metabolism of Isobutanol-1-^{14}C.* Tech. Report ARC-B-20. Stauffer Chemical Co., Agric. Res. Cent., Mountain View, Calif. 94040. (1968).

[33] J. B. McBain, L. J. Hoffman, J. J. Menn and J. E. Casida. *Pest. Biochem. Physiol.* In press.

[34] H. E. Skipper, L. L. Bennet, C. E. Bryan, L. White, M. A. Newton and L. Simpson. *Cancer Res.* **11**, 46 (1951).

[35] J. J. Menn and J. B. McBain. *XIIIth Int. Congress of Entomology, Moscow* (1968).

[36] J. B. McBain, L. J. Hoffman and J. J. Menn. *J. Agr. Food Chem.* **18**, 1139 (1970).

[37] J. B. McBain and J. J. Menn. *Biochem. Pharmacol.* **18**, 2282 (1969).

[38] D. L. Bull. *J. Agr. Food Chem.* **18**, 1134 (1970).

INSTRUMENTATION IN DETERMINATION OF ORGANOPHOSPHORUS TERMINAL RESIDUES

MORTON BEROZA and M. C. BOWMAN

US Department of Agriculture, Agriculture Research Service, Beltsville, Maryland 20705 and Tifton, Georgia 31794, USA

ABSTRACT

The most widely used instruments for the determination of organophosphorus pesticide residues are gas chromatographs with highly specific detectors, e.g. thermionic and flame photometric detectors. With them, pesticides and their metabolites can be determined, amounts in the range of 0.02–0.001 p.p.m. being detectable. Many of these analyses, of which some will be described, do not require 'clean-up'. Thin-layer chromatography, used for semiquantitative analyses, clean-up and confirmation of identities, may be adaptable to quantitative analysis. Use of spectrometric analyses is declining owing to the need for time-consuming clean-up, but some of these analyses are still needed and automated systems are helpful. Significant improvements in a wide variety of instruments have resulted in analyses that are more reliable, sensitive and versatile.

Phosphorus pesticides have been gaining favour and are now in widespread use because they are generally of low persistence and do not tend to accumulate in animal tissue or in the environment. Rapid and reliable means of determining these pesticides and their metabolites have therefore become most important in our efforts to assure a safe and adequate food supply as well as an environment that is free from contamination.

Almost every type of instrumentation that can be applied has been tried for the determination of organophosphorus (P) residues. Thus the methodology used for P residues, listed in *Table 1,* is not only extensive but is heavily dependent on instrumentation. Furthermore, all of the methods are useful, depending on the pesticide(s) being analysed and the type of information desired.

Time-limitation forced our coverage to be selective rather than comprehensive. We therefore selected items from references appearing in the last three years, mainly to highlight current technology and developments. We also took the liberty of including some new items from our own laboratories.

We have come a long way from the time when analytical methods dealt solely with residues of the parent pesticide. Today the determination of P residues is a highly sophisticated endeavour, and though many of our problems have been solved, there remains an extraordinary volume of work to be done. The number of P pesticides is large, and each pesticide may produce several metabolites.

79

Table 1. Methodology for determining organophosphorus residues

I. Chromatography
   A. Gas chromatography
      1. With detectors of P compounds
         (a) Alkali-flame (thermionic)
         (b) Flame photometric
         (c) Microcoulometric
         (d) Emission spectrometry
      2. With detectors not responsive to P
         (a) Electron capture
         (b) Microcoulometric
         (c) Electrolytic conductivity
         (d) Flame ionization
   B. Thin-layer chromatography
   C. Paper chromatography
   D. Column chromatography (liquid–liquid, liquid–solid, gel)
   E. Reaction chromatography

II. Spectrometry
   A. Visual (colorimetric) and ultra-violet
   B. Fluorescence and phosphorimetry
   C. Infra-red
   D. Mass
   E. Nuclear magnetic resonance

III. Polarography

IV. Bioassay—cholinesterase inhibition

V. Combination analyses

VI. Automation of analyses

These residues may be found in an even larger number of crops, soils and other materials which have to be analysed. Steps involved in a residue analysis are shown in *Table 2.* We have to determine whether an extraction is complete. Amount of 'clean-up' (separation of pesticide from interfering extractives) needed will depend on crop, method of extraction and means of determination.

Table 2. Steps in the determination of pesticide
residues

I. Comminution of crop or material

II. Extraction

III. Clean-up

IV. Determination
   A. Individual
   B. Multicomponent
      1. Single pesticide and its metabolites
      2. Several pesticides and their metabolites
   C. Group of pesticides

V. Confirmation of identity

VI. Establishment of quantitative validity

We do not always know which pesticides are present or what the terminal residues are. If we do, which ones shall we determine? The volume and complexity of the problems should keep residue chemists and those in related disciplines rather busy in the future. Fortunately they can be aided immeasurably by improved instrumentation and techniques.

GAS CHROMATOGRAPHY

Unquestionably the most widely used instrumentation for the direct analysis of P residues is the gas chromatograph (GC), and the most important contribution toward the popularity of its use has been the introduction of the highly specific detectors. These devices respond with remarkably high sensitivity to P compounds, and yet do not respond appreciably to extraneous material in the sample. The great advantage of using these selective detectors is that clean-up, which is the laborious or time-consuming part of the analysis, is held to a minimum and often even eliminated. Determinations are therefore speeded and simplified; analyses become more accurate and reliable because losses in clean-up are minimized or avoided.

The highly specific detectors are generally based on the extensive degradation of the sample, e.g. in a flame or in an oven, and the monitoring of the resulting small fragments to which the organophosphates are reduced (e.g. HPO for the flame photometric detector) under precisely controlled conditions.

The alkali-flame or thermionic detector was the first highly specific detector for determining P residues and is probably the most widely used detector for these determinations today. The original version, which consisted of a flame-ionization detector with sodium sulphate on a platinum coil in the vicinity of the flame, responded to nanogramme (ng) amounts of P residues[1, 2] (see *Figure 1*). Its mechanism of operation has not been determined conclusively. Many modifications of the detector have appeared and these have gradually overcome

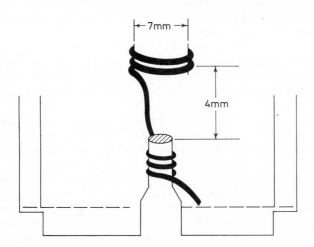

Figure 1. Thermionic detector. The 7-mm Pt–Ir helix is coated with salt and held above burner jet

shortcomings in the original design, which have been noted to be long equilibration time, gradually decreasing sensitivity, excessive noise and short life-time. The halogen response was practically eliminated by replacing sodium sulphate with potassium chloride $(KCl)^3$ or another alkali metal halide. Other alkali metal salts $(RbCl, CsBr, Rb_2SO_4, KBr)$ were found suitable[4, 5]. Some were held on a ceramic bead at the flame jet[4]. In another design a plug of caesium bromide was moulded to the burner tip[6]. A bead of mixed salts (fused Rb_2SO_4–KBr, 1 : 1) has also been used[7]. Precise placement of the electrode above the flame jet[4, 8, 9] and configuration of the electrode[8, 9] were shown to affect response to P compounds. [The Rb_2SO_4 detector responds to compounds with other elements (N, S, halogen) and response to each is optimum at different heights of the electrode above burner and at different flowrates of the gases [10–12]. A comprehensive review of flame detectors using different salt additives has recently appeared[13].] The most recent alkali-flame detectors have sensitivities in the order of 1 to 50 picogrammes (pg), are linear in response, give a selective response to P compounds 5 000 to 10 000 times that of other organics, have low noise levels, have stable baselines for long periods and are usable for months. The latest Varian-Aerograph detector[14] utilizes Rb_2SO_4 in a metal cup through which the effluent gases pass and burn on the salt bed; ions are collected with a loop-shaped electrode positioned about 1 cm above the flame. This detector is said to be sensitive to 1 pg of P compound and about 1 ng of N-, S- or Cl-containing compounds. The Hewlett-Packard Co. markets another version of the detector[15] in which the collector electrode is a platinum cylinder containing a KCl crystal with a bore in its longitudinal axis; the position of the crystal relative to the flame can be adjusted. This detector, unlike the Rb_2SO_4 one, does not respond to halogens and is therefore more specific in its response. It is said to detect less than 10 pg of parathion. Other commercial versions are available; however, the alkali-flame detector is simple enough that many workers prefer to make their own salt-supporting probes[7, 16, 17]. It has been suggested that at weekly intervals the home-made KCl-coated platinum coil probe[2] should be regenerated by heating in a Meker burner for a few seconds[17].

In general, excellent results can be obtained with the alkali-flame detectors if certain precautions are observed. Close control of flowrate, especially hydrogen, is essential; differential flow controllers and capillary flow restrictors are useful for this purpose. The surface of the alkali-metal salt may require cleaning from time to time. Background current, which gives a rough estimate of the concentration of alkali in the flame, should be checked daily to avoid sensitivity shifts.

In a novel variation of the alkali-flame detector, called the chemi-ionization detector[18], CsBr vapour is caused to react in an electrically heated inert gas with a GC effluent containing P compounds. Picogramme amounts of P pesticides are detected, but no data on actual residue analyses are given.

The flame photometric detector of Brody and Chaney[19] is the second most widely used detector for determining P residues. It monitors the light-emission of compounds burning in a hydrogen-rich flame. With a 526 nm filter, it responds to P compounds; with a 394 nm filter, it senses sulphur compounds. The detector is very stable, gives linear response for P compounds over at least three decades of concentration, is not easily contaminated, is insensitive to water, is easily used with temperature programming, is easy to operate and

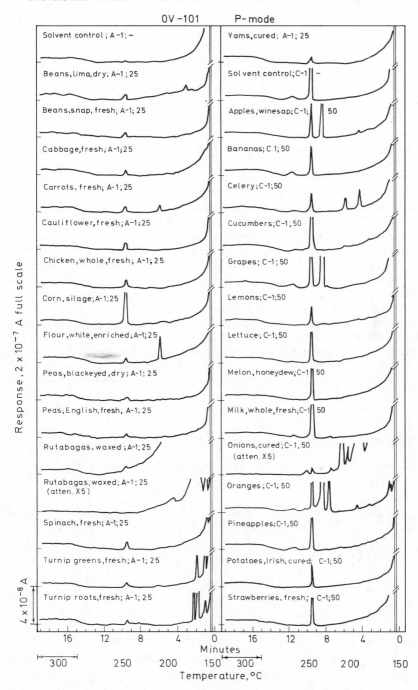

Figure 2. Chromatograms of food extracts with OV-101 packing and the phosphorus flame photometric detector[24]

maintain; its response can be attenuated, results are highly reproducible, and in our hands it has been generally trouble-free. As little as 0.1 ng of a P compound is detectable (twice noise). The main drawback of this detector is its high cost. However, its highly specific response minimizes or eliminates the need for clean-up so that costs of analyses may be less with it than with the alkali-flame detector. In our laboratories more than 100 P compounds have been determined in more than 25 materials. Only extracts of fatty materials have to be subjected to a clean-up, and this was a simple hexane–acetonitrile partition. The clean-up was not applied to eliminate interference with detector response but to avoid shortening the life of the column with non-volatile deposits. Most of this work and specific conditions for analysis were described in a recent review[20]. The detector has been used in some very difficult analyses, e.g. to determine as many as six compounds, a parent insecticide (fenthion) and five of its metabolites[21]. In this instance, the insecticide residue was separated into three fractions by rapid column chromatography, and each fraction was analysed by GC in less than five minutes. The column chromatography was not a clean-up but a separation required to avoid the overlapping of the peaks in GC.

Because clean-up was minimal or unnecessary in the many residue analyses we conducted with the flame photometric detector, we investigated the possibility that the detector might be useful for multicomponent analyses. The relative retention times of 138 pesticides and metabolites containing both P and sulphur were determined both isothermally and by temperature programming on packings containing four thermally stable liquid phases: OV-101, OV-17, OV-210 and OV-225[22]. With temperature programming, extracts containing multicom-

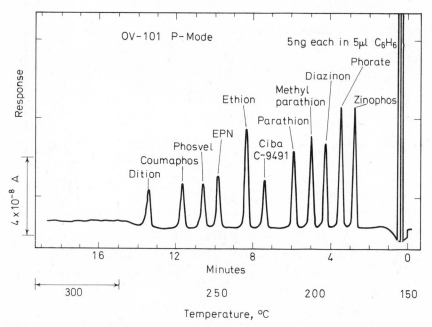

Figure 3. Chromatogram of 11 pesticide standards with same conditions as used for chromatograms of *Figure 2*

ponent residues of pesticides with a wide range of retention times could be analysed with a single injection of sample. This general procedure and the tabulation of retention times should facilitate identification of multicomponent P residues in environmental samples or in samples of unknown or indefinite history.

The requirement of analysing for all P pesticide residues in a food sample is a severe one. The pesticides and metabolites, which may have widely differing polarities, all have to be extracted, and interference from the foods themselves should be absent or minimal. We have found that exhaustive Soxhlet extraction (usually four hours) with ten per cent methanol in chloroform meets this requirement without extracting excessive amounts of extraneous material[23]. This method of extraction (or blending if Soxhlet extraction was not applicable) was then applied to 39 foods, selected to represent as wide a spectrum of types as possible[24]. The extract, subjected only to a hexane–acetonitrile partition if fatty, was then analysed by flame photometric GC with temperature programm-

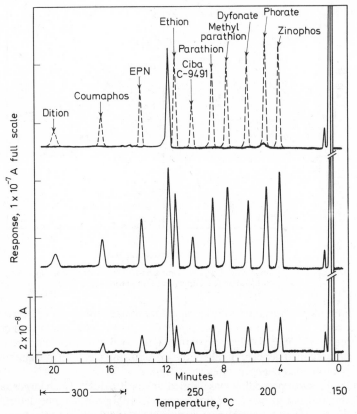

Figure 4. Chromatograms of milk extracts containing pesticide standards, made with Dexsil 300 packing and the phosphorus flame photometric detector. Top: solid line, blank milk extract, equivalent to 50 mg of milk; broken line, blank milk extract to which 0.025 p.p.m. of each pesticide [1.25 ng of each[was added before injection. Centre: milk extract obtained by adding 0.025 p.p.m. of each pesticide to milk sample and then extracting. Bottom: same as centre, but 0.010 p.p.m. of each pesticide added

ing. Typical backgrounds obtained with the foods and pesticide standards for the OV-101 column are shown in *Figures 2* and *3* respectively. The attenuation was adjusted so that compounds present at the 0.01 to 0.05 p.p.m. level would be visible. P residues could be determined in more than 80% of the foods with little or no interference. Since each analysis included the entire temperature-programmed scan from 150° to 300°C, this result is considered satisfactory. Only for the remaining 20% of the foods will a clean-up have to be applied to improve results.

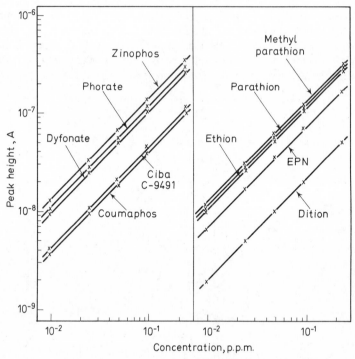

Figure 5. Responses obtained from extracts of milk to which ten organophosphorus pesticides were added at five concentrations before extraction

In our opinion the major criterion in regard to usefulness of a GC detector for residue analysis is not the ratio of pesticide signal to electrical or other noise (ultimate sensitivity), but the ratio of this signal to interference from the sample. With more than 80 per cent of the foods not requiring clean-up in P analyses, the flame photometric detector rates very high.

When the same procedure was applied to S pesticides[24], much larger samples had to be injected to overcome the lesser sensitivity of the flame detector to S compounds. Owing to these larger sample sizes and the lesser selectivity of the detector response to S than to P compounds, background interference was observed with many of the foods, especially after repeated injections of the extracts, when shifts in the retention times of pesticides were noted. We tried to volatilize the interfering material by holding the column at 300°C for prolonged periods, but results were still not satisfactory, and the time lost in purging the column was excessive.

This problem has now been largely solved through the use of a new high-temperature liquid phase called Dexsil 300 (Analabs, Inc. North Haven, Conn.). With it on 80/100 mesh acid washed Chromosorb W, the temperature of the column can be raised to 350° or 400°C and the interferences removed[25].

Typical results with Dexsil column are shown in *Figures 4* and *5*. It is believed that the instrumentation and procedures described constitute a very satisfactory multicomponent analysis. The procedure is rapid, sensitive and to the best of our knowledge reliable when properly used (see original articles).

Other highly specific detectors advanced for the GC analysis of P residues are the microcoulometer[26] and the emission spectrometric detector[27], in which the atomic phosphorus line at 2535.65Å is used. These detectors do not appear to be widely used for determining P residues.

Phosphorus compounds have also been determined by GC using detectors responsive to groupings or elements other than P in pesticide residues. For example, the electron-capture detector might be used to determine residues containing halogen or sulphur (see detectors under IA2 of *Table 1*). Since discussion of these detectors and others used in residue analysis is outside the scope of this presentation, the reader is referred to a recent review of this subject[28].

THIN-LAYER CHROMATOGRAPHY

Although the number of recent references to the use of thin-layer chromatography (TLC) is great, only a few of the items mentioned instrumentation. TLC has been used in the semi-quantitative analysis of P compounds, the clean-up of extracts, for confirmation of identity and in metabolism studies. Most analyses are conducted on glass or plastic 20 cm × 20 cm plates or on microscope slides[29]. The use of a glass plate with channels recessed 2 mm and filled with adsorbent has been suggested for clean-up of pesticide extracts[30]. An apparatus was devised to apply up to nine 1–2 ml samples of pesticide extract to a TLC plate in 20–30 min, during which time the solvent is evaporated and no attention of the analyst is required[31].

The possibility that TLC could be used for the quantitative analysis of P residues has much to recommend it: low cost of apparatus, speed and ease of operation, high capacity of many of the adsorbents, large variety of chromogenic reagents and adsorbents, and good sensitivity, specificity and versatility.

In 1968 we described a simple dual-beam, fibre-optic scanner for TLC plates that measures the reflectance of spots[32]; results with it have been most promising. The heart of the instrument is a fibre-optic scanning head in the shape of a Y (see *Figure 6*). Half of the fibres conduct light from an incandescent source (which can be monochromatic) to a small rectangular area on the plate (20 mm × 1 mm); the other half of the fibres (randomly mixed among the first fibres) carry light reflected from the plate to a CdS photocell that registers its response on a recorder through a simple Wheatstone bridge circuit. A second Y-shaped fibre-optic assembly is set up beside the first head to act as a reference; it monitors the blank area adjacent to the TLC spots and compen-

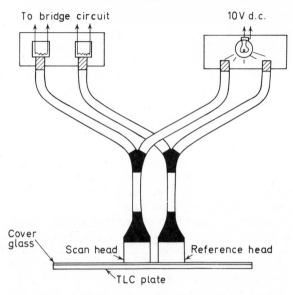

Figure 6. Arrangement of Y-shaped fibre optics for dual-beam scanning of TLC plates

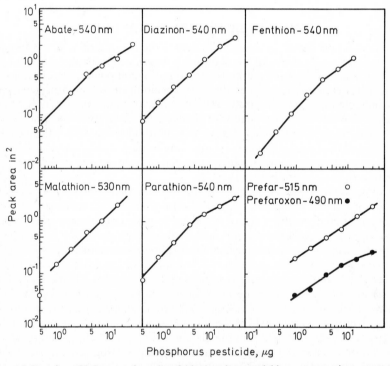

Figure 7. Data from TLC scans of a series of thiophosphate pesticides, concentration versus peak area. Scanning wavelength is given for each pesticide

sates for background differences, such as in chromogenic spraying. In scanning the TLC plate, the two fibre-optic heads are held stationary while the plate moves under the heads at the rate of about 7 cm/min. A sheet of plate glass is set on the TLC plate, and the heads, by resting on this cover glass, are kept a fixed distance from the adsorbent. Scans of a TLC plate furnish chromatograms similar to those from GC. Some typical results with P pesticides are shown in *Figure 7*. In repeated scans of any one spot, the standard deviation was only 1 to 2 per cent. Standard deviations on *different* developed spots of 1 to 2 µg of insecticide were 11 to 16 per cent in our initial tests, but now are much better. We understand the scanner is being made available commercially soon.

Several other TLC scanners are already on the market and should be similarly useful. These usually rely on transmission rather than on reflectance of light.

Because of the need to analyse many samples, especially for regulatory purposes, quantitative TLC should offer a means of getting the less difficult or routine analyses done, especially since unskilled technicians could be trained to conduct the analyses.

Quantitative TLC should also be useful in the analysis of polar materials which cannot readily be determined by GC.

OTHER FORMS OF CHROMATOGRAPHY

Very little new instrumentation for analysis of P compounds with other forms of chromatography has appeared recently. except in liquid–liquid chromatography. A few reports employing paper chromatography with cholinesterase inhibition have appeared. References to column and gel chromatography have dealt with clean-up rather than instrumentation.

Liquid–liquid chromatographs are now commercially available and have been used for pesticide residue analysis[33-35]. These instruments usually operate at high pressures and with narrow-bore columns to achieve rapid analysis and good resolution. The use of controlled surface-porosity supports as column materials has been very helpful[35]. Available detectors include flame ionization, spectrophotometric, heat of adsorption, electrolytic conductivity, refractive index, fluorimetric and polarographic[36]. An ultra-violet-absorption detector has been used to detect 0.5 ng of compound[35]. The future of liquid–liquid chromatography will depend on its ability to compete with other methods of analysis. Use of the technique is very limited at present but is still developing. A highly sensitive specific detector is needed for pesticide residue analysis.

SPECTROMETERS

Several excellent reviews on the use of spectrometry for determining P residues have appeared[37, 38]. The use of this type of methodology (*Table 1*, II) for pesticide analysis has been declining owing to some serious limitations. Spectrometric procedures usually require a thorough clean-up, which can be time-consuming and may result in losses; the clean-up may have to be changed for each crop–pesticide combination; the procedures usually determine only one compound or a single summed value, e.g. total P. Yet spectroscopic methods continue to be important for several reasons. There may be no other way to determine certain pesticides. Expensive equipment, such as for GC, may not be available, and more accessible methods such as colorimetric ones may provide the necessary answers. Spectrophotometric analyses for total phosphorus content or cholinesterase inhibition are of considerable interest to regulatory officials because they provide a rapid screening procedure for P residues; only samples giving positive results need be examined further by more specific methods. Such procedures are still frequently cited. Automated equipment, mostly of the type marketed by Technicon Corp., has been adapted to speed these analyses[39, 40]. Samples are automatically degraded by combustion or wet digestion–oxidation and the resulting orthophosphate determined colorimetrically, usually as phosphomolybdenum blue. Autoanalysis of individual 'spots' from TLC chromatograms can contribute specificity to this non-specific analysis[41]. Automated systems based on cholinesterase inhibition have also appeared[42]. Clean-up of samples for these automated analyses is still done manually.

STRUCTURE DETERMINATION

If the use of spectrometers for the direct determination of P residues is declining, the use of this instrumentation for determining the structure or identity of metabolites is not only very much on the rise, but is proving extremely valuable. Infra-red, ultra-violet, n.m.r. and mass spectrometers are being widely used. Although this instrumentation cannot be discussed in detail, a few comments are in order. Sensitivity of these instruments has been enhanced and new techniques are being devised. Fourier transform techniques, especially with infra-red and n.m.r. spectrometers, have markedly improved sensitivity; however, this instrumentation is expensive and not yet generally available. Mass spectrometers, some costing $20 000 or less, are becoming more popular. These instruments are of special interest to residue chemists because mass spectrometry is inherently a very sensitive technique and therefore dovetails with the needs of residue chemists. GC has been combined with the various spectrometers. With mass spectrometry, GC serves as an inlet system and purification method for minute amounts of chemical. This combination can generate a tremendous amount of data. Computers, which are becoming more generally available, can eliminate much of the drudgery of compiling the data and putting them in an interpretable form. At the same time, computers have been used to improve the sensitivity and accuracy of analyses.

The highly specific GC detectors can be useful for elemental analysis: thermionic for P, flame photometric for P or S, microcoulometry or electrolytic conductivity for Cl, S and N. Reaction chromatography, which is a combination of a chemical reaction and chromatography (usually GC or TLC), is useful for determining the functional groups present. Chromatographic mobility (e.g. Kovats retention indices, R_F value in TLC) can also be informative.

Structure determination is crucial in the development of a pesticide because at an early stage it is essential to determine which are the important metabolites. Failure to do so may eventually require repetition of costly residue studies.

EXTRACTION

No special instrumentation has been advanced recently for extraction of crops. Exhaustive Soxhlet extraction[43] seems to the authors to give the most generally satisfactory results; simpler or faster methods are then adopted when they give equivalent recoveries. In a study of nine extraction procedures for six P insecticides and nine of their metabolites, Soxhlet extraction with 10% methanol in chloroform gave the most complete extraction of the residues (comprising a wide range of polarities) without removing excessive weights of co-extractives[23]. With enough units set up, Soxhlet extraction is not time-consuming. Although the extraction takes time (usually four hours), the attention of the analyst is not required during extraction, the finished extract is already filtered, and its volume is usually smaller than that obtained by other conventional procedures, thus requiring less time to concentrate.

CLEAN-UP

The sweep–codistillation apparatus of Storherr and Watts[44, 45] has proved very useful in the clean-up of extracts for pesticide analysis. An apparatus has been devised[46] for simultaneously distributing up to five samples of pesticide extracts in binary solvent systems for clean-up. The apparatus, which consists of a series of Craig countercurrent-distribution cells modified to permit recovery of one of the phases, is mounted on a shaker unit.

Clean-up by column chromatography or TLC is considered standard and does not usually involve special instrumentation.

CONFIRMATION OF IDENTITY AND QUANTITATIVE VALIDITY

Although GC and other analyses are regularly used to determine P residues, the need to confirm the identity of compounds producing peaks in GC by an independent method has been fully established. In this connection, the use of all of the methodology of *Table 1* and associated instrumentation is applicable. TLC or GC with liquid phases of different polarities are often used to check GC results. Infra-red and mass spectrometry can be used to check the identity of residues after suitable clean-up.

Although not frequently mentioned, quantitative validity is most important. For example, did a peak on a chromatogram result solely from one pesticide, or might a small amount of impurity be under the peak? Separate analyses of a different type giving the same result establish quantitative validity. *p* values (partition distribution values in binary solvent systems) are also used for this purpose and for confirmation of identity[47, 48].

FINAL COMMENTS

The importance of instruments for P and other residue analysis has been widely recognized, and significant improvements in sensitivity, reliability and capability have been realized. Much peripheral equipment has helped upgrade analyses and deserves mention, e.g. better GC supports and liquid phases, GC dual detectors, new and improved chemical reagents and adsorbents, ready-made TLC plates, integrated combinations of instruments, automatic injection for GC and other systems, computer-controlled devices for instrumentation of all kinds. At the moment our greatest need is for an all-purpose method for determining P residues.

REFERENCES
1 A. Karmen and L. Giuffrida, *Nature, Lond.*, **201**, 1204 (1964).
2 L. Giuffrida, *J. Assoc. Offic. Agr. Chem.* **47**, 293 (1964).
3 L. Giuffrida, N. F. Ives and D. C. Bostwick, *J. Assoc. Offic. Anal. Chem.* **49**, 8 (1966).
4 W. A. Aue, C. W. Gehrke, R. C. Tindle, D. L. Stalling and C. D. Ruyle, *J. Gas Chromatogr.* **5**, 381 (1967).
5 J. Miyamoto and Y. Sato, *Botyu Kagaku*, **34**, 3 (1969).
6 C. H. Hartmann, *Bull. Environ. Contam. Toxicol.* **1**, 159 (1966).
7 D. A. Craven, *Analyt. Chem.* **42**, 1679 (1970).
8 H. K. DeLoach and D. D. Hemphill. *J. Assoc. Offic. Anal. Chem.* **52**. 533 (1969).
9 H. K. DeLoach and D. D. Hemphill. *J. Assoc. Offic. Anal. Chem.* **53**, 1129 (1970).
10 M. Dressler and J. Janak, *Coll. Czech. Chem. Commun.* **33**, 3970 (1968).
11 M. Dressler and J. Janak, *J. Chromatogr. Sci.* **7**, 451 (1969).
12 W. A. Aue, *Advances in Chemistry*. (In press).
13 V. V. Brazhnikov, M. V. Gurev and K. I. Sakodynsky, *Chromatogr. Rev.* **12**, 1 (1970).
14 C. H. Hartmann, *Research Notes* (Varian Aerograph), p 6, Summer (1970).
15 J. L. Bernard and J. V. Wisniewski, *Pittsburgh Conf. Anal. Chem. and Appl. Spectry., Cleveland, Ohio*. Abstr. Paper no. 159 (1970). *Also* Operating Note, Phosphorus detector model 15150A, Hewlett-Packard Co.
16 J. R. Wessel, *J. Assoc. Offic. Anal. Chem.* **51**, 666 (1968).
17 R. P. Watts and R. W. Storherr, *J. Assoc. Offic. Anal. Chem.* **52**, 513 (1969).
18 M. Scolnick, *J. Chromatogr. Sci.* **8**, 462 (1970).
19 S. S. Brody and J. E. Chaney, *J. Gas Chromatogr.* **4**, 42 (1966).
20 M. Beroza and M. C. Bowman, *Environ Sci. Technol.* **2**, 450 (1968).
21 M. C. Bowman and M. Beroza, *J. Agr. Food Chem.* **16**, 399 (1968).
22 M. C. Bowman and M. Beroza, *J. Assoc. Offic. Anal. Chem.* **53**, 499 (1970).
23 M. C. Bowman, D. B. Leuck and M. Beroza, *J. Agr. Food Chem.* **16**, 796 (1968).
24 M. C. Bowman, M. Beroza and K. R. Hill, *J. Assoc. Offic. Anal. Chem.* **54**, 346 (1971).
25 M. C. Bowman and M. Beroza. *J. Assoc. Offic. Anal. Chem.* **54**, 1086 (1971).
26 H. P. Burchfield, J. W. Rhoades and R. J. Wheeler, *J. Agr. Food Chem.* **13**, 511 (1965).
27 C. A. Bache and D. J. Lisk, *Analyt. Chem.* **37**, 1477 (1965).
28 W. E. Westlake and F. A. Gunther, *Residue Revs.* **18**, 175 (1967).
29 C. W. Stanley, *J. Chromatogr.* **16**, 467 (1964).
30 M. J. Matherne Jr and W. H. Bathalter, *J. Assoc. Offic. Anal. Chem.* **49**, 1012 (1966).
31 M. Beroza, M. E. Getz and C. W. Collier, *Bull. Environ. Contam. Toxicol.* **3**, 18 (1968).
32 M. Beroza, K. R. Hill and K. H. Norris, *Analyt. Chem.* **40**, 1608 (1968).
33 J. J. Kirkland, *J. Chromatogr. Sci.* **7**, 7 and 361 (1969).
34 J. J. Kirkland, *Analyt. Chem.* **41**, 218 (1969).
35 H. Felton, *J. Chromatogr. Sci.* **7**, 13 (1969).
36 R. D. Conlon, *Analyt. Chem.* **41** (4), 107A (1969).
37 D. J. Lisk, *Science*, **154**, 93 (1966).
38 D. C. Abbott and H. Egan, *Analyst*, **92**, 475 (1967).
39 F. A. Gunther and D. E. Ott, *Residue Revs*, **14**, 12 (1966).
40 F. A. Gunther, *Ann. N.Y. Acad. Sci.* **160**, 72 (1969).
41 D. E. Ott and F. A. Gunther, *J. Assoc. Offic. Anal. Chem.* **51**, 697 (1968).
42 G. Voss, *J. Assoc. Offic. Anal. Chem.* **52**, 1027 (1969).
43 W. B. Wheeler and D. E. H. Frear, *Residue Revs.* **16**, 86 (1966).
44 R. W. Storherr and R. R. Watts, *J. Assoc. Offic. Agr. Chem.* **48**, 1154 (1965).
45 R. W. Storherr and R. R. Watts, *J. Assoc. Offic. Anal. Chem.* **51**, 662 (1968).
46 M. Beroza and M. C. Bowman, *Analyt. Chem.* **38**, 837 (1966).
47 M. Beroza and M. C. Bowman, *J. Assoc. Offic. Agr. Chem.* **48**, 358 (1965).
48 M. Beroza, M. N. Inscoe and M. C. Bowman, *Residue Revs.* **30**, 1 (1969).

THE CHEMISTRY AND METABOLISM OF ORGANOCHLORINE INSECTICIDES

CHEMICAL ASPECTS OF INSECTICIDAL CHLORINATED HYDROCARBONS AND THEIR BEHAVIOUR UNDER ATMOSPHERIC CONDITIONS

F. KORTE

Institute for Ecological Chemistry, Birlinghoven, Germany

ABSTRACT

The incomplete knowledge of the balance of trade products is discussed. Since it is impossible to investigate the full range of environmental chemicals, pesticides offer themselves as adequate models in general. In the field of pesticides there are terms lacking realistic definitions (for instance 'chlorinated hydrocarbons' and 'persistence') causing misinterpretations. Concerning the mechanism of dispersion of pesticides in the atmosphere our knowledge is very limited. Of all reactions in the atmosphere only some reactions in the gaseous phase are known, but nothing when pesticides are adsorbed to particles of air pollutants. Ultraviolet irradiation of cyclodiene insecticides under experimental conditions leads to bridged isomers and dechlorination products. Some of these reactions were confirmed under practical conditions. Sunlight changes p,p'-DDT only slowly to DDE and some other derivatives. Lindane, however, isomerizes to only small amounts of α-hexachlorocyclohexane.

I will discuss some chemical aspects of insecticidal chlorinated hydrocarbons and their behaviour under atmospheric conditions, including certain important aspects of the dispersion tendency of these chemicals in the environment.

When talking about environmental problems caused by technical chemicals, a wide range of chemical, biological and certainly also of meteorological aspects is involved. Today we want to concentrate mainly on chemical and biochemical aspects.

In my opinion in all discussions of these substances so far it is not fully realized that the degree of knowledge of the respective chemical structures varies with the chemical substance involved. Let me begin with some remarks on terms we are using every day without having found clear-cut definitions for them.

It is safe to state that the structures of the active components, as well as the structures of the byproducts, are known of many products used in trade today and consequently the exact composition of the trade product. However, there are also cases in which the structures are unknown, which is very unsatisfactory, naturally at least from the chemical point of view. I do not have to stress that it does not make much sense to talk of residues of these compounds because it is one of the underlying principles of chemistry to be able to measure only that (at least in small concentrations), of which the structure is known. One example that could be cited is toxaphene.

To avoid misunderstandings I would like to point out that the ignorance of the structure of the substance naturally does not mean that such a compound is dangerous from the toxicological point of view. It merely means that such an ignorance is unsatisfactory from the chemical point of view.

During recent months discussions about environmental chemicals in all industrial countries have become more and more heated whether by better or less good arguments. It seems to me that in future it will be considered absolutely necessary that at least the structure and constituents of every substance should be known. More recent discussions persuade me that more attention from the toxicological point of view will also be given to byproducts. Thus, talking of byproducts of pesticides, it is relatively easy to obtain the necessary chemical data when compared with the problem of managing and describing byproducts of general chemical processes and describing the fate of these byproducts. When a fluorination reaction yields, for instance, hexafluoro-butadiene in small quantities, nevertheless amounting to approximately 1 000 tons/year, the question of the fate and conversion of these byproducts arises.

I know very well that it is utterly impossible to investigate the fate of all these products on a worldwide level. Therefore the only alternative will be, in principle, to investigate representative, realistic model substances in some cases more thoroughly, and to draw from the results conclusions on the fate of the other compounds under environmental conditions. Such model substances should have a deep focus point for the following parameters: production level of the compound, its persistence, its dispersion tendency, conversion under biotic and abiotic conditions and possible biochemical consequences.

In order to evaluate the impact of the applied substance on environmental quality, it is required to know not only the balance of the formulation but also the amounts used regionally as well as globally, as well as the quantitative pattern of use. While in certain countries like the USA and Japan the amounts of applied pesticides are being published, there are practically no quantitative data available on the amounts going into specific uses.

The term 'chlorinated hydrocarbons' poses the first problem, because so far no clear definition has been found. From the chemical point of view, for instance, dieldrin with one epoxide group naturally is chlorinated hydrocarbon. However, of the pesticides used today, 40 per cent contain halogen in one form or another and most of them are nevertheless classified for instance as phosphorus acid esters or as belonging to other groups. This problem of classification resides in the fact that on the one hand compounds with similar structures sometimes have similar activities, e.g. cyclodiene insecticides, and on the other, the activities of compounds of completely different substance classes are also similar. This is the reason why biologically active substances frequently are not classified according to their chemical structures but to their activities, e.g. flavourings, fungicides.

But what do we mean by 'persistence'? Persistence can be found in all classes of chemicals. Such a statement is trivial but it seems that the public relates 'persistence' primarily to the term 'chlorinated hydrocarbons'. Indeed, the characteristic feature of some chlorinated hydrocarbons is a chemical persistence and a certain degree of mammalian toxicity, but the chlorinated hydro-

96

carbons also include such compounds as dihydroheptachlor (an experimental insecticide) having pesticidal activity on the one hand, but on the other an extremely low mammalian toxicity, in the range of sodium chloride, and being rapidly metabolized and excreted by animals. In addition, everybody realizes that compounds other than chlorinated hydrocarbons, which are classified as non-persistent (for instance phosphorus insecticides, carbamates), do in fact undergo hydrolysis, oxidation etc. extremely rapidly. Their breakdown products, however, which may also contain chlorine, fluorine and other elements, may even be more persistent than the so-called chlorinated hydrocarbons. In addition, if one uses the term 'persistence' one should clearly differentiate between purely chemical and enzymatical persistence.

Perhaps what we commonly understand by 'undue persistence' could be described as follows. A substance is unduly persistent whenever a measurable quantity thereof continues to exist in some discernable chemical form. Obviously, the most desirable pesticide would be one that has a biological half-life just sufficient to perform its function as a pesticide, with *no* residual residue. Since this is difficult to achieve, the rhythm of use of the pesticides in terms of its function time must always be considered. Therefore, the *'function time rhythm'* of a pesticide must take into consideration not only its biological half-life, but also its presence afterwards in terms of any residual terminal chemical definition.

As far as pesticides are concerned, I am of the opinion that this term should, in principle, not only include parent compounds but also their most persistent degradation products under enzymatic and environmental conditions. Then a relatively high number of persistent final products containing chlorine or halogen, respectively, is formed upon hydrolysis of phosphoric acid esters or other classes of substances. In this connection, in general, with the exception of DDT, nothing is known about the degree of undue persistence of these compounds and their further breakdown.

What do we understand by the term 'residues' which is so often used? The environmental contamination by chemicals is generally identified by 'residue levels'. While this term has been defined by the FAO/WHO Joint Meeting for pesticide residues, it may have various meanings when applied to other environmental chemicals. Sometimes only parent compounds are involved, but sometimes also biotic or abiotic conversion products. It seems to be well accepted that metabolites in general are biologically less active than the parent compounds. Some investigations, however, have shown that a metabolite can be more active than the applied substance (e.g. parathion — para oxon, heptachlor — heptachlorepoxide). Moreover, atmospheric conversion products sometimes can have slightly different biological activities (e.g. cyclodienes and their photois .nerization products). Furthermore, metabolites may be more persistent than the parent compound (DDT — DDE), and there are indications that the influence upon the growth or development of the eggshells of some birds is not caused by the applied DDT but by one of its primary metabolites, and also by other known environmental contaminants such as PCB compounds etc.

Basically we would all be happy to know all metabolites and atmospheric conversion products. But this is for many reasons impossible and probably also not necessary. Our primary effort should be to concentrate on the most persistent products, no matter whether these are parent compounds, their metabolic derivatives or their atmospheric conversion products. These persi-

E

stent chemicals (let us call them final residues) may be able to influence the environmental quality (positively or negatively) in a more effective way than those having short lives.

For pesticides we know the residue levels of the parent compounds in a number of commodities; we have some knowledge of residual conversion products in animals but know almost nothing about conversion products originating from the use of organochlorine pesticides in vegetable food.

As far as the unintentional residues in the atmosphere are concerned, some data are known for the concentrations of the parent compounds (*Figure 1*).

Compound	Air	Rainwater	Rivers
Dieldrin	20 (London, 1966)	9–28 (England, 1964/65)	10 (Scotland, 1966) 0–118 (USA, 1965)
BHC	10 (London, 1966)	12–164 (England, 1964/65)	detected (Scotland, 1966; USA, 1965)
DDT + analogues	10 (London, 1966)	210 (London, 1965)	5 (Scotland, 1966) 190 (USA, 1965)

Figures in p.p. 10^{12}

Figure 1. Concentration of insecticides in the environment

Pesticides are introduced into the air in several ways: by drifting, from aeroplane application, by evaporation from plants and soil as well as via transpiration by plants. For instance, four weeks after foliar application of 1.2 mg of ^{14}C labelled endrine per plant on white cabbage, residues in plants and soil amounted only to six per cent; 94 per cent had disappeared into the atmosphere.

At first, it was assumed that the only cause for the disappearance of residues was evaporation from the surfaces of plants or from the soil. It was found that under the described experimental conditions evaporation from surfaces (glass, silica, paper), macroscopically equal to the surfaces of the leaves, was at most 60 per cent (vapour pressure of endrine $= 2 \times 10^{-7}$ torr, 25°C). It was found that the additional disappearance of about 34 per cent must obviously be caused by the living plants, probably via transpiration, or excretion with the guttation water.

In the atmosphere, pesticides may be converted photochemically. The ratio between the particle form and the gaseous form is not known. It can only be estimated that for DDT, owing to stronger adsorption at particles of air-pollutants, the particle form ratio is higher than that of dieldrin or lindane, and that in polluted areas this ratio is also higher than in unpolluted ones. On the other hand, it has also been estimated that the major part of pesticides in the atmosphere is present in gaseous form (Atkins, Eggleton, 1970). Nevertheless, it seems important to measure photochemical reactions of pesticides when adsorbed to particles, since this may change the reaction velocity. Probably the type of reaction, too, is changed owing to chemical intercession with pollutants adsorbed to the particles. Up to now, no investigations have been carried out in this respect as far as I know.

Concerning the mechanism of dispersion in the atmosphere, we have some data from extensive measurements of the distribution of radioactive isotopes (Junge, 1969; Peterson, 1965; Stewart, 1955). For this dispersion, besides numerous analyses, there are also mathematical models. We know, for instance, that for the troposphere of the Northern Hemisphere there are debris circles within 12 to 25 days and that there is a good mixture in the first circuit. On the other hand, transfer across the Equator to the Southern Hemisphere is slow. There are some indications that the relatively constant levels of chlorinated hydrocarbons found in rainwater at different stations are representative for the Northern Hemisphere.

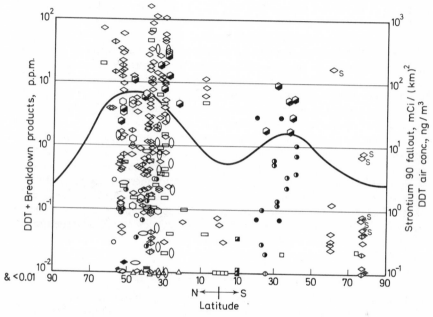

Figure 2. Fallout — ^{90}Sr, DDT and breakdown products (after W. G. Appleby, 1969). Residue values less than 0.01 p.p.m. plotted at 0.01 p.p.m. including non-detected values

Figure 2 (Appleby, 1969) gives a survey at which latitudes DDT-residues are present in the human and wildlife populations and other parts of the environment. It reveals that residues prevail in zones where DDT has been extensively used in the past and in zones with dense population. In the Southern Hemisphere there may be a similar distribution pattern, but owing to the lack of data (there are sufficient data only for Australia and New Zealand) the graph is not complete for this half of the earth.

What chemical changes do organochlorine compounds undergo after they have disappeared into the atmosphere? Owing to the difficulties involved in simulating the atmosphere, experiments in the laboratories allow for only indirect conclusions as to the behaviour of a chemical in the environment. However, preparative–photochemical experiments lead to an understanding of the general reactivities of the environmental chemicals in question and to the synthesis and identification of photoproducts, which can occur in low concentrations. Photochemical reactions in solution reveal the conversion of these compounds when dissolved in plant waxes.

How difficult it is to predict the conversions under atmospheric conditions can best be shown by the following example: It is generally believed that with wavelengths below 280 mm the sunlight spectrum has no considerable energy on the earth's surface owing to absorption in the atmosphere. Therefore the irradiation experiments with u.v. lamps, which emit mainly 254 nm, permit no conclusions on the reactions in sunlight.

On the other hand, aldrin is easily photolysed in sunlight, although it absorbs at considerably shorter wavelengths than 280 nm. So far it is not known whether this photolysis is due to a small portion of the sunlight of wavelengths below 280 nm which penetrates through the atmosphere, or to the photosensitization with singlet-oxygen or with other air pollutants. A catalysing effect of particulate matter in the atmosphere, which under practical conditions is possible, has also to be considered when the pesticides are adsorbed to this matter.

CYCLODIENE INSECTICIDES

It has been known for some years that the insecticides endrin and dieldrin undergo chemical changes under the influence of sunlight. Photodieldrin (the bridged isomer of dieldrin) has been found as a residue in vegetable and animal products. Δ-Keto-endrin (the bridged, endrin-isomeric ketone) was found on plants as a residue.

Upon irradiation under various conditions, aldrin isomerized to photoaldrin, dieldrin to photodieldrin. The corresponding isomerization products of the other cyclodienes, endrin, heptachlor, heptachlorepoxide, chlordane and *trans*-chlordane are also known (*Figures 3* and *4*). Most of these isomerization reactions were confirmed under practical conditions.

For these same compounds reductive photodechlorinations have also been found. So far under field conditions, however, only the dechlorinated endrin isomer has been found. The same reductive dechlorination has also been demonstrated for endosulphane under laboratory conditions.

Irradiation of dieldrin in perfluorinated hydrocarbons, which are the only inert solvents for such photochemical reactions, resulted in the presence of nitrogen dioxide in a number of photoproducts. These photoproducts are different from the ones we know so far; however, they have not yet been identified.

100

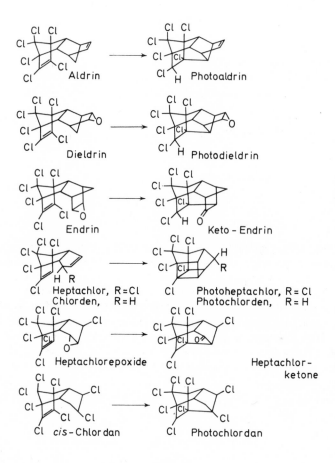

Figure 3.

101

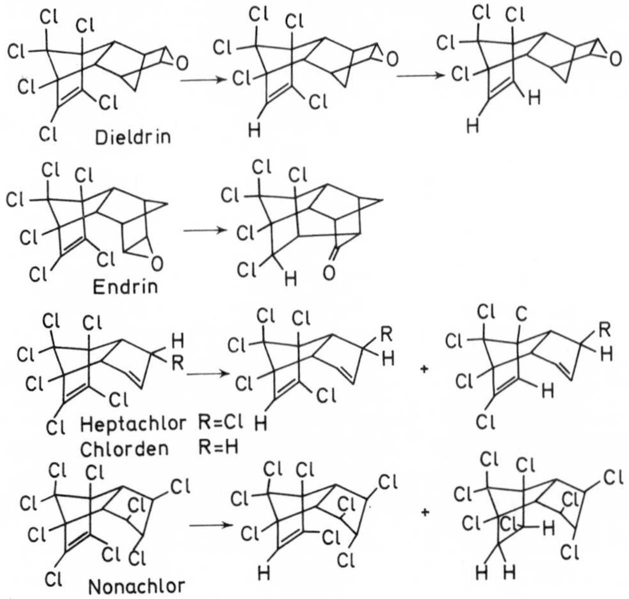

Figure 4.

DDT

Sunlight changes *pp'*-DDT only slowly to DDE, *pp'*-dichlorobenzophenone, *p*-chlorobenzoylchloride, *p*-chlorobenzoic acid and *p*-chlorophenyl-*p*-chlorobenzoate (*Figure 5*). With a considerably higher rate of photolysis, methoxychlor yields analogous products. Since DDE is sometimes called a global pollutant, its degradation in the inanimate environment is of particular interest. Upon sensitized irradiation as well as upon irradiation as solid (Pyrex filter) DDE forms *pp'*-dichlorobenzophenone, 1-chloro-2,2-bis-(*p*-chlorophenyl)ethylene, as well as an isomer of DDE, namely (1-chloro-2-*p*-chlorophenyl-2-*p*-*o*(*m*)-dichlorophenylethylene). Upon irradiation in methanol

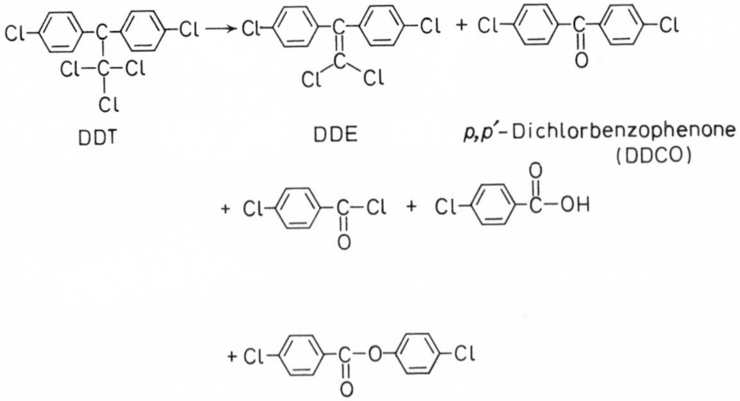

102

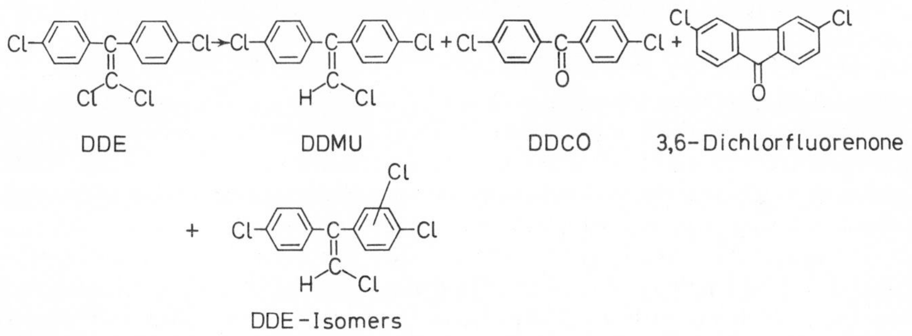

DDE   DDMU   DDCO   3,6–Dichlorfluorenone

DDE–Isomers

Figure 5.

with wavelengths of below 260 nm, DDE yields 3,6-dichlorofluorenon. Upon irradiation as solid (Pyrex filter) in the presence of chlorophyll, there is a high yield of the DDE isomer mentioned, which had been found also upon irradiation in the gaseous phase (air).

HEXACHLOROCYCLOHEXANE ISOMERS

Even upon irradiation with wavelengths down to 230 nm the photolyses of the hexachlorocyclohexane isomers contained in the insecticide used in forestry yield no compounds that can be identified. The β- and δ-isomers, as solid particles, after several days of the experiment yield merely traces (approximately one per cent) of the α-isomer. Lindane (γ-hexachlorocyclohexane) isomerizes to only small amounts of the α-isomer. Besides lindane, admitted for use in agricultural plant protection, there also occurs in foodstuffs the α- and β-isomer. Since the β-isomer is not formed at all under environmental conditions, and only traces of the α-isomer, there should be no doubt that these isomers become part of the foodstuffs by the use of technical BHC.

REACTIONS WITH γ-IRRADIATION

For the reason that pesticides can also reach higher layers of the stratosphere, their behaviour under γ-irradiation is also of interest, since, for instance, the CO-level of the atmosphere remains constant owing to reactions in the stratosphere. Therefore investigations ought to be made to see whether the stratosphere is also a sink for organochlorine compounds. So far we know nothing about these questions and we have no knowledge about the catalytic effects of particles on reactions of adsorbed organic compounds in the troposphere and the stratosphere.

REACTIONS ON SOIL SURFACES AND ATMOSPHERIC PARTICLES

We know nothing about reactions of organochlorine compounds when adsorbed to the soil, whereas for some other pesticides reactions by the soil have been described (Crosby, 1970). We only know the residual behaviour in

103

various soil types, the influence of humidity, of organic matter, of temperature and micro-organisms. Certain photolyses at the soil surface are also known, for instance, of dieldrin, methoxychlor and 4-CPA (Pesticides in the Soil Symposium, Michigan State University, 1970). Chemical changes of these compounds when adsorbed to the soil and when adsorbed to atmospheric particles have to be investigated separately, since the reactants are quite different in soil and atmosphere. It is probably impossible to make mathematical models allowing conclusions on reactions from the one medium to the other.

In conclusion I would like to summarize the most serious gaps which in my opinion we have in our knowledge of the impact organochlorine pesticides have on the environment: the chemical balance of active compounds and trade products; the chemical structure of a number of byproducts and also of some active compounds; the metabolism in plants and, to a less extent, in the soil; the reactions in the atmosphere and the soil.

ORGANOCHLORINE COMPOUNDS IN THE ENVIRONMENT IN JAPAN

M. Goto*

Department of Chemistry, Gakushuin University, Tokyo

ABSTRACT

The most important organochlorine pesticide in Japan was technical BHC until 1968. It was applied mainly in paddy fields, where it decomposed rapidly in summer time. The environmental contamination due to technical BHC will be discussed in detail.

PCP is now the most important organochlorine herbicide. It is mainly used during the season of rice-transplantation, and it has not yet given rise to any serious problems in Japan. It is detected in almost all river waters in concentrations between 0.01 and 0.1 p.p.b.

Table 1 shows the production, exports and imports of organochlorine insecticides in Japan. Up to 1968 the most important organochlorine compound was technical BHC. Production has increased yearly and it reached 45000 tons in 1968. The amount of DDT and cyclodiene insecticides consumed in Japan were about six per cent and two per cent of that of BHC respectively. Technical BHC is a mixture of various isomers of BHC, and the composition is about 68 to 70 per cent of α-, 9 per cent of β-, 13 to 15 per cent of γ- and 8 per cent of δ-isomers. The β-isomer has the lowest vapour pressure, the lowest solubility in water and the greatest toxicity towards human beings.

Table 1. Production, exports and imports of organochlorine insecticides in Japan

(In metric tons)

	BHC		DDT		Cyclodienes
	Production	Exports	Production	Exports	Imports
1960	15426	—	1308	83	681
1961	16917	584	1392	35	499
1962	17547	544	1746	142	463
1963	20272	480	1826	12	533
1964	27537	207	1694	16	703
1965	33231	6922	2391	773	498
1966	34568	9871	3881	1047	674
1967	41742	2130	4199	2149	776
1968	45695	2462	4936	2237	767

* Present address: Organisch-Chemisches Institut der Universität Bonn, 53 Bonn, Germany.

105

In Japan, annual statistics for pesticides are published by the Japan Plant Protection Association[1]. The production and shipment of pesticides are summarized in detail. This Association's handbook, together with annual meteorological statistics, annual river water statistics, and the statistics for farming, facilitates the study of environmental pollution by pesticides in large degree.

Figure 1 shows the amount of BHC applied to cultivated fields in 1968 in Japan[1]. The amount is expressed as the amount of γ-BHC/ha per year. Since γ-BHC is included in technical BHC in the concentration of only 13 to 15 per cent, the actual amount of technical BHC used amounts to seven to eight times those indicated in *Figure 1*. The amount of γ-BHC applied, for example, in Fukuoka, in the northern part of the Kyushu Island, in 1968 reached more than 4 kg/ha. This means about 28 kg of technical BHC was applied/ha in one year. If this amount were distributed uniformly in the soils at a depth of 10 cm, the concentration of γ-BHC would be approximately 3 p.p.m., i.e. 21 p.p.m. in total BHC. Actually one can often detect total BHC in a concentration of more than 10 p.p.m. in orchard soils. It was fortunate that BHC was applied mainly to rice fields

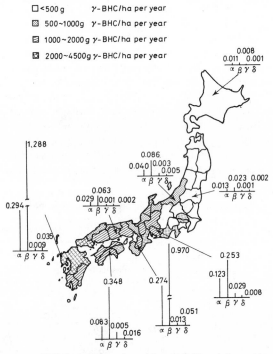

Figure 1. The amount of BHC applied to the cultivated field and the residues in cow milk.

in the summer time in Japan, because γ-BHC decomposes rapidly in paddy soils with sufficient water at 25° to 37°C. This situation was also more or less true for DDT.

Table 2 shows the average values of BHC residues in the environment in Japan[2]. The relative amounts of BHC isomers are given as percentages in parentheses. The reason for the high concentration β-BHC observed in paddy soil may be as follows: (1) β-BHC has the lowest vapour pressure and its co-distillation with water is lower; (2) β-BHC is decomposed by soil bacteria with difficulty. β-BHC residues are also very high in rice straw, rice grain, tomatoes and rain water in comparison with the ratio of original BHC applied. β-BHC has the least concentration among its isomers in air, i.e. four per cent. The reason is again that β-BHC has the lowest vapour pressure among the isomers. The β-BHC concentration is increased in rain water; this is probably due to the fact that in the upper part of the atmosphere the BHC isomers, except for β-BHC, are readily decomposed by sunlight and β-BHC is dissolved in rain water at a higher concentration.

Table 2. Some examples of BHC residues

Sample no.	α-BHC	β-BHC	γ-BHC	δ-BHC	total BHC
Paddy soil 18	0.539 (27)	1.029 (51)	0.231 (11)	0.220 (11)	2.019 p.p.m.
Rice straw 25	1.914 (13)	8.146 (56)	0.989 (7)	3.635 (25)	14.684 p.p.m.
Rice grain 10 unpolished	0.152 (41)	0.079 (21)	0.044 (12)	0.097 (26)	0.372 p.p.m.
Tomatoes 5	0.234 (55)	0.061 (14)	0.105 (25)	0.026 (6)	0.426 p.p.m.
Air (Tokyo) 3	0.105 (42)	0.010 (4)	0.076 (31)	0.058 (23)	0.249 µg/m^3
Rainwater (Tokyo) 7	0.454 (37)	0.220 (18)	0.388 (31)	0.171 (14)	1.233 p.p.b.
Market cow milk 5	0.055 (19)	0.229 (78)	0.002 (1)	0.006 (2)	0.292 p.p.m.
Technical BHC	(68 ~ 70)	(9)	(13)	(8)	

( ): Ratio (%) of each isomer to total BHC

Attention should be paid to the following facts: paddy soil, rice straw and market cow milk have the highest concentrations of β-BHC. The increasing order of the percentages of β-BHC is: paddy soil, rice straw and market cow milk. β-BHC is concentrated from paddy soils to cow milk. This is in accord with the natural sequence. Rice plants are grown in the paddy soils and the cow is fed with the rice straw. Thus if one sprays technical BHC over a paddy field, the cow milk is contaminated with β-BHC, and β-BHC is concentrated step by step.

The pathway for the contamination of cow milk by β-BHC was investigated by Fukunaga and his co-workers[2].

Table 3. BHC residues (p.p.m.) of foodstuffs

Foodstuff	BHC total	γ-BHC	β-BHC
Rice straw A	10.597	0.935	5.130
Rice straw B	2.328	0.275	0.820
Rice straw C	0.998	0.114	0.477
Hay	0.161	0.040	0.039
Italian rye grass	0.073	0.007	0.040
Silage	0.047	0.019	0.006
Combined foodstuff	0.117	0.045	0.014

Table 3 shows BHC residues in cow foodstuffs. A higher amount of β-BHC was detected in rice straws. A means that BHC was applied to rice plants until a later stage of cultivation, B means it was applied until a middle stage of rice cultivation and C means it was applied only at an early stage or not applied at all. It is now clear that the origin of β-BHC in cow milk was residual β-BHC in the rice straw, which was used as a foodstuff for cows. Hay, Italian rye grass, silage and combined foodstuff had very low residues. The highest residue of β-BHC was observed in the rice straw, especially when technical BHC was applied until a later stage of rice plant cultivation. This situation will be illustrated in more detail.

Rice seeds are first planted in a bed in the middle of May. In July, small rice plants are transplanted into the paddy fields. About one week after rice-transplantation, fine BHC granules, which easily dissolve in water, are sprayed over water surfaces. γ-BHC is absorbed by the roots of the rice plants, reaches the leaves and kills rice-borers on the plants. At this stage rice plants grow rapidly and require much water. The highest concentration of BHC in river water can be observed at this stage. It sometimes amounts to about 30 p.p.b. in a small river, but never exceeds 2–3 p.p.b. in a larger river. The maximum concentration will appear and disappear within a week after spraying.

At the end of August, when the rice plants develop ears, BHC is again sprayed over the paddy water to kill the rice-borers. Rice plants again require enough water at this stage.

The last application of BHC is from September to October. This is to kill leafhoppers and other insects. At this stage, the paddy field has little water. Thus BHC is difficult to decompose and remains in the paddy soils; this is absorbed into the straws.

Figure 1 shows the β-BHC residues in cow milk, as determined in February 1970; these were determined by the Ministry of Health and Welfare, which has about 45 monitoring stations throughout Japan. (In November 1969, the production of BHC and DDT for domestic consumption was stopped, and in November 1970, the application of BHC and DDT to paddy fields was prohibited in Japan.)

There are extensive works of Tatsukawa[3,4,5] on organochlorine pesticides in river water. The concentrations of total BHC in river water in the northern part of Shikoku Island are usually between 0.01 and 10 p.p.b. (July 1970). The Inland Sea of Japan is a closed system and BHC residues in the sea water reach a maximum value of 0.1 p.p.b. from summer to autumn. Usually BHC residues in river water do not exceed 10 p.p.b. However, Tatsukawa observed higher concentrations of BHC in rain water. In 1970 he found four times the values, of more than 10 p.p.b., in Matsuyama, Shikoku Island. In July 1970, he observed 144 p.p.b. of BHC and the ratio of β-BHC to γ-BHC was about five.

When BHC is sprayed in a rural community, about 50 μg of BHC/m^3 on average in 24 h can be observed. Tatsukawa detected 0.05 to 0.1 μg of BHC/m^3 in nine cities of Western Japan in the summer of 1970.

PCP is also a very important herbicide in Japan (production in 1969 was 16344 tons as sodium salt), and the use of PCP is similarly distributed throughout Japan. PCP is detected in almost all river water in Japan. It is mainly used during the season of rice-transplantation to inhibit the growth of weeds. The greatest concentration of PCP in river water is observable this season. *Figure 2* shows the concentration of PCP in July 1969. In another season 0.01–0.1 p.p.b. is observed, and these concentrations do not seem to be dangerous from an ecological point of view.

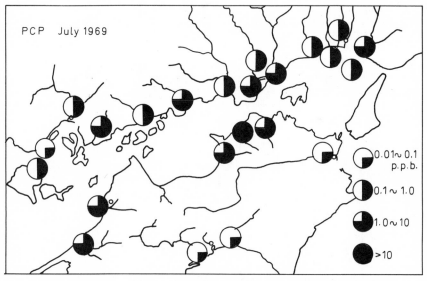

Figure 2. PCP residues in river water in south-western Japan (Tatsukawa).

BHC and PCP are the main pollutants in Japan. However, DDT and its decomposition products are also detected in the environment often to the degree of one-tenth of the concentration of BHC. Quite recently high residues

109

of dieldrin and endrin were found in cucumbers by several monitoring stations in Japan. The residues range from 0.01 to 0.05 p.p.m. for dieldrin and 0.002–0.02 p.p.m. for endrin. According to the established tolerance for cucumbers endrin should not be detected and dieldrin must be less than 0.02 p.p.m. Moreover, it was found that the average dieldrin residue of adult abdomen fat of 74 Japanese was 0.46 p.p.m. The reason for these high residues of cyclodiene insecticides is still unknown. Investigations are in progress by the Ministry of Health and Welfare.

REFERENCES

1 *Pesticide Handbook*. Edited and published by the Japanese Plant Protection Association: Tokyo, Japan (1970).
The Problem of the BHC Residues, Japan Plant Protection Association: Tokyo (1970).
[2] K. Fukunaga. Unpublished work.
[3] R. Tatsukawa. *Kagaku to Seibutsu*, **8**, 539 (1970).
[4] R. Tatsukawa, T. Wakimoto and T. Ogawa. *J. Food Hyg. Soc., Japan*, **11**, 1 (1970).
[5] R. Tatsukawa. *Kagaku Asahi*, **12**, 45, (1970).

THE FATE OF CHLORINATED HYDROCARBONS IN LIVING ORGANISMS

G. T. Brooks

Agricultural Research Council Unit of Invertebrate Chemistry and Physiology, University of Sussex, Brighton, UK

ABSTRACT

Tracing the origin of problems attending the use of organochlorine insecticides, it is evident that the basic difficulties arise from (a) insect resistance to these compounds, (b) the early notion that they were completely inert biologically, and (c) analytical developments permitting their detection in minute amounts. Increasing awareness of the complexity of the chemistry of these compounds and lack of knowledge of their mode of action adds emotional overtones to the basic problems, which seem really to centre around insect resistance, since there is now much evidence that organochlorine compounds, although frequently persistent, are not completely inert. Considering the 'organochlorine problem' in relation to the other formidable problems that presently confront mankind, it is difficult to escape the conclusion that, resistance excepted, these compounds have been entirely beneficial. The paper considers current information regarding the biodynamics and biotransformation of mainly DDT, hexachlorocyclohexane and the diene-organochlorine (cyclodiene) insecticides in living organisms.

INTRODUCTION

I want to confine my attention mainly to the classical organochlorine insecticides DDT, Lindane {γ-hexachlorocyclohexane (γ-HCH)} and the cyclodienes. Looking back on the past fifteen years or so, it seems paradoxical that the use in pest control of such apparently simple molecules as these should lead to so many difficulties. The first major problem was undoubtedly insect resistance. Then came the electron-capture technique and the ability to detect (or suspect!) the presence of minute amounts of these compounds in almost every commodity we handle. Since public awareness of pollution problems seems to spring from the publicity given to organochlorine insecticides, events following from this ability suggest that the electron-capture technique may prove to have almost as much influence on the course of history as the advent of nuclear weapons! Thirdly, recent work has shown that the chemistry of these compounds, especially the photochemistry of DDT and the cyclodienes, is more complex than was formerly realized, and this must be a nightmare for those involved in residue problems,

111

if, however, fascinating for chemists. Fourthly, we are only now beginning to find small clues concerning the way in which these compounds affect the function of the nervous system. In fact, sterically well-defined molecules such as these are being used to probe the nature of the nervous system itself[1-6], so we know that they exert at least some of their acute effects on biological membranes, but at the present state of the art how can we possibly predict the long-term effects, if any, of their presence on such membranes at sub-lethal levels? From what has been done so far, it seems clear that when we know how these compounds act, we shall also know a great deal about the mode of action of anaesthetics and natural toxins that act on the nervous system.

The resistance problem seems to me to be the most serious one of all, and here we have a good example of the way in which the presence of chemicals in the environment can alter, often irreversibly, the nature of living organisms. I say 'irreversibly' because we know quite well that once organochlorine resistance has arisen, it may decline on removal of the selecting agent, but usually re-appears more quickly than before if the chemical is used again. In other words, we cannot return to the situation existing before the chemical was first used.

Now we certainly know that organochlorine resistance arises by selection of insect populations containing naturally resistant insects, but recent work also indicates that insect enzymes which metabolize insecticides can be induced, just as those of mammals can. Organochlorine compounds, probably partly on account of their persistence, appear to be particularly good enzyme-inducers, and their induction of microsomal mixed-function oxidases might contribute to resistance toward other toxicants that are also metabolized by these enzymes. It must be emphasized that much of the work done so far on induction in insects has involved high dietary levels of organochlorines[7] or other inducers[8], and some idea of the 'no-effect' dietary level is required; there are indications that for houseflies this is significantly lower for Dieldrin than for DDT[7]. [The major pure components of Aldrin (HHDN) and Dieldrin (HEOD) are used in most laboratory experiments; see footnote, *Table 3*]. Microsomal epoxidase activity is induced in DDT-resistant houseflies by topically applied doses of DDT greater than about half (0.1 µg) the LD_{50} to the WHO susceptible strain of *Musca domestica*, and Dieldrin induces epoxidase activity in three Dieldrin-resistant housefly strains when topically applied at some twenty times (0.5 µg) the LD_{50} to susceptible strains[9]. Such doses would select normal insects for 'classical resistance' to these toxicants, so that only in insects already resistant to them would resistance, or additional resistance, be observed toward other toxicants through enzyme induction. Exposures of this sort seem likely to arise only when insects are being killed in areas newly treated with toxicants, rather than from residue levels. Thus in an improbable situation, which nevertheless serves to put the matter in perspective, a normal housefly would need to absorb all the Aldrin from nearly 60 mg of carrot tissue containing the 0.35 p.p.m. residue, found by Hulpke[18] after seed application, to receive the LD_{50}. Nevertheless, we should not lose sight of the fact that this is an area where the problems of terminal residues and resistance may occasionally overlap. Moriarty[10] has provided a useful review of the sub-lethal effects of synthetic insecticides on insects.

BIODYNAMICS

Higher plants

Although the number of investigations of the fate of pesticides in plants has increased considerably during the last ten years, especially in relation to the behaviour of systemic pesticides, there were very few detailed investigations of the distribution of organochlorine compounds until fairly recently. This is probably because these compounds are non-systemic, and their penetration into plants is of little importance in pest control, although barley plants were shown in 1964 to take up DDT and a number of experiments have indicated the translocation of Aldrin and Heptachlor (as their epoxides) and the endosulphan isomers. The need for more detailed information concerning the nature of organochlorine residues in plants has resulted in a recent series of investigations by the Bonn group[11].

DDT and analogues—There is little information about the behaviour in plants of compounds such as methoxychlor [1,1,1-trichloro-2,2-bis-(*p*-methoxyphenyl)ethane] or the acaricidal derivative kelthane [dicofol; 2,2,2-trichloro-1,1-bis-(*p*-chlorophenyl)ethanol] but experiments in Bonn[11] indicate that 20 to 30 per cent of the total residues recovered after the application of DDT to leaves of cabbage, or in carrots after soil application, are biotransformation products consisting of DDE [1,1-dichloro-2,2-bis-(*p*-chlorophenyl)ethylene], DDD [1,1-dichloro-2,2-bis-(*p*-chlorophenyl)ethane] and more polar compounds not yet identified. Recent work[12] has shown that a large number of photo-oxidation products, including compounds derived from chlorinated biphenyls and chlorinated fluorenes, are produced when DDT or DDE are irradiated in methanol with ultra-violet light (> 260 nm) in the presence of oxygen. *pp'*-Dichlorobenzophenone is a significant photo-oxidation product of DDE under these conditions and has been detected as a DDT residue on leaves. Such products, if formed from DDT or DDE on plant surfaces, or in the soil, may enter the plant and add to the residues formed by biotransformation of DDT in the plant, or may themselves be further transformed in the plant. For a number of compounds, photo-oxidation products formed by ultra-violet irradiation resemble the products of oxidative biotransformation *in vivo*, and some of the compounds recently identified[12] may indicate the possible nature of hitherto unrecognized metabolites of DDT.

γ-HCH and the cyclodienes—The results of experiments in which γ-HCH and various cyclodiene insecticides[11, 13–17] were applied to the leaves of white cabbage are summarized in *Table 1*, in which the order of increasing persistence of total residues is from left to right (that is, from γ-HCH to photodieldrin [(3,6-*exo*-4,5,13,13-hexachloro-10-oxahexacyclo-(6,3,1,1$^{3, 6}$, 1$^{9, 11}$,0$^{2, 7}$,0$^{5, 12}$)tridecane]. The relatively low total residues of γ-HCH, technical Heptachlor, Aldrin and Endrin undoubtedly relate to loss of these compounds from the leaves by volatilization, and residues contain the highest proportion of unchanged toxicant when the latter cannot undergo epoxidation. *trans*-Chlordane and the constituents of technical Heptachlor penetrate the leaf surface rapidly and the residues of *trans*-Chlordane appear to be considerably more persistent than those from technical Heptachlor, measurements with the latter being difficult because of its heterogeneity. Because of the recognized sequential conversions Aldrin → Dieldrin

Table 1. Total residues of [14C]-labelled γ-HCH and various [14C]cyclodienes after application to the leaves of growing cabbage plants[11,13-17]

	γ-HCH	Technical Heptachlor	Aldrin	Endrin	trans-Chlordane	Isodrin	Dieldrin	Photo-dieldrin
Amount applied (mg/plant)	1	1	1	1.3	1	1	1	2.5
% of applied 14C recovered	8.3(4)†	15[a]	17(4)	11(4)	35(4)[a]	30(10)[d]	40(4)	75(4)[c]
	4.7(6)		12(6)	*	20(10)[b]		29(6)	
% of recovered 14C as unchanged toxicant	30-40(4)[h]		4(4)[e]	90(4)[g]		5(4)[d]	75(4)[f]	
	30-40(6)		6(6)[e]			Nil(10)	79(6)[f]	

† Time (weeks) after application is given in parentheses.
* Tobacco plants treated with 2.08 or 1.04 mg of 14C-labelled Endrin/plant under various conditions contained a total residue of 32-47 per cent of the applied 14C six weeks after application.
[a] 90 per cent of this in the leaves.
[b] 80 per cent of the residues in leaves consisted of mainly three unidentified metabolites.
[c] 30 per cent of this inside the leaves, of which 15-33 per cent consists of at least three metabolites.
[d] Remainder of 14C at four weeks and whole of 14C at ten weeks are conversion products: mainly Endrin and Δ-keto-Endrin plus other, more hydrophilic, compounds.
[e] Remainder of recovered 14C consists of six conversion products, including one very hydrophilic metabolite and small amounts of Dieldrin and photodieldrin.
[f] Remainder of recovered 14C consists of photodieldrin plus more hydrophilic metabolites.
[g] Remaining ten per cent consists of a very polar metabolite together with a small amount of Δ-keto-Endrin.
[h] Remaining 14C consists of five more polar metabolites.

(*Figure 3*) → photodieldrin (VI; *Figure 3*), and Isodrin → Endrin → Δ-keto-Endrin (1,8-*exo*-9,10,11,11-hexachloropentacyclo-(6,2,1,1$^{3, 6}$,0$^{2, 7}$,0$^{4, 10}$)dodecan-5-one; VII; *Figure 3*), the behaviour of both photodieldrin and Δ-keto-Endrin in plants is of interest. It appears that, like Dieldrin but unlike Aldrin, photodieldrin penetrates the leaf surface slowly and, in contrast to Aldrin, Dieldrin and Endrin, neither it nor its metabolites translocate in the plant[15], so that there is no contribution to dissipation from this factor and the residues are rather persistent (*Table 1*). Total residues of Δ-keto-Endrin also disappear more slowly than those arising from Endrin, although the ketone itself is transformed, mainly into one hydrophilic product, rather more rapidly than is Endrin[17].

Once absorbed by the cabbage plant, Endrin is rather more persistent than Dieldrin (*Table 1*), although the pattern of metabolite distribution and the consistent appearance of hydrophilic metabolites in the soil after foliar application of Endrin indicates that translocation to the roots and soil contributes to its elimination from the plant. Although Aldrin and Isodrin are transformed about equally rapidly (*Table 1*) the former produces hydrophilic metabolites rather than much Dieldrin or photodieldrin, whereas Isodrin produces Endrin (up to 30 per cent) and Δ-keto-Endrin (up to 20 per cent), a sequence of increasing persistence. As a result, the Aldrin–Dieldrin combination is somewhat more readily metabolized by cabbage plants than the Isodrin–Endrin pair, in marked contrast to the situation observed in some mammals.

Clearly, plant structure will have a profound influence on the uptake and distribution of toxicants and the higher residues of Endrin found in tobacco plants, in contrast to cabbage plants, after foliar application, are believed to result from lower penetration through the leaf surface coupled with restricted evaporation due to its hairy nature[16]. An unidentified, very hydrophilic, metabolite found in the plant tissue (as much as 30 per cent of the recovered radioactivity after six weeks) behaves like the one found in cabbages and, once again, there is evidence that metabolite(s) pass through the roots into the soil.

Table 2. Distribution of residues after application of ^{14}C-labelled Lindane to soil containing growing spinach and carrots[13]

	Spinach		Carrots	
Soil application rate (p.p.m.)	0.4	0.7	0.35	0.7
Time of exposure (weeks)	2	8	8	10
% applied ^{14}C in soil†	60	58	51.1	44.8
% applied ^{14}C {Leaves	1.5	0.81	0.5	0.7
in plant }Roots	0.2	0.17	6.4	5.4
% unchanged* Lindane in internal ^{14}C	43.5	55.8	52.1	54.2

† Unchanged Lindane (γ-HCH).
* Remainder consists of five unidentified metabolites.

When spinach is grown in soil treated with ^{14}C-labelled γ-HCH, the label is carried into the roots and leaves (*Table 2*) and consists of unchanged γ-HCH (44–56 per cent), together with five metabolites that are also produced in cabbage[13]. Most of the residue, about half of it unchanged γ-HCH, is found in the leaves, in contrast to the situation with carrots, which at equivalent soil dosage take up three to seven times more γ-HCH and retain most of this in the root, again converting about the same proportion (39–43 per cent) into a similar series of metabolites. With carrots grown in soil treated with ^{14}C-labelled-*trans*-Chlordane a different distribution was found; more residues were found in leaves (0.06 p.p.m.) than in roots (0.01 p.p.m.) twelve weeks after application, the root residues consisting mainly of metabolites, whilst in leaves 66 per cent of the labelled material was present as unchanged *trans*-Chlordane. The roots and leaves of carrots grown in Isodrin-treated soil contain Isodrin, even twelve weeks after the application. Endrin appears fairly quickly and is still present in the leaves twelve weeks after treatment; at this time 90 per cent of the activity in the leaves consists of degradation products, including Δ-keto-Endrin.

Because its root has a high affinity for lipophilic substances, the carrot can be used as a test plant to indicate the presence of soil residues. Hulpke[18, 20] recently examined the distribution of ^{14}C-labelled Aldrin during the germination and development of carrot and onion seeds treated with the toxicant at a practical level. In the carrot variety 'Juwarot', radioautography reveals radioactivity in the root and in the growing cotyledons. At full development the average residue content of the carrot roots is 0.35 p.p.m., whereas the edible part of the onion (variety 'Zittauer Gelbe') contains only 0.03 p.p.m., with highest concentration (1 p.p.m.) in the roots (i.e. at the base of the bulb) and a small residue (0.003 p.p.m.) in the green shoots. The basis of the distribution seems to be that with this type of application the lipophilic toxicant is 'fixed' in the older parts of the plant, so that the relatively newer tissue contains little residue. With the onion, green shoots contain Aldrin (44 per cent), Dieldrin (16 per cent) and unidentified polar materials (40 per cent); roots contain Dieldrin (76 per cent) and Aldrin (24 per cent); the edible part contains only Dieldrin. The presence of hydrophilic conversion products only in the green shoot suggests that the Aldrin initially associated with the appropriate part of the seed, or Dieldrin formed in or later transported into the shoot from other areas, is metabolized during its development.

The difference in behaviour of Aldrin in different varieties of carrot is very interesting. When seeds of the varieties 'Bauers Kieler rote' and 'Juwarot' develop after equal treatment with ^{14}C-labelled Aldrin, the mature root of the former contains residues of 0.07 p.p.m. and the green plant 0.06 p.p.m., whereas the corresponding residues for 'Juwarot' are 0.41 p.p.m. and 0.21 p.p.m. Furthermore, roots of 'Bauers Kieler rote' contain 80 to 90 per cent of the residue in the periderm and 10 to 20 per cent in the inner layers of the cortex, whereas 'Juwarot' residues are confined to the periderm and may therefore be removed by peeling. There must also be a striking difference in the distribution of enzymes effecting Aldrin epoxidation, since in these experiments both root and shoots of 'Bauers Kieler rote' contained Aldrin and Dieldrin in the ratio 55:45; although shoots of 'Juwarot' contained both Aldrin and Dieldrin, the roots contained only Aldrin. An earlier supposition that differences in residue content and distribution of the kind found with these two varieties is due to differences in the content of essential oils seems not to be valid, since the levels of essential oils are similar in both.

A study of the behaviour of ^{14}C-labelled Aldrin in lettuce[19] shows that absorption occurs by transportation through the vascular bundles and by evaporation from the soil followed by condensation on the plant. Seed coating (10 g/100 g of seed) resulted in a 0.002 p.p.m. residue in the edible parts, whereas with soil treatment the residue is approximately proportional to the applied dose, ten times the recommended dose resulting in a residue of 0.2 p.p.m. Dieldrin was found in all parts of the plants.

Most of the investigations discussed were conducted under greenhouse conditions, and although they provide much valuable information they cannot reproduce field conditions. However, field trials are currently in progress to determine, for example, the residues produced by Aldrin after the application of ^{14}C-labelled Aldrin at 3 kg/hectare to soil under various conditions of climate and agricultural practice[11]. The 0.055 p.p.m. residue found in sugar beets grown in the treated soil in Germany consisted of Aldrin (0.001 p.p.m.), Dieldrin (0.004 p.p.m.) and hydrophilic metabolites (0.05 p.p.m.). Maize grown in Californian soil treated at the same rate contained no detectable ^{14}C in the grain or cobs, and the husks of the ears contained 0.004 p.p.m. of Aldrin, 0.004 p.p.m. of Dieldrin and 0.032 p.p.m. of metabolites. The residue of 0.35 p.p.m. in the leaves consisted of Aldrin (0.02 p.p.m.), Dieldrin (0.05 p.p.m.) and metabolites (0.28 p.p.m.). By planting new crops at later intervals it will be possible to assess the effect of factors such as bacterial activity in the soil on the nature of the residues found in both crops and soil. The foregoing account shows that organochlorine insecticides undergo biotransformation in plants to compounds not yet identified in many cases. The toxicological significance of these products cannot be evaluated until they are first identified, and then synthesized in sufficient quantity to enable such evaluations to be made.

Insects and micro-organisms

When considering the biodynamics of organochlorine compounds and their residues in higher plants and vertebrates, we are usually concerned with amounts which are, hopefully, very sub-lethal. On the other hand, a great many investigations with insects have involved the measurement of whole-body levels of toxicant after a single dose at or near the toxic level, without much regard for details of distribution. However, the detailed mechanism has been examined[21] of absorption of DDT from minute, externally applied, lanolin spheres by adult *Phormia terraenovae*, and some recent investigations of the dynamics of Dieldrin in relation to toxic action in the housefly are also worthy of note[22-25]. Slightly toxic compounds (a term frequently depending strictly on the species studied) are not often investigated, but the dynamics of certain cyclodienes of this type and the influence of synergists have been examined in connection with structure–activity relations in the housefly[26]. The number of investigations of this sort is likely to increase in future because of ecological problems, and insects should be ideal for investigating the possible effects of sub-lethal levels of organochlorines on vigour, reproductive capacity etc. Apart from the influence of differences in morphology, especially the large surface/volume ratio, on the rate of entry of the insecticide, the behaviour of a single dose of an organochlorine is frequently similar in general pattern to that found in vertebrates. This is to be expected, since, comparing topical application of a toxicant to an insect with oral administration to a mammal, the critical factors of uptake, storage and excretion that determine the internal level apply in both cases. It is, of course, the difference in the balance of these factors which can be so important for selective toxicity.

The versatility of micro-organisms in their ability to degrade organic molecules is well known, and it is clear that we are highly dependent upon them for the final degradation of many molecules that may have been modified in the direction of increased polarity during their passage through the biosphere, but still retain their basic structure. Most reports on the interaction of micro-organisms with organochlorine compounds relate to attempts to demonstrate metabolic degradation, with only incidental information regarding the dynamics of toxicant distribution.

A number of reports have indicated the rapid anaerobic conversion of DDT into DDD by soil micro-organisms. This conversion (92 per cent after 86 h in still culture) does not occur via the unsaturated molecule DDE in *Aerobacter aerogenes* and conversion into further products is slow[27]. The growth of streptococci and micrococci associated with cheese is not inhibited by Lindane, DDT or DDE, and the levels of these compounds are not reduced by these organisms in culture. However, various *Geotrichum* and *Brevibacterium linens* isolates from cheese reduce the levels of added DDE and DDT, without DDD formation with the former species[28]. Lindane levels appear to be unaffected by cheese micro-organisms in culture and the earlier investigations of Bridges[29] demonstrated the stability of this compound in intact cheese.

Cells of the yeast *S. cerevisiae* absorb the HCH isomers in the decreasing order $\alpha > \gamma > \delta > \beta$, which deviates from the order of their solubility in organic solvents and also from the order of their toxicity, which is $\delta > \gamma > \beta > \alpha$. The intracellular concentrations of the α, γ, δ and β-isomers reach plateau levels corresponding to uptake of 60, 40, 24 and 18 per cent respectively of the available material (concentration of each isomer 3×10^{-5} M in the medium). Thus the most biologically active isomer (δ) is only slightly more readily taken up than the slightly toxic β-isomer and the most readily absorbed isomer (α) is least toxic[30]. These observations indicate that the stereochemistry of the isomers is the important factor for their toxic action, which may involve interaction with phosphoinositides in the cytoplasmic membrane.

Some information is available concerning the dynamics of conversion of Aldrin into Dieldrin by soil micro-organisms. Fungi able to effect this conversion have been classified[31] as (a) rapid Dieldrin producers after an initial lag phase, (b) linear producers of Dieldrin, (c) low producers, and (d) producers that also appear to metabolize Dieldrin, since the amount produced passes through a maximum and then declines. Similar behaviour is observed with a number of actinomycetes and bacteria and there are also indications in some cases that Aldrin is degraded directly, without the intermediate production of Dieldrin[31, 32], a situation that may also occur in plants.

Whilst it is not always easy to compare the conditions of the metabolism experiments so far conducted with micro-organisms, it does seem that the biotransformation of most cyclodienes, except Dieldrin, can be demonstrated fairly readily. Thus Dieldrin added at 0.15 p.p.m. in the medium to growing cultures of *Aspergillus niger* and *flavus*, and of *Penicillium notatum* and *chrysogenum*, was not metabolized in two to three weeks, in which time Aldrin was substantially converted into other compounds, as well as Dieldrin[33]. In contrast, *A. flavus* and *P. notatum* converted 38 and 23 per cent respectively of the available radioactive material in three weeks after exposure to ^{14}C-labelled-photodieldrin at 0.059 p.p.m. in the culture medium[15], so that the photo-isomer is apparently more labile than Dieldrin in these organisms. More recently, Matsumura *et al.*[34] demonstrated the slow metabolism of Dieldrin (1–6 per cent in four weeks) by a *Pseudomonad* at a much higher concentration (10 p.p.m.) in the medium and also the extensive conversion of Endrin by several soil micro-organisms. Concentration effects seem important, at least with the cyclodienes, since quite large increases of toxicant added to the culture medium result in a relatively slow increase in metabolite formation; in an experiment with isobenzan (Telodrin; 1,3,4,5,6,7,8,8-octachloro-1,3,3a,4,7,7a-hexahydro-4,7-methano-isobenzofuran) in *Aspergillus niger* a 500-fold increase in concentration in the medium effected only a 20-fold increase in metabolite production, with indications that the converting systems approached saturation at the upper concentration[35]. Many of the metabolic products indicated in these studies are still unidentified and there is, as yet, no evidence for the total degradation of the hexachloronorbornane nucleus.

Vertebrates

Since living organisms are essentially particles of lipid–protein complex located in an inorganic environment, it seems clear that they must eventually come into equilibrium with lipid–soluble materials distributed in their environment. Therefore, with constant exposure to an organochlorine compound, absorption will continue until the solubility limits of the organism are reached, unless an elimination process is also present, in which case the internal level will rise until intake is balanced by elimination. This is a form of consecutive reaction $A \rightarrow B \rightarrow C$, where A is the external concentration of organochlorine, B is the tissue concentration and C is the organochlorine eliminated, either intact or as metabolites.

It seems clear that the distribution behaviour is not related in a simple manner to physical properties such as fat solubility, and detailed analysis of exposure to organochlorine compounds must consider the relationship between rate of intake and concentration in the tissues, the relationship between the concentrations in different tissues (of importance for estimating total exposure from measurements of levels in a single tissue), the changes in tissue concentration with time of exposure and the changes in tissue levels when exposure ceases. There is experimental evidence that continuous exposure to a cyclodiene insecticide results in a limiting upper level of accumulation in biological systems that depends on the level of exposure, and that this level falls exponentially with time when exposure ceases. Whilst emphasizing the limitations of the mathematical treatment, Robinson (for example, ref. 36) considers that for vertebrates the experimental observations are generally consistent with those expected if the animal is regarded as a two-compartment system of the mamillary type used in investigating the pharmacodynamics of drugs.

Whilst it is emphasized that the compartments are conceptual and cannot necessarily be equated with particular tissues, a system consisting of a central compartment (the blood), which receives insecticide at a constant rate, can transform or eliminate it, and is in contact with another, otherwise isolated, inert storage compartment, provides a useful basis for interpretation of the available data. Assuming rapid equilibrium between the storage compartment and the central compartment, the concentration c at time t in the latter, when toxicant is entering at a constant rate α, is given, in simplest terms, by $c = (\alpha/k)(1 - e^{-kt}) + c_0 e^{-kt}$, where k is the rate constant for elimination from the central compartment and c_0 the level of toxicant present at zero time. This equation requires an eventual approach to a plateau level of toxicant in the central compartment, and the decline in toxicant level in this compartment when exposure ceases may be represented by a similar equation, $c = c_\infty + (c_0 - c_\infty)e^{-kt}$, where c_0 is the concentration at termination of exposure and c_∞ that at $t = \infty$. This simple expression requires an asymptotic approach to a low concentration (c_∞), which may be finite or zero, and neglects the effect of transfer of toxicant from the storage compartment.

The conclusions that tissue concentrations of cyclodiene insecticides are related to the rate of intake, that a constant rate of ingestion of insecticide will result in finite concentrations in the various tissues as the time of exposure increases indefinitely, that the concentrations in the blood and other tissues are correlated and that tissue levels decline logarithmically when exposure ceases, appear to be applicable also to DDT for man and some experimental animals, with some reservation regarding the phase of concentration decline[37].

Information for other vertebrates and for important residues such as DDE and the HCH isomers (mainly β and γ) is scanty, although β-HCH has highest chronic toxicity among the HCH isomers and appears to be the most persistent one, appearing for example as a prominent constituent of HCH residues in human fat and breast milk, presumably through the use of technical HCH. For Dieldrin[38], DDT, DDE, DDD, DDMU and DDMS[39, 40] (*Figure 1*), half-lives of 47, 28, 250, 24, 27 and 8 days respectively have been indicated in the pigeon and there are indications from various sources[41, 42] that birds, and also fish and other marine organisms, exposed to organochlorines accumulate plateau levels of these compounds and that the levels decline when exposure ceases. Plateau levels attained will clearly change if the level of exposure changes and the amounts accumulated can be relatively high, especially in marine organisms at the end of food chains. Recent investigations[43] indicate that polychlorinated biphenyls (PCB) are now widespread in the environment and the distribution and levels in predatory British birds resemble those of DDE and Dieldrin, highest values occurring in some fish-feeders. Some molluscs have exceptional capacities for concentrating organochlorine compounds in their tissues and, like carrots, may be used as indicators of the presence of organochlorine residues in their environment.

A detailed analysis[44] of the decline in Dieldrin concentration in various tissues of male rats after cessation of dietary administration indicates a biphasic decay for blood and liver, with similar decay constants and half-lives (*Table 3*) for the corresponding phases in each tissue. The experimental observations are best fitted by the inclusion of a second exponential term

Table 3. Pharmacokinetic characteristics of some cyclodiene insecticides and DDT

Compound[a]	Dose/time[b]	Tissue	Time to saturation level (days)	Biological half-life (days)	Reference
HEOD (Dieldrin)	10 p.p.m.[c]/56	Rat liver[e]		1.3 (m); 10.2 (m)	44
HEOD	10 p.p.m./56	Rat blood[e]		1.3 (m); 10.2 (m)	44
HEOD	10 p.p.m./56	Rat adipose		10.3 (m)	44
HEOD	10 p.p.m./56	Rat brain		3.0 (m)	44
HEOD	20 p.p.m./250	Rat adipose		10 (m); 12.7 (f)	69
Photo-dieldrin	10 p.p.m./26	Rat adipose		1.7 (m); 2.6 (f)	69
HEOD	75 p.p.m./365	Rat adipose		14.7 (m)	36
Telodrin	5–25 p.p.m. (various times up to 224 days)	Rat adipose Rat adipose	∼170 (m) ∼200–250 (f)	10.9 (m) 16.6 (f)	70 70
Dieldrin	211 µg daily/550	Human blood	∼365	84–112 (m)	72
Endrin[d]	0.8 p.p.m./1	Rat[f]		1–2 (f)	71
	1.6 p.p.m./1	Rat[f]		6 (f)	71
Endrin	0.4 p.p.m./12	Rat[f]	6 (m); 6 (f)	3 (m); 3 (f)	71
Endrin	200 µg/kg (i.v.)	Rat[f]		2–3 (m); 4 (f)	71
HHDN (Aldrin)	0.2 p.p.m./84	Rat[f]	53 (m); 200 (f)	11 (m); 100 (f)	66
β-DHC	50 µg (single i.v.)	Rat[f]		1 (m)	73
DDT	5 p.p.m./168	Rat adipose	140–168 (m)		37
DDT	Various/7 years	Rhesus monkey adipose	365–465		37
DDT	35 mg daily/600	Human adipose	365 (m)	1–2 years	37

[a] Dieldrin is not less than 85 per cent of 1,2,3,4,10,10-hexachloro-6,7-*exo*-epoxy-1,4,4a,5,6,7,8,8a-octahydro-1,4-*endo,exo*-5,8-dimethanonaphthalene (HEOD: the pure component used here). Aldrin is not less than 95 per cent of 1,2,3,4,10,10-hexachloro-1,4,4a,5,8,8a-hexahydro-1,4-*endo,exo*-5,8-dimethanonaphthalene (HHDN: the pure component used here).
[b] Times in days unless otherwise indicated.
[c] Concentration in the daily diet.
[d] Single administration at these concentrations in the diet.
[e] Half-lives for fast and slow phases of biphasic elimination are given.
[f] Data based on pattern of excretion of ^{14}C-labelled compounds from intact rat; other data shown are based on measurement of toxicant in the tissues.
(m) = male: (f) = female.

in the decay equation, and it is interesting that the decay constant and half-life (10.3 days) for Dieldrin in adipose tissues, for which elimination is adequately expressed by a single exponential term, are similar to those found for the slower phase of decline in blood and liver. On this basis it is considered that there is rapid interchange of toxicant between blood and liver, which constitute the central compartment, while adipose tissue belongs to a second compartment from which transfer of toxicant to the central compartment is rate-limiting for its further elimination after the initial rapid decline in the central compartment. This suggestion may be relevant to the observations of Street[45], who showed, without conclusive evidence that microsomal enzyme induction is responsible, that dietary DDT increased the metabolism of Dieldrin. If release of Dieldrin from adipose tissue to the microsomal enzymes, rather than their level, is the factor limiting metabolism, then the inability of inhibitors of enzyme induction to prevent the increased metabolism may be explained and the effect of DDT may be somehow to accelerate the release of Dieldrin from adipose tissue to the enzymes in the central compartment.

Some of the principles discussed above are illustrated by the data of *Table 3*. Worthy of note are the short half-lives of photodieldrin, β-DHC (2-*exo*-4,5,6,7,8,8-heptachloro-3a,4,7,7a-tetrahydro-4,7-methanoindane) and Endrin. In rats urinary excretion is much more important for the elimination of photodieldrin than for Dieldrin, regardless of sex, so that the two compounds appear to be treated rather differently in the body. As found with Dieldrin, a greater proportion of hydrophilic metabolites of photodieldrin is found in female urine than in male urine, although the total excretion of males is greater than that of females in the same time, so that the usual sex difference is present. Very high levels of labelled material are found in the kidneys of males after administration of ^{14}C-labelled photodieldrin, and it is of great interest that about 70 per cent of the material excreted in male urine is the ketonic derivative 'Klein's metabolite' (V, *Figure 3*), whereas the ether-extractable fraction of female urine contains, in contrast, at least four other metabolites but no ketone[46,47].

There is clearly a remarkable contrast between the dynamics of Dieldrin and Endrin in the vertebrates so far investigated; most of the latter compound is excreted as metabolites within a week after a single dose or after cessation of chronic dosing. Δ-Keto-Endrin is also readily eliminated as metabolites, so that in vertebrates the stability of photodieldrin, Endrin (therefore Isodrin) and Δ-keto-Endrin is opposite to that found in the higher plants examined. The low persistence of β-DHC is related to its very rapid conversion into hydrophilic metabolites, in contrast to the much slower conversions found with Isobenzan and Heptachlor. As a somewhat similar chlorinated cyclic ether, Isobenzan may be expected to have some of the properties of the persistent epoxides such as Dieldrin and Heptachlor epoxide, and the formation of the latter from Heptachlor *in vivo* undoubtedly accounts for its slow elimination compared with β-DHC.

An obvious difference between animals and plants lies in the ability of the former to dispose of metabolic products by excretion. Whether there are fundamental differences in the nature of the metabolic processes is unknown since the structures of so many of the metabolites remain to be determined.

BIOTRANSFORMATIONS

Aromatic compounds, DDT and γ-HCH

The foregoing account has considered the biodynamics of organochlorine compounds with only incidental reference to the nature of the biotransformation products, which will now be considered.

Although aromatic compounds in general appear to be eliminated fairly readily *in vivo*, many organochlorine pesticides contain a chlorinated aromatic nucleus, which sometimes appears to be the factor limiting their final biodegradation. Thus, an organophosphate ester containing such a nucleus may be rapidly hydrolysed *in vivo*, and the phosphate moiety eliminated by the normal metabolic pathways, so that only the chlorinated phenol produced by hydrolysis remains. Chlorinated phenols may also arise by direct aromatic hydroxylation and so it is often the fate of these that one has to consider, except where the nucleus is so highly chlorinated as to make hydroxylation difficult. Cornish and Block[48] found, for example, that the excretion of chlorinated naphthalenes as *S*-conjugates by rabbits decreased with increasing chlorination, so that during a four-days period there was little or no significant excretion of tetrachloro- and higher chlorinated naphthalenes. These observations are relevant to the biodegradation of PCB compounds and DDT analogues and also HCH (hexachlorocyclohexane) isomers, since the last-named are potential precursors of aromatic molecules. Since chlorinated phenols can be retained in plants as glycosides and can be excreted as various conjugates by vertebrates,

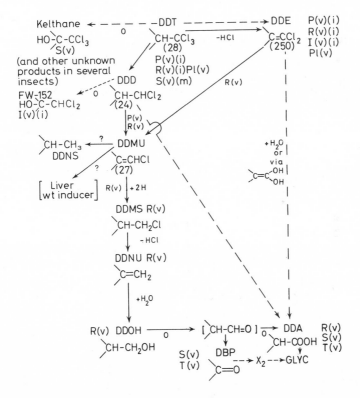

Figure 1. Postulated routes of biotransformation of DDT in pigeons, rats, micro-organisms and some insects. The pathway for pigeons differs from that in rats beyond DDMU. Broken lines indicate mainly insect pathways. Figures in parentheses are biological half-lives in the pigeon. m = micro-organisms; Pl = plants; P = pigeon; R = rat; S = *Sitophilus granarius*; T = *Triboleum castaneum*; I = insect; v = *in vivo*; i = *in vitro*. See text for references

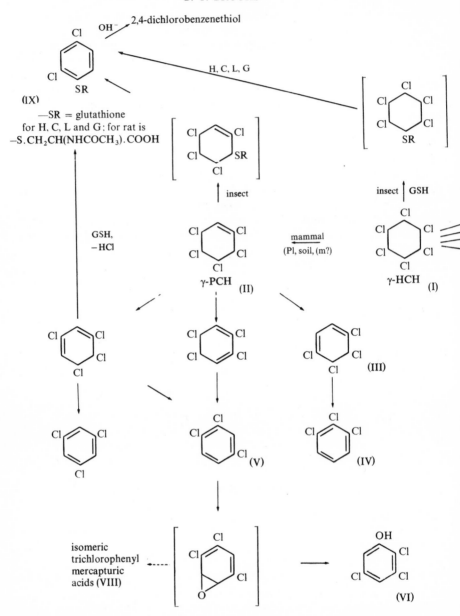

Figure 2. Probable pathways and some products of γ-HCH metabolism. Pathway (I) → (IV) has been indicated for both insects and mammals. Pathways (I) → (VI) and (VII), (II) → (VI) and (VII), have been indicated for the rat, with (VII) and its derivatives predominating. Pathways (I) → (II) → (IX) and (II) → (IX) have also been indicated for the rat and (V) is converted into (VI), (VII) and (VIII) in rabbits. Thus (II) and (V) are indicated intermediates in mammalian

124

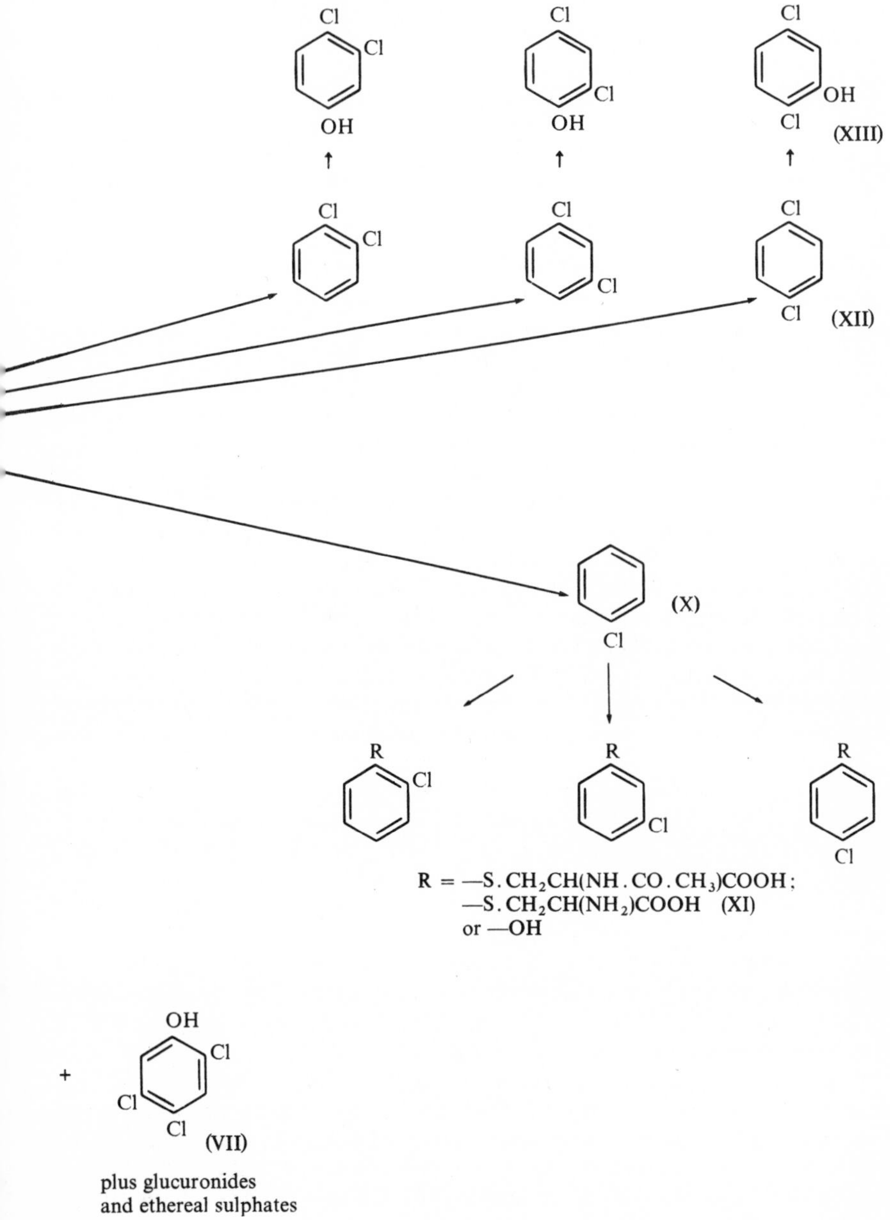
Cl
Cl
OH
Cl
Cl
OH
Cl
OH
Cl
(XIII)
Cl
Cl
Cl
Cl
Cl
Cl
(XII)
(X)
Cl
R
Cl
R
Cl
R
Cl
R = —S.CH₂CH(NH.CO.CH₃)COOH;
—S.CH₂CH(NH₂)COOH (XI)
or —OH
+
OH
Cl
Cl
Cl
(VII)
plus glucuronides
and ethereal sulphates

metabolism. There is evidence that monochloro- (X) and dichloro-benzenes (XII) are metabolites in insects. The formàtion of acid–labile precursors of the cysteine conjugates (XI) from monochlorobenzene has been demonstrated in the locust and the formation of conjugates of the phenols (XIII) from dichlorobenzene has been found in the rabbit. H = housefly; C = cattle tick; L = locust; Pl = plant; m = micro-organisms; G = grass grub. GSH, glutathione.

they may still be potentially available to the biosphere by conjugate cleavage, so that final breakdown is very dependent on exposure to light and air, and especially on the ability of micro-organisms to degrade aromatic rings.

It seems surprising that aromatic ring hydroxylation has not been demonstrated as a common feature of the metabolism of DDT and its analogues (*Figure 1*), although the grain weevil *Sitophilus granarius* excretes a complex glycoside containing labelled 4-hydroxy- and 3-hydroxy-4-chlorobenzoic acids after treatment with ^{14}C-labelled DDT[49]. The unidentified metabolic products produced by several insects possessing effective microsomal mixed-function oxidase enzymes may result from ring hydroxylation, with or without NIH shift of the *p*-chlorine atoms; in fact there is some indication of the loss of *p*-chlorine in certain houseflies[50].

DDD and DDE appear to arise by separate pathways in several organisms, and the latter is frequently only slowly metabolized, so that little is known about its further metabolism. However, Datta[51] has indicated that, in rats, DDE is slowly converted into DDMU and thence to DDNU and DDA via the sequence of *Figure 1*, but without DDMS formation; from which it appears that the conversion of DDMU into DDNU can occur either directly by reductive dechlorination or by reduction to DDMS and then dehydrochlorination. According to recent work[52] on the pathway in the pigeon, DDMS is converted (half-life about eight days) into DDMU, and DDNU is very rapidly transformed into DDNS, an additional, unidentified metabolite being formed in each case. DDA is not found after feeding with any DDT metabolite. Thus DDT biotransformation in the vertebrates so far examined involves dehydrochlorination, reductive dechlorination and saturation reactions, which may or may not be followed by double bond hydration in liver and kidneys leading to DDOH and eventually to DDA. The ability of rabbit and rat liver microsomes to hydrate the epoxide ring system (having some analogy with a double bond) of certain cyclodiene epoxides is 10000 and 1000 times, respectively, greater than that of pigeon liver microsomes[53], which may have some reflection upon the general ability of pigeons to effect hydration reactions. Investigations on the photochemistry of DDT previously referred to indicate the availability of molecular rearrangements, although the formation of such products *in vivo* has not been indicated so far. A major problem with insects has been the difficulty of isolating sufficient of the oxidative metabolites for characterization and the lack of reference compounds derived from the intact DDT molecule by oxidation.

Problems of metabolism of the HCH isomers concern firstly the mechanisms of aromatization and secondly the fate of the chlorinated benzenes and their derivatives so produced. There is evidence that all the isomers are metabolized by mammals and insects, but the pathways for isomers other than γ-HCH remain obscure. The β-isomer is known to be particularly persistent, a property probably largely related to a lack of *trans*-relationships between adjacent hydrogen and chlorine atoms in this molecule, which makes dehydrochlorination difficult; the other isomers all contain *trans*-related adjacent hydrogen and chlorine atoms, so that dehydrochlorination is facilitated. The left side of *Figure 2* shows some probable pathways of γ-HCH metabolism and the right side shows additional products that either actually occur or should be considered as possible metabolic products.

Several aspects of the aromatization process remain obscure. Thus, a number of experiments with whole insects and insect homogenates, including the housefly, indicate 2,4-dichlorophenylglutathione as a terminal metabolite from γ-HCH, γ-PCH (γ-2,3,4,5,6-pentachlorocyclohexene) and δ-PCH[54], corresponding to the replacement of one chlorine atom in each by glutathione (GSH), followed by further loss of chlorine and aromatization (pathways I→IX and II→IX; *Figure 2*). On the other hand, another report[55] indicates, without reference to the nature of the products, that soluble supernatant preparations from houseflies liberate appreciable amounts of chlorine from γ-HCH without enzymic loss of glutathione or conjugate formation. In this investigation, the glutathione conjugate formed by these housefly preparations from γ-PCH was indistinguishable (paper chromatography) from the conjugate formed with rat liver soluble enzymes by replacement of one chlorine atom[56]. Clearly, much depends on the value of the chromatographic identities, but in view of the results with whole insects and homogenates, it seems strange that soluble housefly preparations liberate appreciable amounts of chlorine from γ-HCH without conjugation, whilst replacing only one chlorine atom in γ-PCH with conjugation. It may be that the soluble enzyme preparations can produce only intermediate chlorinated alicyclic structures, whereas homogenates or whole insects contain the necessary enzyme systems to complete the aromatization. The metabolic pathway via S-pentachlorocyclohexylglutathione is currently favoured for insects.

The production has been indicated of mono-, di- and tri-chlorobenzenes (X, XII and IV; *Figure 2*) from α-HCH and of 1,2,3- and 1,2,4-trichloro-, 1,2,4,5- and 1,2,3,4-tetrachloro-, and pentachloro-benzenes from γ-HCH in houseflies[57]; of 1,2,3,5-tetrachlorobenzene from γ-HCH in micro-organisms. 1,2,4-Trichlorobenzene is a probable intermediate in rats, as indicated in *Figure 2*. Mono-, di- and tri-chlorobenzenes seem unlikely to present any persistence problems since they are metabolized to mercapturic acids, cysteine conjugates (XI; *Figure 2*) and/or phenols and phenolic conjugates in insects and mammals. 4-Chloropyrocatechol is formed from monochlorobenzene in locusts and, since pyrocatechol formation is frequently the first stage in the complete degradation of aromatic rings by microorganisms, the excretion of such products should present no indefinite environmental problem. Since cleavage of the ether linkages of some chlorinated phenoxyalkanoic acids affords phenols similar to those likely to arise from Lindane, the metabolic fate of these herbicides is likely to be relevant to this discussion; for example, 2,4-dichlorophenol (from 2,4-dichlorophenoxyacetic acid) suffers ring degradation by soil bacteria after its initial conversion into 3,4-dichloropyrocatechol. It is not clear whether tetrachlorobenzenes and pentachlorobenzenes, which might present residue problems, are formed to any extent from Lindane in plants or mammals.

Diene-organochlorine (Cyclodiene) compounds

At first sight the cyclodiene compounds appear to be unique from the point of view of biotransformation, since they contain neither an aromatic nucleus nor a simple aliphatic structure that is obviously vulnerable to

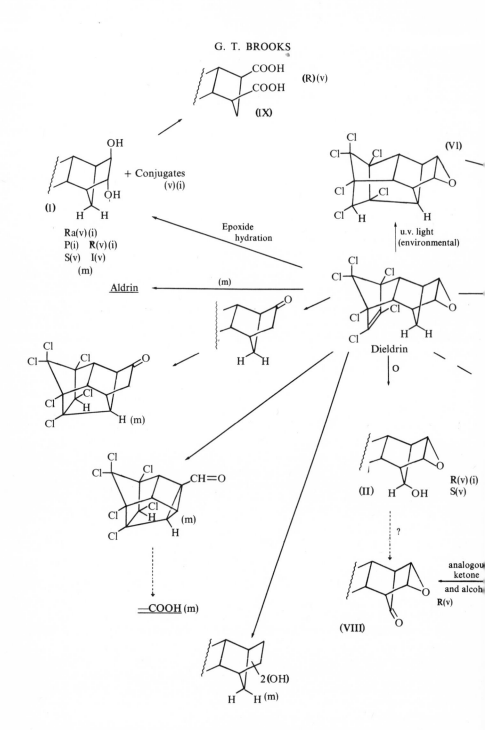

Figure 3. Biotransformations of Dieldrin, photodieldrin and Endrin in mammals, insects and micro-organisms. Structure (III) and the structures of some of the compounds produced by micro-organisms are tentative. e = environmental; H = housefly; I = some insects; mo =

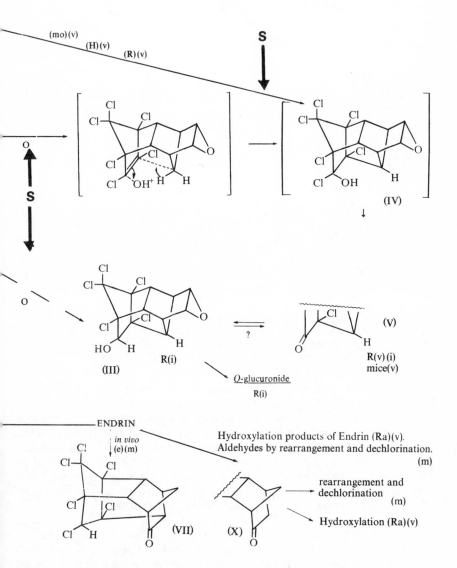

mosquito; m = micro-organisms; P = pig; Ra = rabbit; R = rat; S = sheep; v = *in vivo*; i = *in vitro*. S→; sesamex inhibits. For references see text. The use of a partial structure implies that the remainder of the molecule is unchanged.

129

F

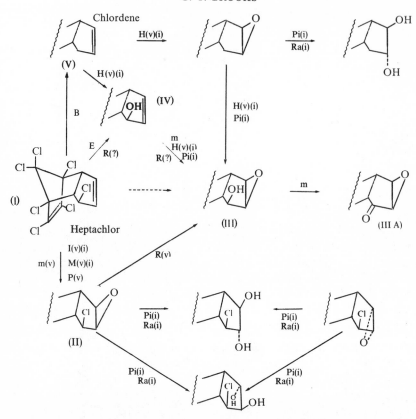

Figure 4. Summary of the biotransformations of heptachlor and related compounds. The use of a partial structure implies that the remainder of the molecule is unchanged. B = bacteria; H = housefly; I = some insects; P = plants; M = mammals; Pi = pig; R = rat; m = micro-organisms; Ra = rabbit; E = environmental conversion; v = *in vivo*; i = *in vitro*

enzymic attack. However, it is now fairly clear that even the more persistent cyclodienes differ only quantitatively from other reduced polycyclic systems in their susceptibility to attack by the drug-metabolizing enzymes, and it is interesting that progress in research on the latter almost exactly parallels the development of knowledge about cyclodiene metabolism[58]. The diversity of the metabolic pathways available, *in vivo* and *in vitro*, is illustrated in *Figures 3–5*, which summarize information available for the commonly used persistent cyclodienes and for some related compounds. Information regarding less familiar compounds is referred to elsewhere[41, 58].

Aldrin, Isodrin and Heptachlor—Since these compounds are normally rapidly converted into their respective epoxides, Dieldrin, Endrin and Heptachlor epoxide, it is usually the fate of the last-named that has to be considered in relation to residue problems. However, there are indications, especially with Aldrin and Heptachlor, that in plants and micro-organisms metabolic pathways are available which do not involve intermediate

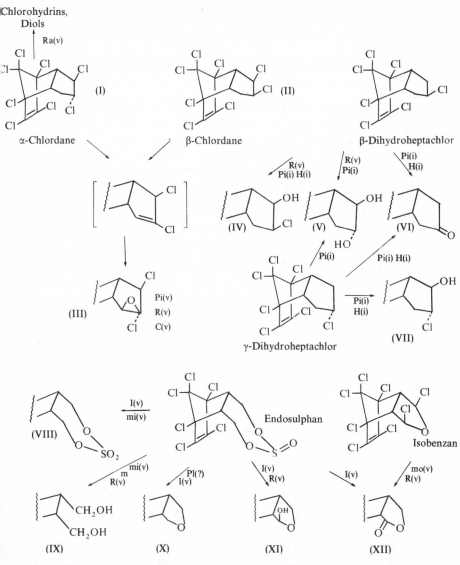

Figure 5. Biotransformation products established or postulated for α- and β-chlordane, β- and γ-dihydroheptachlor, the endosulphan isomers (the molecule shown is the α-isomer but should be taken to represent the β-isomer also), and isobenzan (Telodrin). C = cow; H = housefly; I = insects; m = micro-organisms; mi = mice; mo = mosquito larvae; Pi = pig; R = rat; i = *in vitro*; v = *in vivo*. The use of a partial structure implies that the remainder of the molecule is unchanged.

formation of the persistent epoxides, so that use of the precursors rather than their epoxides in pest control provides additional opportunity factors for detoxication. For Aldrin and Isodrin, the additional metabolites have not yet been identified; it may be noted that photoisodrin, although apparently

131

not yet indicated as an Isodrin conversion product, is less toxic to insects than Isodrin or Endrin and if formed may be a general detoxication product. With Heptachlor, bacterial or environmental replacement of the allylic chlorine atom by hydrogen to give chlordene (V; *Figure 4*) or by hydroxyl (IV; *Figure 4*) drastically reduces toxicity and exposes the molecule to attack by the oxidizing enzymes of micro-organisms[59] and higher forms[60].

Dieldrin, Endrin and Heptachlor epoxide—Metabolic products from these compounds have been identified, some positively and some tentatively, mainly in mammals and micro-organisms, and with higher organisms they appear to arise by oxidation, or oxidative dechlorination with rearrangement in the case of Dieldrin. It is not clear at present whether the hydroxy-epoxide (III; *Figure 4*), indicated to be a transformation product of Heptachlor epoxide (II; *Figure 4*) in rats[61], arises by hydrolytic or oxidative replacement of chlorine. However, the latter route would be analogous to the conversion of photodieldrin (VI; *Figure 3*) via intermediate (IV) into the ketone (V), and would lead to the hydroxy-epoxide via reduction of the ketone IIIA (*Figure 4*); formation of the latter has not so far been indicated from Heptachlor epoxide. Although the Heptachlor epoxides have been shown to hydrate to the *trans*-diols *in vitro* (*Figure 4*), no such conversion has yet been demonstrated *in vivo*. Cleavage of the epoxide ring of Dieldrin has also been demonstrated *in vitro*[62, 63] and is now well recognized to occur in several organisms (*Figure 3*); the further conversion of the *trans*-diol (I) into the dicarboxylic acid (IX; *Figure 3*) in rats[11] (six per cent conversion of a 210 mg dose administered during five days) is the first instance of the cleavage of a norbornane nucleus of a cyclodiene compound by a living organism.

The remarkably rapid elimination of Endrin by rats appears to be associated entirely with oxidative biotransformation, there being no evidence so far for hydration of the epoxide ring[63a]. Excretion is mainly in faeces and consists of Endrin, together with the product of its methylene-bridge hydroxylation (compare II; *Figure 3*), and another, unidentified, monohydroxylation product, while tissues contain the bridge-ketone analogous to compound VIII (*Figure 3*). Hydroxylation without skeletal rearrangement also occurs in rabbits, which excrete in the urine four metabolites, including a hydroxy-Endrin conjugate, a free hydroxy-Endrin (believed to be hydroxylated at the junction of the norbornane rings) and a hydroxy-derivative of the ketone X (*Figure 3*)[11]. This remarkable example of the effect of stereochemistry on biological stability (contrast Dieldrin) is presumably related to the greater exposure of the Endrin skeleton to attack by microsomal oxidases.

Soil micro-organisms effect transformation of Dieldrin (*Figure 3*) and Endrin by, *inter alia*, rearrangement of the epoxide ring, with or without skeletal rearrangement, or by skeletal rearrangement to give aldehydes. Some of the products from Endrin apparently resemble those obtained by its thermal rearrangement and further conversion of these may occur by reductive dechlorination[34]. The toxicological and residue significance of most of these compounds is unknown at present.

Dihydroheptachlor, Chlordane, endosulphan (Thiodan) and isobenzan (Telodrin)—The high toxicity and persistence of Aldrin, Isodrin and Heptachlor in insects is undoubtedly related to their conversion into the stable toxic epoxides rather than into detoxication products; the corresponding compounds lacking reactive double bonds owe their reduced toxicity to the availability of methylene groups that can be hydroxy-lated[26, 60, 64]. Thus, in contrast to Heptachlor, the dihydroheptachlor isomers can be hydroxylated *in vivo*, so that their biotransformation results in detoxication[11]. For example, the influence of these detoxication processes on dihydroheptachlor toxicity to the housefly is made evident by the synergism observed when they are suppressed by appropriate enzyme inhibitors *in vivo*[65]. The metabolites of β-DHC excreted by rats include[11] the chlorohydrin IV and the *trans*-diol V (*Figure 5*), so that as far as is known at present, detoxication produces compounds with the intact cyclodiene skeleton. Further chlorination of the cyclopentane ring increases persistence, as with the chlordane isomers (*Figure 5*), although the α-isomer at least is converted into chlorohydrins and diols in rabbits and unidentified metabolites in plants[11, 66]. The recent demonstration that both isomers are converted into the epoxide III (*Figure 5*)[67] *in vivo* implies double-bond formation before epoxidation and shows that completely reduced polycyclic systems are not necessarily excluded from epoxidation. This epoxide attains storage levels, depending on the level of Chlordane isomers fed, in the fat of rats, dogs and pigs and its further fate (with regard to epoxide ring cleavage, for example) is at present unknown.

There is a marked contrast between endosulphan and isobenzan in regard to persistence in living organisms, although similar metabolic pathways are available, in principle, for both compounds (*Figure 5*). Isobenzan stability is clearly related to the protection against enzymic attack afforded by chlorine substitution in the furan ring, whilst the endosulphan structure presents opportunities for detoxication that are unique among cyclodiene compounds. Nevertheless, the detoxication products demonstrated so far still retain the intact hexachloronorbornene nucleus.

CONCLUDING COMMENTS

In spite of the evident complexity of the problem, much progress has been made in elucidating the behaviour and fate of organochlorine insecticides in living organisms, although the identities of a number of metabolites, especially those produced by plants and micro-organisms, remain to be determined. The modifications identified so far are mainly peripheral, involving hydroxylation and the reductive, hydrolytic and oxidative removal of chlorine, with or without molecular rearrangement in the cyclodienes. Although conjugation mechanisms are evidently available for some of these primary products, their nature is still generally obscure, except for the phenolic compounds produced from Lindane, and the primary products are frequently excreted unchanged. Final removal from the environment must depend on microbial activity and it remains to be seen whether the cyclodienes and their rearrangement products can be completely degraded, although the *Pseudomonas* sp. called Shell 33 by Matsumura[34] can apparently use Dieldrin as the sole carbon source.

It is not easy to develop highly biodegradable pesticides that retain really high toxicity to the target organism, and this is especially true with organo-chlorine compounds, which display strict structural requirements for toxicity. There are, however, indications that this can be done with DDT analogues[1], and to some extent with cyclodiene[53, 68] compounds (requiring the use of a synergist), by providing sites for oxidative or hydrolytic degradation in the molecules. This approach has the advantage that any development of resistance may involve the enhancement of the mechanism already provided by molecular design and so can be overcome by the use of appropriate synergists.

Earlier reference was made to possible inductive effects of organochlorine residues on insect microsomal enzymes. A similar discussion is applicable to mammals. While it is impossible to say whether increased microsomal enzyme activity has resulted from the basal body burden already established, it has been shown that induction does not occur in male rats until the dietary cyclodiene content is raised more than 25 times above the background dietary level. Further, the background concentration of pp'-DDE in the blood did not decrease when the background body burden of HEOD was increased ten times in human volunteers, indicating that enzyme activity, at least for pp'-DDE degradation, was not induced under these conditions.

Insecticide resistance apart, it is difficult to escape the conclusion that, within the bounds of our present knowledge, the use of these compounds has been entirely beneficial. Ironically, an additional benefit is that awareness of their distribution characteristics has reminded us of the existence of more serious pollution hazards. What is very clearly needed is some means by which the persistence of compounds of this sort can be controlled at will to suit individual insect control problems.

REFERENCES

[1] G. Holan, *Nature, Lond.*, **221**, 1025 (1969).

[2] T. Narashi and H. G. Haas, *J. Gen. Physiol.* **51**, 177 (1968).

[3] T. Narashi and J. W. Moore, *J. Gen. Physiol.* **51**, 93s (1968).

[4] D. E. Weiss, *Austral. J. Biol. Sci.* **22**, 1337 (1969).

[5] D. E. Weiss, *Austral. J. Biol. Sci.* **22**, 1355 (1969).

[6] D. E. Weiss, *Austral. J. Biol. Sci.* **22**, 1373 (1969).

[7] F. W. Plapp Jr and J. Casida, *J. Econ. Ent.* **63**, 1091 (1970).

[8] N. Ahmad and W. A. Brindley, *Toxicol. Appl. Pharmacol.* **15**, 433, (1969).

[9] C. R. Walker and L. C. Terriere, *Entomologia Exp. et Appl.* **13**, 260 (1970).

[10] F. Moriarty, *Biol. Rev.* **44**, 321 (1969).

[11] Institut für Okologische Chemie, Schloss Birlinghoven, *Jahresbericht* 1969; Gesellschaft für Strahlenforschung m.b.H.

[12] J. R. Plimmer, V. I. Klingebiel and B. E. Hummer, *Science*, **167**, 67 (1970).

[13] H. Itokawa, A. Schallah, I. Weisgerber, W. Klein and F. Korte, *Tetrahedron*, **26**, 763 (1970).

[14] I. Weisgerber, W. Klein, A. Djirsarai and F. Korte, *Liebigs Ann. Chem.* **713**, 175 (1968).

[15] W. Klein, R. Kaul, Z. Parlar, M. Zimmer and F. Korte, *Tetrahedron Letters*, 3197 (1969).

[16] I. Weisgerber, W. Klein and F. Korte, *Liebigs Ann. Chem.* **729**, 193 (1969).

[17] W. Klein. Paper presented at the IUPAC Symposium on 'Chemistry of Pesticides under Metabolic and Environmental Conditions', Bonn/Birlinghoven (September 1970).

[18] H. Hulpke. *Qual. Plant. Mater. Veg.* **18**, 331 (1969).

[19] H. Hulpke, *Qual. Plant. Mater. Veg.* **19**, 333 (1970).

[20] H. Hulpke and W. Schuphan, *Qual. Plant. Mater. Veg.* **19**, 347 (1970).

[21] C. T. Lewis, *J. Insect Physiol.* **11**, 683 (1965).

[22] C. H. Schaefer and Y. P. Sun, *J. Econ. Ent.* **60**, 1580 (1967).

[23] Y. P. Sun, C. H. Schaefer and E. R. Johnson, *J. Econ. Ent.* **60**, 1033 (1967).

[24] Y. P. Sun, *J. Econ. Ent.* **61**, 949 (1968).

[25] P. Gerolt, *J. Insect Physiol.* **15**, 563 (1969).

[26] G. T. Brooks, *Wld Review Pest Contr.* **5**, 62 (1966); and unpublished results.

[27] J. R. Plimmer, P. C. Kearney and D. W. Von Endt, *J. Agric. Food Chem.* **16**, 594 (1968).

[28] R. A. Ledford and J. H. Chen, *J. Food Sci.* **34**, 386 (1969).

[29] R. G. Bridges, *J. Sci. Food Agric.* **7**, 305 (1956).

[30] H. Lyr and G. Ritter, *Zeitschrift F. Allg. Mikrobiologie*, **9**, 545 (1969).

[31] C. M. Tu, J. R. W. Miles and C. R. Harris, *Life Sci.* **7**, 311 (1968).

[32] F. Korte, G. Ludwig and J. Vogel, *Liebigs Ann. Chem.* **656**, 135 (1962).

[33] F. Korte, G. Ludwig and J. Vogel, *Liebigs Ann. Chem.* **656**, 135 (1962).

[34] F. Matsumura, G. M. Boush and A. Tai, *Nature, Lond.*, **219**, 965 (1968); and personal communication (1970).

[35] F. Korte and M. Stiasni, *Liebigs Ann. Chem.* **673**, 146 (1964).

[36] J. Robinson and M. Roberts, 'Accumulation, distribution and elimination of organochlorine insecticides by vertebrates'; Society of Chemical Industry *Monograph No.* 29, p 106. London (1968).

[37] *Report of the Secretary's Commission on Pesticides and their Relationship to Environmental Health*, US Department of Health, Education and Welfare, Washington D.C. (December 1969).

[38] J. Robinson and V. K. H. Brown, *Nature, Lond.* **213**, 734 (1967).

[39] S. Bailey, P. J. Bunyan, B. D. Rennison and A. Taylor, *Toxicol. Appl. Pharmacol.* **14**, 13 (1969).

[40] S. Bailey, P. J. Bunyan, B. D. Rennison and A. Taylor, *Toxicol. Appl. Pharmacol.* **14**, 23 (1969); and personal communication.

[41] G. T. Brooks, *Residue Rev.* **27**, 81 (1969).

[42] *Third Report of the Research Committee on Toxic Chemicals*, Agricultural Research Council: London (1970).

[43] I. Presst, D. J. Jefferies and N. W. Moore, *Environ. Pollut.* **1**, 3 (1970).

[44] J. Robinson, M. Roberts, M. Baldwin and A. I. T. Walker, *Food Cosmet. Toxicol.* **7**, 317 (1969).

[45] J. C. Street, In *Enzymatic Oxidations of Toxicants*. Ed. by E. Hodgson, North Carolina State University, Raleigh N.C. (1968).

[46] R. E. Dailey, M. S. Walton, V. Beck, C. L. Leavens and A. K. Klein, *J. Agric. Food Chem.* **18**, 443 (1970).

[47] A. K. Klein, R. E. Dailey, M. S. Walton, V. Beck and J. D. Link, *J. Agric. Food Chem.* **18** 705 (1970).

[48] H. H. Cornish and W. D. Block, *J. Biol. Chem.* **321**, 583 (1958).

[49] D. G. Rowlands and C. J. Lloyd, *J. Stored Prod. Res.* **5**, 413 (1969).

[50] F. J. Oppenoorth and N. W. H. Houx, *Entomologia Exp. et Appl.* **11**, 81 (1968).

[51] P. R. Datta, *Ind. Med.* **39**, 49 (1970).

[52] S. Bailey, P. J. Bunyan and A. Taylor. Paper presented at the *IUPAC Symposium on 'Chemistry of Pesticides under Metabolic and Environmental Conditions'*. Bonn/Birlinghoven (September 1970).

[53] G. A. El Zorgani, C. H. Walker and K. A. Hassall, *Life Sci.* **9**, 415 (1970).

[54] A. G. Clark, S. Murphy and J. N. Smith, *Biochem. J.* **113**, 89 (1969).

[55] P. Sims and P. L. Grover, *Biochem. J.* **95**, 156 (1965).

[56] P. L. Grover and P. Sims, *Biochem. J.* **96**, 521 (1965).

[57] W. T. Reed and A. J. Forgash, *J. Agric. Food Chem.* **18**, 475 (1970).

[58] G. T. Brooks. Paper presented at the *IUPAC Symposium on 'Chemistry of Pesticides under Metabolic and Environmental Conditions'*, Bonn/Birlinghoven (September 1970).

[59] J. R. W. Miles, C. M. Tu and C. W. Harris, *J. Econ. Ent.* **62**, 1334 (1969).

[60] G. T. Brooks and A. Harrison, *Nature, Lond.* **205**, 1031 (1965).

[61] R. Kaul, W. Klein and F. Korte, *Tetrahedron*, **26**, 331 (1970).

[62] G. T. Brooks and A. Harrison, *Bull. Env. Contam. Toxicol.* **4**, 352 (1969).

[63] G. T. Brooks, A. Harrison and S. E. Lewis, *Biochem. Pharmac.* **19**, 255 (1970).

[63a] A. Richardson, J. Robinson and M. K. Baldwin, *Chem. and Ind.* 502 (1970).

[64] R. I. Krieger and C. F. Wilkinson, Personal communication (1970).

[65] G. T. Brooks and A. Harrison, *Life Sci.* **6**, 1439 (1967).

[66] F. Korte, *Botyu-Kagaku*, **32**, 46 (1967).

[67] B. Schwemmer, W. P. Cochrane and P. B. Polen, *Science*, **169**, 1087 (1970); and personal communication.

[68] G. T. Brooks, *Proc. 5th Br. Insectic. Fungic. Conf.* 472 (1969).

[69] V. K. H. Brown, J. Robinson and A. Richardson, *Fd. Cosmet. Toxicol.* **5**, 771 (1967).

70 J. Robinson and A. R. Richardson, Internal Rept., Shell Research Ltd., Sittingbourne, England (1963).
71 W. Klein, W. Muller and F. Korte, *Liebigs Ann. Chem.* **713**, 180 (1968).
72 C. G. Hunter and J. Robinson, *Arch. Environ. Health*, **15**, 614 (1967).
73 R. Kaul, W. Klein and F. Korte, *Tetrahedron*, **26**, 99 (1970).

FATE OF INSECTICIDAL CHLORINATED HYDRO-CARBONS IN STORAGE AND PROCESSING OF FOODS

PERCY B. POLEN

Velsicol Chemical Corporation, Chicago, Ill. 60611, USA

ABSTRACT

Susceptibility to volatilization and localization of organochlorine pesticide residues in outer layers of treated plants favours a reduction of the residues during food preparation, both in home and commercial processing. As a result of preparation, finished foods of plant origin usually contain substantially less residues than the raw agricultural products from which they are derived. Processing wastes and some byproducts carry the residues out of the human food chain, except where they are re-introduced as feed components for animals being raised to produce human food. Such products ordinarily contain organochlorine residues localized in the fat and, generally, processing would merely redistribute the fat (and residues) between various derived foods. Where fat is removed, as in trimming, baking or broiling of meats, a net reduction of residues results.

Introduction of pesticide residues to the human food chain is less likely directly from foods of plant origin treated for pest control than from the indirect route: consumption of foods of animal origin derived from animals which have consumed food-processing wastes and certain byproducts.

This presentation highlights fairly extensive documentation on the fate of pesticide residues in typical food processing, both commercial and in the home, with special attention to the organochlorine insecticides, parent compounds and metabolites. It will become evident that normal food preparation practices, as an incidental effect, physically remove substantial amounts of pesticide residue from the 'stream' of agricultural products as they are converted into prepared human food. On the other hand, the same residues may be reintroduced to the 'stream' with process byproducts that are fed to food-producing animals.

Regulatory agencies, both national and international, seeking to limit the human intake of pesticide residues through consumption of food, have established systems of 'tolerances'. A legal tolerance is the maximum concentration of pesticide allowed in a particular dominion on a crop or food product. Its value is generally no higher than that residue level likely to result from 'good agricultural practice', and the pattern of established tolerances must in all cases

137

be judged as 'safe' in that it controls the probable daily pesticide intake by humans below an acceptable upper limit.

Conceptually tolerances apply to human food, but in actual practice this is not so. Most raw agricultural commodities or food products moving in commerce, the items on which tolerances are established, are subjected to further processing or cleansing and preparations at home before they become human food. For very practical reasons tolerances are enforceable on food products moving in commerce, but not for food on the dining table. It is found that there is a substantial difference between organochlorine pesticide residue intake inferred by some from existing tolerance patterns and the probable actual intake from human consumption of finished foods.

As a class, the organochlorine compounds lend themselves particularly well to studies of their fate in food processing. They are distinctly 'visible', especially during the past fifteen years after the introduction of gas chromatography as a routine analytical technique. Their detectability is further enhanced by their tendency to localize in the lipid phase and at the outer surface of plants to which they are applied as insecticides.

The properties which cause these residues to localize in plants also make their removal easier in home preparation of food and in the unit processes of commercial food manufacture. One other property that should be mentioned as an aid to removal is the susceptibility of the organochlorine pesticides to co-distillation with water under certain conditions.

First, let us look at the tendency of organochlorine pesticides to concentrate in outer layers and peels of fruits and vegetables. Several studies appear in the literature for potatoes and other root crops grown in soils treated with chlorinated cyclodienes.

In about 80 per cent of the observations on potatoes, residues were detected only on the peel, not in the pulp. The ratio of residue level on peel compared to that in pulp is a good index of separation. Aldrin, heptachlor and chlordane are found 20 to 300 times more concentrated on the peel than in the pulp. The epoxides, dieldrin and heptachlor epoxide, were 3 to 15 times more abundant on the peel than in the pulp.

Other root crops display similar effects. Beets grown in soil treated with technical chlordane carried all of their detectable residues on the peels, none being detected in the pulp. Carrots grown in the same soil carried roughly 24 times as much residue in the peel as in the pulp.

There is, of course, a difference among varieties in their pesticide penetrability. When five varieties of carrots were compared, four coloured varieties of carrots grown in soil treated with aldrin or heptachlor at massive doses generally carried at least 70 per cent of their combined detectable residues in the peel; a fifth, white variety had only 55 per cent in the outer layer.

The depth of penetration of the constituents of technical heptachlor into rutabagas grown in heptachlor-treated soil was remarkably small. Almost 70 per cent of the total residue was retained in the thin waxy layer at the surface of the rutabaga and 91 per cent could be removed by scraping away the waxy layer and 2 mm of outer tissue.

It would be expected, then, that with the residues of organochlorine compounds lying so close to the surface, substantial removal of these would result typically by washing, peeling or abrasive peeling of the surface. This was

138

confirmed by studies carried out on typical unit processes used in home and commercial preparation of food. One study demonstrates substantial reductions of the DDT complex of residues. Residues in potatoes grown in DDT-treated soil were reduced approximately 20 per cent by washing alone, 90 to 94 per cent by peeling alone, and over 96 per cent when cooking was also performed. On the other hand, boiling potatoes with skins intact effected no appreciable reduction in the residues.

Chlordane residues on whole potatoes were reduced 15 to 25 per cent by boiling alone, and 50 to 80 per cent by baking. Peeling plus cooking was most effective. No chlordane residues were detected in the pulp of potatoes which had been first peeled and then boiled. Likewise, turnips and beets grown in chlordane-treated soil were freed of detectable residues by peeling and boiling; carrots under the same conditions were freed of 98 per cent of their total measured chlordane residues.

Although washing alone does remove some organochlorine residues, effectiveness depends on several factors: character of the surface (that is whether smooth or rough, waxy or non-waxy); surface to volume ratio (the bigger the fruit, the more effective is washing); the level of residue (the higher the level, the easier to remove). These factors can be sensed in results of studies of unit canning operations. DDT residues were reduced 91 per cent by washing tomatoes, but only 48 per cent by washing spinach. When detergent was added to the wash water for spinach, the reduction rose from 48 per cent to 73 per cent.

It is interesting to compare these figures with those for parathion residues on spinach, when water washing alone removed only 9 per cent and detergent washing 24 per cent. This evidence implies a greater potential for penetration of the tissues by the more polar compound.

Commercial preparation of fruits or vegetables sometimes includes blanching, that is, immersion in hot water or exposure to steam. About one-half of the DDT residues on green beans were removed by blanching alone. DDT residues on spinach, which had been reduced one-half by washing alone, were reduced an additional 10 per cent by blanching for a total of 60 per cent removal. One may conclude that the waxy surfaces are only moderately affected by blanching.

The combined effect of the total canning process of DDT residues may be seen in the following figures. Operations in which peeling was one step resulted in the greatest diminution of residues: reductions were 99 per cent for tomatoes and 96 per cent for potatoes. Where the epidermis is not removed, the results are less quantitative. The total canning process removed DDT residues to the extent of 91 per cent from spinach and 83 per cent from green beans.

Pesticide residues in citrus fruits also have been shown to be localized in the rinds, and therein concentrated mostly in the oils. Typically the citrus distributed through the fresh fruit market would be freed of the rind (and hence the pesticide residues) before being consumed by humans. Commercial processing also separates the rind from its major food products: canned and frozen juices and juice concentrates. While the oils, potentially high in residues, are mainly excluded from commercial juice products, the completeness of the separation is an important consideration in limiting residues in the final product. Residue studies on minor citrus-rind products, marmalade and candied rind, have been reported only to a limited degree. A recently published report on studies carried out in the 1950s shows DDT residues near 1 p.p.m. in dried orange-rind products. Surprisingly, parathion withstood the marmalade-making process and residues were found in the same order of magnitude as for DDT, that is between 0.2 and 1.3 p.p.m. in eight brands of orange marmalade. This remained in spite of cooking in syrup to about 222°F (106°C). More modern studies on rind products do not appear to be published, and the levels implied by the earlier data are not evident in recent reports on total diet studies.

Little published data are available on the effects of storage on reduction of residues. One published study reports no significant decrease in DDT or carbaryl in 7-days storage of tomatoes at 55°F (13°C). A decrease in malathion residue was observed, but it is not clear whether the analysis included possible hydrolysis products as well as the parent compound.

The total diet studies of the US Food and Drug Administration offer ample additional evidence that the pesticide residues of organochlorine compounds are substantially lower than the levels of the tolerances imply. The contribution of home processing was especially highlighted in the most recent report, wherein residue levels for compounds found six or more times per food group were compared, 'before' and 'after' processing by a dietician. The author states: 'The data indicate a loss in residue when food is prepared for eating through peeling, stripping outer leaves, cooking, etc.' The conclusion was based on observations for the food categories designated as: potatoes, leafy vegetables, legume vegetables, root vegetables, garden fruits, fruits. Average reduction of residues in preparation of the foods was 45 to 68 per cent for the organochlorine group consisting of DDT, DDE, toxaphene and endrin; kelthane, observed in fruits only, diminished about 24 per cent of the initial residues. Compounds for which no significant reduction in residues was observed in this test were TDE, dieldrin and lindane. It is difficult to assess the report for the last three compounds since most of the analytical values reported are below the declared limit of detectability of the method.

Concern over the fate of organochlorine pesticides in the treatment of oil-seed crops often arises from the belief that, being non-polar, these compounds may concentrate in the oil and thus be introduced to the human diet in concentrated form via salad oils, margarines or shortenings etc. Substantial documentation now exists that normal commercial manufacturing processes for edible vegetable oils remove virtually all of the residues of organochlorines that may result from good agricultural practice, and the risk of direct introductions of residues to human diet by this route is negligible.

The production of edible oil follows this course. Oil-producing seeds (or beans) are either pressed or solvent-extracted to isolate the crude oils. These oils, generally inedible at this point, are subjected to a multistage treatment to produce the finished edible oil or shortening. They are alkali-refined, bleached, deodorized and, if hardening is desired, hydrogenated in that order.

Crude oils, even though themselves inedible, receive considerable attention with respect to their pesticide content. Frequently the finishing processes are performed at plants that are far from the extraction facilities, and crude oils may be transported across political boundaries. Inspections here may reveal residues of organochlorine compounds, which, being lipophilic, are extracted with the crude oil. Tolerances established for pesticides in crude oils should take into account the substantial changes in levels which result from typical processing to convert the oils into edible form.

Whereas organochlorine levels may be increased in the oils (compared to the source crop), they are decreased in oil seed (or bean) meals by the extraction process. Since the meals are used in animal feeds, risk of transmitting these pesticides to the human food chain via animal products is diminished.

Accumulating evidence now shows that residues of organochlorine pesticides are removed from the oils themselves in commercial refining. Such observations contributed to the basis for establishing tolerances in the United States for residues of DDT and toxaphene in soybeans, as well as in crude soybean oil moving in inter-State commerce. Pilot-plant and commercial-scale production studies have demonstrated that 15 organochlorine pesticides (including one miticide and one herbicide) are removed in the deodorization and hydrogenation stages of vegetable oil processing. (These compounds are: aldrin, BHC, chlordane, DDT, dieldrin, endrin, heptachlor, heptachlor epoxide, kelthane, lindane, methoxychlor, sesone, strobane, TDE or DDD, and toxaphene.) Neither alkali-refining nor bleaching stages of processing have major effects on the organochlorine insecticide levels of the oils.

Two properties of chlorinated hydrocarbons make them susceptible to removal by commercial edible oil treatment: volatility and susceptibility to dechlorination in the hydrogenation process. Deodorization, which is a vacuum–steam distillation, removes the organochlorine pesticides with the volatile fraction. During hydrogenation organochlorines are probably converted into chlorine-free organic compounds. This hypothesis, although not demonstrated specifically for pesticides, has been shown to be true for structurally similar organochlorine compounds. Adsorption by activated carbon in the hydrogenation catalyst has also been suggested as the mode of removal of pesticides.

Pesticide monitoring confirms that finished vegetable oil products have lower levels of organochlorine pesticide content than crude oils and that there is no disproportionate occurrence in vegetable oil, fats and shortenings when compared with other food groups. United States food surveys showed that this group contributes a maximum of 0.002 to 0.004 mg daily intake of combined organochlorine compounds, representing 2.5 per cent to 3.7 per cent of total daily intake from all foods. The diet composite (1964–7), consisting of salad oil, mayonnaise, shortening and peanut butter, averaged a combined organochlorine pesticide level of about 0.02 p.p.m. The surveys showed that finished oil (and oil-seed meals) contains significantly lower levels of chlorinated hydrocarbons than do the crude oils. None of the chlorinated hydrocarbons (except DDT and BHC occasionally) were found in oleomargarine, which is largely hydrogenated oil. The exceptions are likely to have been introduced as a result of non-agricultural use of pesticides—after processing.

In dairy and other animal products processing of foods typically will take a different course. Keeping in mind that the organochlorines are lipophilic, we see that they remain with the fats, and total physical separation from food is less likely than in plant products. Most dairy processing involves a redistribution of residues with butter fat. Cream, butter or cheese will generally have the same organochlorine residue level in fat as the milk from which they are produced.

141

Some milk products, such as condensed milk or dried milk, may lose a proportion of their initial organochlorine residues in the condensing processes by forced co-distillation with water vapour at elevated temperatures. Steam deodorization under high vacuum has been shown to remove dieldrin and heptachlor epoxide from butter oil completely. This process is comparable to deodorization, which was referred to as a unit process in the manufacture of edible vegetable oils.

Separation of fat is probably responsible for reduction of organochlorine residues observed in preparing poultry. Cooking in water for three hours at 190° to 200°F (about 90°C) removed up to 90 per cent of DDT, dieldrin, heptachlor epoxide and lindane residues. The drippings contained about the same level of residues as abdominal fat. Frying and baking removed 50 to 75 per cent for lindane and DDT. Some conversion of DDT into DDD was observed, more at higher temperatures. Cooking chicken at 121°C removed 63 per cent of chlordane and all Telodrin, but Ovex (p-chlorophenyl p-chlorobenzenesulphonate) residues remained.

The reduction of residues in preparing beef is dependent to a larger extent on trimming of fat and discarding of fat drippings from broiling or frying. Frying and pressure-cooking was found to remove 35 per cent to 50 per cent of DDT residues from the prepared beef, but otherwise little residue reduction occurs at lower temperatures of preparation.

Process studies on meat and dairy products indicated that, although some residue reduction is possible, the proportions and frequencies of such loss are likely to be much smaller than for plant products. Total diet survey seems to show consistently that dairy and animal products are the major source of residues in human diet. But organochlorine compounds are not used on animals. Why are animal products the greatest source? It seems that the answer lies in the practice of incorporating into animal feed the waste products of agriculture and food processes, discarded fractions which carry most of the residues from 'good agricultural practice' but in a relatively concentrated form.

You will recall that in reviewing canning operations we observed that peels of potatoes, tomatoes and other fruits and vegetables carry most of the pesticide residues. They comprise a waste product of commercial plants that may be incorporated into animal feed. Citrus rind and pulp discards also may find their way into animal feed. The same is true of dried sugar-beet pulp, a byproduct of sugar manufacture.

The potential is great for introducing pesticide residues into human diet via incorporation of process wastes into animal feeds and, from our review of the fate of residues, it seems that this source is probably of more moment than all others.

BIBLIOGRAPHY

D. C. Abbott. 'Pesticide residues in food'. *Report of the Government Chemist*, pp 72–75 (1968).
J. W. Cook. *Effects of washing, cooking, and other processing on residues of organochlorine pesticides. IUPAC report on terminal residues. J. Assoc. Offic. Analyt. Chem.* **53** (5), 999 (1970).
P. E. Corneliussen. *Pesticides Monit. J.* **4** (3), 89 (1970).
R. P. Farrow, E. R. Elkins, W. W. Rose, F. C. Lamb, J. W. Ralls and W. A. Mercer. *Residue Revs.* **29**, 73 (1969).

R. P. Farrow, F. C. Lamb, R. W. Cook, J. R. Kimball and E. R. Elkins. *J. Agr. Food Chem.* **16** (1), 65 (1968).

C. J. S. Fox, D. Chisholm and D. K. R. Stewart. *Canad. J. Plant. Sci.* **44**, 149 (1964).

F. A. Gunther. *Residue Revs.* **28**, 1 (1969).

F. C. Lamb, R. P. Farrow, E. R. Elkins, R. W. Cook and J. R. Kimball. *J. Agr. Food Chem.* **16** (2), 272 (1968).

E. P. Lichtenstein, G. R. Myrdal and K. R. Schulz. *J. Agr. Food Chem.* **13** (2), 126 (1965).

B. J. Liska and W. J. Stadelman. *Residue Revs.* **29**, 61 (1969).

P. B. Polen. 'Fate of organochlorine pesticides in vegetable oil processing'. *IUPAC Report on Terminal Residues, J. Assoc. Offic. Analyt. Chem.* **53** (5), 997 (1970).

J. G. Saha and W. W. A. Stewart. *Canad. J. Plant Sci.* **47**, 79 (1967).

J. G. Saha, R. H. Burrage, M. A. Nielson and E. C. R. Simpson. Canadian Department of Agriculture, *Pesticide Progress*, **6** (5), 117 (1968).

J. G. Saha. Unpublished work (1970).

D. K. R. Stewart, D. Chisholm and C. J. S. Fox. *Canad. J. Plant Sci.* **45**, 72 (1965).

H. Stobwasser, B. Rademacher and E. Lange. *Residue Revs.* **22**, 45 (1968).

J. C. Street. *Canad. Med. Ass. J.* **100**, 154 (1969).

K. C. Walker, J. C. Maitlen, J. A. Onsager, D. M. Powell, L. I. Butler, A. E. Goodban and R. M. McCready, *Bull. US Dept. Agric.* ARS 33–107 (1965).

143

OCCURRENCE OF INSECTICIDAL CHLORINATED HYDROCARBONS AND THEIR BREAKDOWN PRODUCTS IN MAN AND THE RESULTING TOXICOLOGIC CONSEQUENCES

R. Fabian, T. B. Griffin and F. Coulston

Institute of Experimental Pathology and Toxicology,
Albany Medical College, Albany, NY 12208, USA

ABSTRACT

The intake, subsequent metabolism and storage of chlorinated hydrocarbon insecticides are discussed, as well as the endogenous and environmental factors affecting the dynamic equilibrium under which these residues are stored in man. In addition the toxicological methods, by which the consequences of these residues are evaluated, are reviewed. There is at present very little evidence to indicate that these residues are harmful to man.

INTRODUCTION

When historians of the year 2500 come to review the scientific and technicological developments of our time, will they judge us to be homicidal maniacs bent on the destruction of all life on this planet? We have contaminated our environment with automobile exhausts, synthetic detergents, atomic radiation, industrial wastes and pesticides of many types. Millions of fish and birds have died as a result of this environmental pollution and in some instances certain species have become extinct.

Or will the future historians label this 30-year period, since the introduction of DDT, as the beginning of a chemical revolution that brought great benefit to mankind? There is no question about the use of pesticides having saved millions of lives that would otherwise have been lost to disease and starvation. The present dilemma is that we cannot feed these millions saved by the use of pesticides without further use of these chemicals in agriculture.

After the introduction of DDT in 1941 there was a rapid rise in the production and use of organic pesticides[1] (*Figure 1*). There arose among the people of many countries of the world the belief that all pests, whether insect, animal or plant, could be eliminated if only sufficient quantities of these chemicals were used. This utopian dream resulted in the indiscriminate use of huge quantities of these chemicals within limited geographical areas. Examples of such usage were the attempts to eradicate the gypsy moth and the fire ant in the USA. These insects were not eliminated, but the results of

145

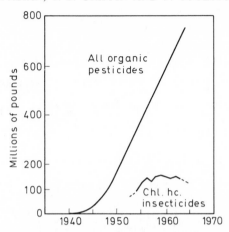

Figure 1. Trend of organic pesticide usage in the USA. Values in millions of pounds of technical products (Reproduced with permission from *Organic Pesticides in the Environment,* 1966, see ref. 1)

these unwise uses of insecticides soon became apparent by the death of fish and birds. These incidents aroused the people to demand restriction and curtailment of the use of insecticides.

Superimposed on the chart illustrating the rise in production of organic pesticides is the story of the chlorinated hydrocarbon insecticides. The use of the organochlorine compounds in the USA reached a peak of about 150 million pounds per year in 1959, and has steadily declined since that time. Figures recently published by the US Department of Agriculture[2] (*Table 1*)

Table 1. Organochlorine insecticides: producers' domestic disappearance of selected kinds by crop year, USA, 1955–68 (Reproduced with permission from *The Pesticide Review,* 1969, see ref. 2)

Crop year*‡	Aldrin–toxaphene group† 10^3 lb	DDT 10^3 lb	BHC 10^3 lb	Total 10^3 lb
1955	54 400	61 800	7 800	124 000
1956	61 570	75 000	9 450	146 020
1957	52 500	71 000	6 600	130 100
1958	78 834	66 700	5 500	151 034
1959	73 331	78 682	4 276	156 289
1960	75 766	70 146	5 111	151 023
1961	78 260	64 068	4 577	146 905
1962	82 125	67 245	2 404	151 774
1963	79 275	61 165	1 299	141 739
1964	83 161	50 542	‡	133 703§
1965	80 568	52 986	‡	133 554§
1966	86 646	46 672	‡	133 318§
1967	86 289	40 257	‡	126 546§
1968	38 710	32 753	‡	71 463§

* Ends 30 September.
† Includes aldrin, chlordane, dieldrin, endrin, heptachlor, Strobane and toxaphene.
‡ Not published separately to avoid disclosure, but probably less than in 1963.
§ Includes only the aldrin–toxaphene group and DDT.

indicate a steep decline in the use of these chemicals in recent years. For the year 1968 the total use of pesticides in the chlorinated hydrocarbon group amounted to only 71 million pounds. This reduction can be attributed to use of other types of insecticides such as the organophosphates, and much more restricted use of the organochlorine compounds resulting from public alarm and the pressure from conservationists.

The chlorinated hydrocarbon insecticides, because of their persistence in the environment and in the adipose tissues of animals and man, pose some very difficult problems in the assessment of their safety. When compared with other insecticides, such as the organophosphates, the chlorinated hydrocarbons have relatively low acute toxicities, giving these chemicals a high safety index when properly applied for short-term usage. However, their persistence in the environment, concentration in the biological food chain, and storage in adipose tissues of man creates questions concerning their long-term use for which we still do not have answers.

Numerous studies of the metabolism of the major chlorinated hydrocarbon insecticides and the occurrence of their breakdown products in man have been made in the past decade. The results of attempts to correlate tissue levels with specific diseases have been equivocal. In some studies no correlation was found between tissue levels and the occurrence of a wide variety of pathological states. In others an association of pathological states with high residue levels was demonstrated, but it is not clear whether these high residues were a cause of disease or a consequence of a lowered ability to eliminate the residues.

Information regarding the effects of pesticides on man are derived from three major sources. First there are the data from experience of use in the population of a limited geographical area. These studies entail determinations of blood and tissue levels, or in certain instances urinary excretion products, combined with attempts to correlate tissue residue levels and specific disease conditions, such as blood dyscrasias, as was described above. Determining the level of exposure is a major problem in these studies. Further complications arise by concomitant exposure to several other chemicals in addition to the one that is being studied. More meaningful data may perhaps be derived from the study of the personnel involved in the manufacture and application of a particular insecticide. These people are subject to exposure levels far above that of the general population; hence the chances of making reliable correlations between exposure and specific disease conditions is greatly improved.

The second major source of information is from cases of acute poisoning resulting from exposure in manufacture or field use, suicide attempts and accidental ingestion. These cases provide us with information of the acute effects in man which could not be obtained by any other means. Determination of dosage is again a major problem.

The third source is from studies in human volunteers. In these exposure to a single specific compound can be more closely controlled and the exact dosage is known. With a background of data derived from animal experiments specific objectives can be established to determine whether certain effects observed in animals will also occur in man. In most cases dosages in the volunteers are not high enough to produce these effects unless some very

147

sensitive parameter is affected, such as cholinesterase inhibition. Nevertheless, because the dosages are often several hundred to a thousand times the exposure levels resulting from use of the chemical in agriculture, unusual effects peculiar to man may be uncovered. Studies of this type carried out over long periods provide the best evidence of safety in man. An example of this type of study will be presented.

METABOLISM AND RESIDUES

The metabolism and fate of chlorinated hydrocarbon pesticides in man, animals, plants and the environment in general has proved to be a complex problem and it is not our intention here to trace these often rather involved pathways. Instead, it is our aim to examine the toxicologic significance of terminal residues found in human tissues. These terminal residues frequently are not chemically identical with the pesticides taken into the body, but are the products of dynamic physical and chemical changes that occur in living tissues. It must also be emphasized that when we cite examples of the metabolic consequences of pesticide ingestion they cannot be taken as generalities for all organochlorine pesticides. The term 'pesticide' is not a chemical classification but rather an economic designation for certain poisonous materials. There are many types of organochlorine pesticides and the metabolic pathways and products are equally varied. The importance of individual study of each chemical, in human volunteers if at all possible, cannot be overstated.

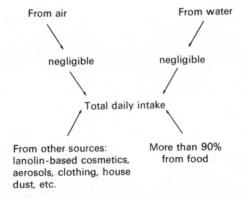

Figure 2. Total daily intake of pesticide chemicals (after K. W. Jager, *Aldrin, Dieldrin, Endrin and Telodrin*. Elsevier: Amsterdam (1970)

The beginning of the sequence of events leading to the occurrence of pesticide residues in man is the intake of the materials into the body and it may be enlightening to examine this. The total daily intake of pesticide chemicals results from a combination of sources[3] (*Figure 2*). By far the largest source is from the food we eat and this is to be expected since the largest applications of pesticide chemicals are to the crops themselves or on the soil in which they are grown. The other sources, particularly the air and water with which we are so concerned of late, represent only negligible intakes of pesticides insofar as humans are concerned. While these sources do not appear to offer any current threat to humans we must not relax our concern, because, of all the sources, air and water represent the most difficult sources to control. We must also continue to be concerned with the intake of pesticides from food and every effort made to reduce this intake so long as we try to anticipate fully the consequences of each reduction.

The detection and measurement of organochlorine chemicals in the environment is a remarkable achievement, considering the minute quantities involved, and is a tribute to the modern means developed over the past decade. These highly sensitive methods have done much to aid the investigation of our environment. These investigations have proved that certain pesticide chemicals are indeed widely distributed throughout the environment. DDT and certain of its degradation products and some cyclodiene residues (dieldrin, endrin etc.) can be found in virtually all samples of recent biological origin.

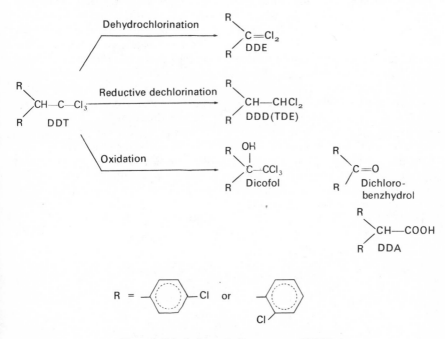

Figure 3. Principal metabolic processes of DDT

The metabolism of DDT has proved to be very complex: only the principal processes are shown in Figure 3. Both DDT and DDE have been identified as residues in the tissues of the general population[4] and DDD is well established as an excretory product in humans after the ingestion of DDT[5]. DDD is also known to be formed from DDT in mammalian tissues where it is also further metabolized to DDE[6].

The metabolism of the cyclodiene insecticides is probably even more complex than that of DDT and no attempt will be made to review the fate of these chemicals. Suffice it to say that epoxidation leads to the principal terminal residues—aldrin, for example, being converted into dieldrin, which is stored. It is known that further metabolism occurs and this leads to compounds which are more hydrophilic and which are more rapidly excreted[7].

Concentrations of DDT, DDE and dieldrin in human tissues have been rather widely studied. In the USA, studies[4, 8, 9] have indicated that the tissue concentrations of these residues have very little dependence on geographic distribution and that levels within a given locality have not changed during the five-year period from 1963 to 1968. Taking adipose tissue as an example, the average concentration of DDT ranged from 1.3 to 2.8 p.p.m.; DDE ranged from about 4.5 to 6.7 p.p.m.; and dieldrin ranged from 0.04 to about 0.22 p.p.m. The concentration of these residues in liver tissue was about one-tenth of that found in the adipose tissue. In fact, it has been shown that levels of these three residues are distributed in human tissues in a highly predictable fashion. This is exemplified in *Figure 4* taken from the studies of D. P. Morgan and C. C. Roan[4] from the Community Studies Pesticides Project. In *Figure 4*, the relationship between whole tissue pesticide concentrations of DDT, DDE and dieldrin in human tissue and the lipid content of these tissues is shown. The tendency for tissue pesticide storage to increase with lipid content is evident. The authors note that the approximate parallelism of DDT and DDE (on the logarithmic scales) indicates a fairly stable proportionality between these compounds. They also think that the flatter curve for dieldrin implies a basically different distribution. *Figure 4* also implies that knowledge of the pesticide content of one tissue, say adipose, would permit estimation of the pesticide concentrations of other tissues from measurements of their lipid content. This is not exactly true, however, and deviations from the indicated regressions may be as significant as those cases

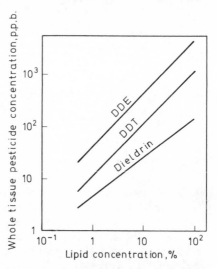

Figure 4. Distribution of residues in human tissues [after D. P. Morgan and C. C. Roan, *Arch. Environ. Health*, **20**, 452 (1970)]

where the prediction is followed. Brain tissue, for example, contains DDT, DDE and dieldrin at levels only about one-ninth of what would be estimated from the lipid content. Brain contains a variety of lipid materials but virtually no neutral fat, and the lower values may reflect differences in solubility, chemical affinity, tissue penetration or a combination of these factors.

The concentration of pesticides in the tissues of those who become chronically ill has been of interest on the grounds that mobilization of fat stores may result in dangerous levels of the pesticides in tissues of the patient. The estimated total dosage available from tissue storage indicates that toxic levels would be exceedingly difficult to reach from such processes. Other studies[10] have failed to show correlations between tissue pesticide levels and disease processes.

Another point worth stressing is that the levels of chlorinated hydrocarbon pesticides in tissues are not static stores but are subject to the normal metabolic processes of the organism. The levels at any given time are a reflection of a dynamic equilibrium between intake of the pesticide, metabolism, storage and elimination of the pesticide or products of its metabolism. For example, in humans, accurate knowledge of the intake of dieldrin permits an accurate prediction of the blood level of the chemical, i.e. in a logarithmic plot of intake versus blood level there is a nearly perfect linear regression[11]. This equilibrium between man and his environment is also observable in the data from the previously cited Community Studies Pesticide Project. That the levels in human tissues have not changed in five years (actually they have been reasonably constant for about 20 years) is a reflection of a similarly constant intake for the same period. This situation is a demonstration of a general principle of toxicology—that a steady state of storage will be reached as a result of continued non-lethal intake of a chemical. At the steady state, the dynamic equilibrium between intake, metabolism and excretion will be maintained. This contradicts the popular misconception that pesticide residues will continue to accumulate in human tissues until intoxication or death occurs. This is clearly not so and from this viewpoint members of the general population need not fear intoxication from their present body burdens of organochlorine insecticides.

What about the 'long-term effect' of this very small but still measurable exposure to chlorinated hydrocarbons? Effects from low-level, long-term exposure have yet to be demonstrated in man if they exist at all. This does not mean we can relax our guard and assume there are no effects whatsoever. Man must be ever vigilant whenever he employs any chemical materials for his purposes.

POSSIBLE CONSEQUENCES OF RESIDUES

Although the kinetics of the tissue storage of chlorinated hydrocarbon insecticides have been intensively studied in animals and man, the interpretation of the toxicological significance of these residues continues to be a complex problem. These chemicals and their metabolic products reside in the tissues in a dynamic equilibrium which can be altered by a variety of exogenous and endogenous factors. Assessment of the toxicological consequences of these residues depends therefore upon a knowledge of how factors such as nutrition, disease and exposure to other chemicals and drugs affect this equilibrium. Further complications are introduced when an attempt is made to assess the long-term effects. Over the lifetime of an individual the equilibrium may be altered many times and some of these alterations may result in permanent changes whose effects require years or even generations for their expression. These potential effects are in the area of carcinogenesis and mutagenesis.

First let us briefly discuss the effects of nutrition upon the toxicity of the organochlorine insecticides. In general, dietary deficiencies tend to increase the toxicity of most chemicals. For example, a low protein diet increased the toxicity of dieldrin as measured by increased mortality, increased liver lipids, and more marked histopathological changes in the liver[12]. However, the relationship between amount of dietary protein and toxicity of dieldrin is not as straightforward as this experiment would lead us to believe, as sex differences also affect the relationship. In rats fed with labelled dieldrin increases in dietary protein up to 25 and 50 per cent resulted in increased excretion of radioactivity in the urine and faeces with decreased mortality in male rats. Female rats, on the other hand, excreted more radioactivity and survived longer on the ten per cent protein diet than on the 25 and 50 per cent diet[13]. With DDT, very low or very high protein diets increased susceptibility of rats to the toxic effects of this insecticide[14].

The quantity of fat, either in the diet or in an individual, can influence toxicity of the chlorinated hydrocarbon compounds. The toxicity of benzene hexachloride was augmented by a high fat diet[15]. Also, increased toxic effects to DDT were observed in rats and mice when the amount of fat in the diet was increased[16]. The amount of body fat present can markedly influence toxic effects. Rats with little body fat are more susceptible to DDT toxicity than those with normal amounts of adipose tissue. Furthermore, starvation of rats with significant storage of DDT in the body fat can mobilize sufficient quantities of the stored DDT to produce tremors[17].

These are just a few examples of how diet and nutritional state can affect the toxicity of the chlorinated hydrocarbons in animals. When this information is extrapolated to man, it would appear that persons in affluent societies with high dietary fat intake are subject to possible toxicities from these chemicals as well as the populace from the underdeveloped countries

Table 2. Chemical–chemical interactions in biological systems

One chemical modifies effects of second by producing changes in:		
Absorption	Distribution and metabolism	Excretion
Change intestinal pH	Competition for plasma protein binding	Competition for conjugation
Alter intestinal motility	Modify cellular uptake	Alter pH of urine
Competition for membrane carriers	Inhibition of esterases	Block tubular secretion
Alter metabolism of intestinal flora	Stimulation of microsomal drug-metabolizing enzymes	—

whose diet might be deficient in protein. But this is at present just speculation.

The possibility of unexpected toxic effects occurring as a result of chemical interactions has received much attention in the last two decades and the subject is particularly germane to the problem of the safety of pesticides. Since everyone is exposed to varying amounts of these chemicals the possibility of undesirable effects resulting from interactions with constituents of food, drugs and other chemicals to which we are exposed, remains one of the major problems of research in toxicology.

The mechanisms by which one chemical may modify the effects of a second have been studied intensively. We now know that one chemical can alter effects of a second by producing changes in the absorption, distribution, metabolism or excretion of the second chemical (*Table 2*). With the chlorinated hydrocarbons the most likely point of interaction is in metabolism because these chemicals are potent inducers of the processing-metabolizing enzymes. Induction of these enzymes accelerates the biotransformation of a wide variety of lipid-soluble substances. Whether this acceleration will increase or decrease the toxic effects of a chemical depends on how that chemical is transformed. If it is converted into a more toxic material, speeding up its metabolism may increase toxic effects.

Although instances of increased toxicity of pesticides resulting from enzyme induction have been reported, such cases seem to be relatively few. For example, in one study designed to test the effect of pretreatment of rats and mice with phenobarbital upon the toxicity of fifteen organophosphorus compounds, increased toxicity was observed for only one compound[18]. For the others induction of microsomal enzymes produced no change, or reduced toxicity. Pretreatment of rats with aldrin, dieldrin or DDT provided marked protection to the acute effects of parathion, increasing the LD_{50} value approximately seven times the pretreatment value[19]. These findings suggest that low levels of chlorinated hydrocarbons may even be beneficial in man by protecting against the acute effects of certain chemicals. The enzyme-inducing ability of DDT has been used therapeutically in the treatment of familial unconjugated non-haemolytic jaundice[20].

One aspect of the problem of chemical interactions, pertinent to our discussion of enzyme induction, is the possibility of increased risk from certain carcinogens. Some carcinogenic chemicals must undergo transformation into an active product before they can induce neoplasia. A continued state of activation of the microsomal enzymes may therefore increase the hazard from exposure to these carcinogens.

The carcinogenic potential of the chlorinated hydrocarbons remains uncertain because there is still a lack of methodology by which these evaluations can be made. Several of these chemicals have been judged positive for tumour induction in animal studies, but the significance of these observations in terms of human exposure levels is very uncertain. The controversy resulting from the recent report[21] of increased hepatomas in mice, after administration of DDT, exemplifies this situation. On the basis of these results, some scientists think that sufficient carcinogenic potential has been demonstrated to ban further use of DDT. Others, however, question the validity of the test procedures. They point out that administration of DDT to newborn mice by intubation at very high levels has no parallel in human exposure. Some doubt has even been voiced concerning the significance of 'hepatomas' as an index of carcinogenicity.

Another potential effect, closely related to carcinogenicity, i.e. mutagenicity, has received relatively little attention. Several assay systems have been developed with bacteria, bacteriophage, *Drosophila*, *Neurospora* and higher plants. Although these systems are excellent screening procedures their relevance to man is not clear. However, chemicals giving positive results in these systems can be studied further in mammalian cell cultures and also *in vivo* in animals such as the hamster by making intensive studies of bone marrow, spleen and testes. Little information is available concerning the mutagenic potential of the chlorinated hydrocarbons, but this aspect of their potential biological effects will undoubtedly receive more attention in coming years.

The last potential effect to be considered is that of embryotoxicity and teratogenesis. Interference with reproductive processes in wildlife, particularly birds, has been well documented. Embryotoxic effects in rats and dogs have been reported for dieldrin and chlordane. These effects are to be differentiated from teratogenesis. Almost any chemical, given in sufficiently high dosage, can produce embryotoxicity. In a recent review of epidemiological studies, no adverse effects upon reproduction in man were detected that could be attributed to the chlorinated hydrocarbons[22].

HUMAN STUDIES

The uncertainties in the extrapolation of animal data to man are so numerous that the critics of our methods of toxicological evaluation have often questioned the relevance of animal experimentation. The extremists among these critics point out our failures, such as occurred with thalidomide, or our failure to predict the retinopathies that occurred with chloroquin, and they label all animal studies as worthless. Retrospective examination of these failures suggests two basic reasons for their occurrence. With thalidomide it was a lack of testing, for subsequent to the finding of congenital malformations in man similar deformities were produced in rabbits and monkeys. With chloroquin it was a difference in response; it is extremely difficult to produce similar lesions in animals. However, in defence of the toxicologists, in both instances the chemicals were used under conditions that were not anticipated at the time that toxicologic evaluations were made. Nevertheless, these two examples do point out the danger of complete reliance upon animal testing. Man is sometimes unique in his responses and the final assessment of a chemical's safety must be made in man himself.

One approach to the problem of evaluating the safety of insecticides is to combine extensive animal testing with carefully controlled human studies. Drugs are evaluated in this manner. Animal studies are carried out in a variety of species to disclose species differences in sensitivity resulting from differences in metabolic and excretory pathways. Dosages sufficiently high to produce toxic effects are administered in acute and chronic experiments to identify target organs and to uncover possible differences in the effects of short- and long-term exposures. When the maximum no-adverse-effect levels have been established, and the toxic effects that are produced at dosages in excess of these levels are defined, experiments in man can be designed to search for these specific effects.

Studies of the effects of methoxychlor conducted by the Institute of Experimental Pathology and Toxicology of Albany Medical College exemplify this type of approach. Detailed experiments were carried out in rats, mice and monkeys, which utilized the classical methods of toxicology supplemented by various special techniques. To produce toxic effects very high doses of methoxychlor, up to 2 500 mg/kg per day, had to be given to the animals. At high dosages such as this the following effects were observed in the animal studies.

(1) Inhibition of testicular maturation, as evidenced by lower testis weights than in the control rats and delay in spermatogenesis, was observed when methoxyclor was given to immature rats. Testicular inhibition was not observed when administration was begun in mature rats. Other scientists had reported a decrease of spermatogenesis in rats and dogs after feeding with the chemical for relatively short periods.

(2) Quantitative studies of the lipid distribution in mice and monkeys revealed a decrease in the amount of triglycerides and an increase in the amount of cholesterol and diglycerides.

(3) Studies in vitro with isolated gut segments indicated changes in the rates of sodium transport. Electron-microscopic examination of the intestinal epithelium revealed swelling of the mitochondria and distention of the intercellular spaces.

(4) Swelling of the mitochondria, distention of the vesicles of the endoplasmic reticulum and increase in the amount of smooth vesicles were observed in the liver. In the acute studies these changes were associated with an increase in demethylase activity. These changes were not seen after several weeks of administration, indicating that adaptation occurred in the face of continued high-level exposure.

Table 3. Human volunteer study on methoxychlor

Volunteer No.	Weeks on test											
	1	2	3	4	5	6	7	8	9	10	11	12
1	P	P	P	P	P	P	P	P				
2	P	P	P	P	P	P	P	P				
3	0.5	0.5	0.5	0.5	0.5	0.5	0.5	0.5				
4	0.5	0.5	0.5	0.5	0.5	0.5	0.5	0.5				
5	0	0	1.0	1.0	1.0	1.0	1.0	1.0	1.0	1.0		
6	0	0	1.0	1.0	1.0	1.0	1.0	1.0	1.0	1.0		
7	0	0	0	0	2.0	2.0	2.0	2.0	2.0	2.0	2.0	2.0
8	0	0	0	0	2.0	2.0	2.0	2.0	2.0	2.0	2.0	2.0
9	0	0	0	0	0	0	P	P	P	P	P	P
10	0	0	0	0	0	0	P	P	P	P	P	P
11	0	0	0	0	0	0	0.5	0.5	0.5	0.5	0.5	0.5
12	0	0	0	0	0	0	0.5	0.5	0.5	0.5	0.5	0.5
13	0	0	0	0	0	0	1.0	1.0	1.0	1.0	1.0	1.0
14	0	0	0	0	0	0	1.0	1.0	1.0	1.0	1.0	1.0
15	0	0	0	0	0	0	2.0	2.0	2.0	2.0	2.0	2.0
16	0	0	0	0	0	0	2.0	2.0	2.0	2.0	2.0	2.0

P – Placebo.

With the observations from the animal experiments in mind studies were performed in human volunteers to search for evidence of similar changes in man. A few words concerning the conditions under which the volunteers participated in these studies is appropriate here. Before any potential subject is accepted he is fully informed of the possible hazards involved by his participation and he is free to withdraw at any time that he feels his well-being is threatened. Some small rewards are offered for taking part in the study, but these are purposely kept at a minimum to ensure that the subject will not neglect his own welfare in order to collect the rewards.

Every effort is made to minimize the risks to the subjects. Before acceptance each volunteer is given a thorough physical examination to disclose any conditions that might be aggravated by his participation. The study is conducted under close medical supervision with frequent examination of the usual clinical parameters and each participant is interviewed daily for subjective complaints.

Thirty-two volunteers, 16 men and 16 women, were used in the methoxychlor study that was carried out at the Alabama State Penitentiary in Montgomery, Alabama. The volunteers were divided into four groups of four men and four women each. Methoxychlor was given by capsule at doses of 0.5, 1.0 and 2.0 mg/kg. The control group received placebo capsules containing starch and lactose. These doses were administered in a staggered schedule (*Table 3*), so that only the lowest dose, 0.5 mg/kg, was given for the first two weeks. Since no ill-effects were observed the second group was started at a higher dose (1.0 mg/kg) while the first group continued. After two more weeks the third group was started at 2.0 mg/kg. This staggered schedule was followed to provide a relatively long-term time/dose response with a small dose to provide some protection from an unexpected toxic effect from the higher doses.

Before administration of methoxychlor, clinical, haematological and serum biochemical values were determined on each subject. Haematological and serum biochemical determinations were repeated weekly. Blood pressure, temperature, pulse and respiration were checked and recorded six times per

Table 4. Fatty acid distribution in adipose tissue. The percentage fatty acid distribution for C-14 to C-20:5 was determined by GLC on each adipose aspirate biopsy of No. 2 placebo, No. 8 high dose IN 3, No. 9 placebo, and No. 15 high dose IN 3

Acid	15	2	8	9
C14	3.3	5.4	2.8	1.0
C16	18.6	25.4	16.1	19.6
C16:1	6.8	5.1	6.8	4.8
C18	3.2	3.3	2.3	2.7
C18:1	50.5	37.3	46.1	30.8
C18:2	8.6	7.0	5.9	6.0
C18:3	1.8	1.1	TR	TR
C20:4	2.0	5.0	7.0	12.4
C20:5	3.2	5.0	7.40	8.3

No significant differences in the percentage fatty acid distribution in adipose fat of the control or high dose patients was observed.

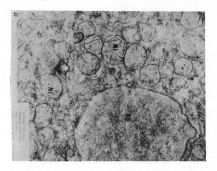

Figure 5. Electron micrograph—control liver

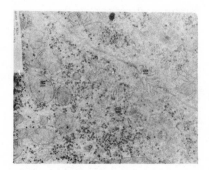

Figure 6. Electron micrograph—human liver from subject given 2.0 mg/kg of methoxychlor

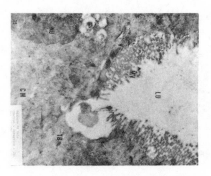

Figure 7. Electron micrograph—human intestine (control)

157

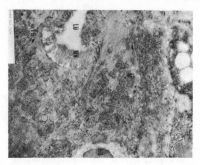

Figure 8. Electron micrograph—human intestine from subject given 2.0 mg/kg of methoxychlor

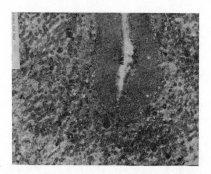

Figure 9. Electron micrograph—human testis from subject given 2.0 mg/kg of methoxychlor

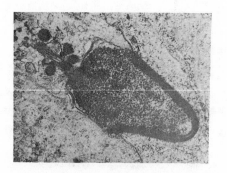

Figure 10. Electron micrograph—human sperm from subject given 2.0 mg/kg of methoxychlor

week. Semen examinations were made before starting administration and at 28 and 56 days.

At the end of the study biopsies were performed on three control and three high-dose subjects to obtain specimens of liver, small intestine, bone marrow, fat and testicle. These tissues were examined by light and electron microscopy and distribution of fatty acids in the subcutaneous fat was determined by gas–liquid chromatography.

No indications of toxic effect were observed in any of the subjects. The clinical parameters remained normal in all and examination of the biopsy specimens did not reveal any significant differences between the subjects given the placebo and those given 2.0 mg methoxychlor/kg. Fatty acid distribution in the subcutaneous fat was similar in both groups (*Table 4*). Electron micrographs of the liver, intestine and testis were normal (*Figures 5–10*). Bone marrow specimens had normal cellularity and distribution of cell types. No effect was observed upon spermatogenesis in the males or on menstrual cycles in the females.

When methoxychlor was given in daily doses 100 to 200 times the levels permitted in the diet by the Federal Food and Drug Administration of the US Government, no toxic effects were found. Prior animal studies at extremely high dosages pointed out the areas where changes might occur, namely, changes in fatty acid distribution, inhibition of spermatogenesis and alterations in the ultrastructure of the intestine and liver. These specific effects were sought in the human study and were not found; nor were there any unexpected indications of toxic effects.

From these results it can be concluded that small residues of methoxychlor taken in the diet are indeed safe for man.

CONCLUSION

Except for instances of acute intoxication, evidence of toxic effects in man resulting from exposure to the chlorinated hydrocarbon insecticides is sparse indeed. Epidemiological studies and experiments in human volunteers have failed to reveal any specific toxic effects that might occur in man from the wise use of these chemicals in agriculture or the control of insect vectors of disease. If properly used the chlorinated hydrocarbons are probably the most economical and safest insecticides available at the present time.

The occurrence of tissue residues from these chemicals continues to be an area of concern because we are unable to assess fully the long-term effects of these residues. Present information indicates that the residues are directly related to intake: so if intake is controlled tissue storage will also be controlled. In fact, storage levels appear to be declining, at least in some countries. Besides there is no evidence that low levels of these residues are harmful.

For the present, much suffering would result if governmental agencies were to ban the use of the chlorinated hydrocarbons, but it is prudent to use them wisely and only for those purposes for which no suitable alternatives exist.

REFERENCES

[1] L. E. Mitchell, In *Pesticides: Properties and Prognosis*. Advances in Chemistry Series No. 60, p 7. American Chemical Society Publications (1966).

[2] *The Pesticide Review.* US Dept of Agriculture (1969).
[3] K. W. Jager, *Aldrin, Dieldrin, Endrin and Telodrin,* Elsevier: Amsterdam (1970).
[4] D. P. Morgan and C. C. Roan, *Arch. Environ. Health,* **20**, 452 (1970).
[5] W. J. Hager, W. E. Dale and C. I. Pirkle, *Arch. Environ. Health,* **22**, 119 (1971).
[6] F. M. Whiting, S. B. Hagyard, W. H. Brown and J. W. Stull, *J. Diary Sci.* **51**, 1612 (1968).
[7] G. Ludwig, J. Weiss and F. Korte, *Life Sci.* **3**, 123 (1964).
[8] L. J. Casarett, G. C. Fryer and W. L. Yauger Jr, *Hawaii. Arch. Environ. Health,* **17**, 306 (1968).
[9] V. Fiserova-Bergerova, J. L. Radomski and J. E. Davies, *Industr. Med. Surg.* **36**, 65 (1967).
[10] W. S. Hoffman, H. Adler and W. I. Fishbein, *Arch. Environ. Health,* **15**, 758 (1967).
[11] C. C. Hunter, *Human Exposures to Aldrin and Dieldrin. Symposium on the Science and Technology of Residual Insecticides in Food Production with Special Reference to Aldrin and Dieldrin.* Shell Oil Co. Publication (1968).
[12] M. Lee, K. Harris and H. Trowbridge, *J. Nutr.* **84**, 136 (1964).
[13] G. S. Stoewstand, E. J. Broderick and J. B. Bourke, *Dietary Protein and Dieldrin Toxicity. Pesticides Symposia,* p 139. Halos and Associates, Miami, Florida (1970).
[14] E. M. Boyd and E. S. DeCastra, *Toxicity of Dicophane (DDT) in Relation to Dietary Protein Intake. Pesticides Symposia,* p 33. Halos and Associates, Miami, Florida (1970).
[15] J. P. Frawley and O. G. Fitzhugh, *Fed. Proc.* **9**, 273 (1950).
[16] H. E. Sauberlich and C. A. Baumann, *Proc. Soc. Expt. Biol. Med.* **66**, 642 (1947).
[17] O. G. Fitzhugh and A. A. Nelson, *J. Pharmacol. Expt. Therap.* **89**, 18 (1947).
[18] K. P. DuBois and F. K. Kinoshita, *Proc. Soc. Expt. Biol. Med.* **129**, 699 (1968).
[19] W. B. Deichmann, *Protection against the Acute Effects of Certain Pesticides by Pretreatment with Aldrin, Dieldrin, and DDT. Pesticides Symposia,* p 121. Halos and Associates, Miami, Florida (1970).
[20] R. P. H. Thompson, C. W. T. Pilcher, J. Robinson, G. M. Stathers, A. E. McLein and R. Williams, *Lancet,* **ii**, 4 (1969).
[21] J. R. M. Innes, B. M. Ulland, M. G. Valerio, L. Petrucelli, L. Fishbein, E. R. Hart, A. J. Pallotta, R. R. Bates, H. L. Falk, J. J. Gart, M. Klein, I. Mitchell and J. Peters, *J. Nat. Cancer Inst.* **42**, 1101 (1969).
[22] K. S. Khera and D. J. Clegg, *Canad. Med. Ass. J.* **100**, 167 (1969).

TERMINAL
RESIDUES OF CARBAMATE INSECTICIDES

META   D DEGRADATION OF
TE INSECTICIDES

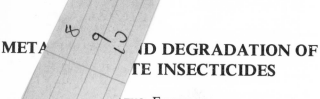

AZUO FUKUNAGA

*Division of   icals, National Institute of Agricultural Sciences,
Nishigah   ), and Laboratory of Insect Toxicology, The Institute   hemical Research, Wako-shi, Saitama, Japan*

ABSTRACT

The relation between the chemical structure and biological activities of alkyl-substituted nitrophenyl N-methyl- and NN-dimethyl-carbamates is discussed. Nitrophenyl NN-dimethylcarbamate is stable and alkyl substituents in the C-3 position cause higher anticholinesterase activity. N-Methyl- and NN-dimethyl-carbamates are metabolized by the microsomes–reduced nicotinamide–adenine dinucleotide phosphate (NADPH) system (mammalian and insect). In this system, N-demethylation, conversion of N-methyl into N-formamide and into N-hydroxymethyl groups; aromatic ring hydroxylation or formation of a dihydrodihydroxy derivative; o-dealkylation; alkyl hydroxylation of an aralkyl substituent and sulphoxidation occurs. By enzymatic hydrolysis, 1-naphthol is always found. The microsome–NADPH system usually forms one or more anticholinesterase metabolites from methyl- and dimethyl-carbamate insecticides, and certain of these metabolites are more potent inhibitors than the carbamate from which they are derived.

The conjugation *in vivo* of naphthyl- and methyl-carbaryl in several mammals is shown; 1-naphthyl methylimidocarbonate O-glucuronide and 4-(methylcarbamoyloxy)-1-naphthyl glucuronide are the major urinary metabolites in urine. The oxidative products from systemic carbamates, Termic and Furadan, in plants are considerably more active as anticholinesterases and it appears that these systemic carbamates are further examples of the importance of both oxidative activation and the delay factor in promoting prolonged systemic activity in the leaves of treated plants. Evidence on the metabolism of carbamate has accumulated that in microsomes from the liver of various mammals and organs of several insects there exists a carbon monoxide-binding pigment designated as cytochrome P-450. In the light of this theory the role of phenolase in the metabolism of carbamate is discussed. On the mechanism of carbamate-resistant insects, the significance of altered aliesterase and oxidative reaction processes is discussed.

INTRODUCTION

The toxic carbamates are usually fairly potent inhibitors of cholinesterase, and the symptoms resulting from their action in intact animals are typically cholinergic, involving lachrymation, salivation, myosis, convulsions and death. The insecticidal carbamates show anti-enzyme properties which differ from

163

those of eserin. Perhaps the most important is that whereas eserin inhibits only cholinesterase[1], some and perhaps all of the insecticidal carbamates can inhibit insect aliesterase both *in vivo* and *in vitro*[2].

Chemical structure and biological activities

Earlier investigations in Dr Metcalf's laboratory regarding the relationship between chemical structure, anticholinesterase activity and insecticidal properties of substituted phenyl *N*-methyl-carbamates have been based on the premise that these compounds inhibit the cholinesterase in a reversible manner by non-covalent bonding of the ring substituent and carbamyl moiety with the anionic and esteratic site of the enzyme, to form a tight enzyme–carbamate complex[3]. In work by Fukuto *et al.*[4], a number of alkyl-substituted nitrophenyl *N*-methyl- and *NN*-dimethyl-carbamates were prepared and examined for alkaline hydrolysis, anticholinesterase activity and toxicity to insects. The nitrophenyl *N*-methyl-carbamates are generally exceedingly unstable under alkaline conditions and their poor anticholinesterase activity may in part be attributed to this high hydrolytic instability. The alkyl-substituted nitrophenyl *N*-methyl-carbamates were slightly more stable and generally possessed higher anticholinesterase properties. Nitrophenyl *NN*-dimethyl-carbamates are stable under the same alkaline conditions, and alkyl substituents in the C-3 position caused higher anticholinesterase activity. Practically all of the compounds used alone were poor in housefly and mosquito larva toxicity, but several were strongly synergized by co-treatment with piperonyl butoxide.

A detailed kinetic study of the alkaline hydrolysis of 4-nitrophenyl *N*-methyl-carbamate was undertaken and mechanisms for the hydrolytic process and for the carbamylation of cholinesterase consistent with the hydrolytic mechanism were proposed. Recently, Fukunaga's group investigated the insecticidal activities of substituted phenyl *N*-methyl-carbamates and *NN*-dimethyl-carbamates against several species of insects[5]. Insecticidal activities of 81 substituted phenyl *N*-methyl-carbamates and 24 substituted phenyl *NN*-dimethyl-carbamates were evaluated with six species of insects. Most of the compounds tested showed low toxicity to the almond moth and the rice stem borer. LC_{95} values to the corn leaf aphid are higher than those to the green peach aphid. The relationship between toxicity to the housefly and the chemical structure of compounds is the same as those reported by Metcalf *et al.*[1] and Fukuto *et al.*[2]. A similar relationship was observed for the adzuki bean weevil. Insecticidal activities of cyano-substituted phenyl *NN*-dimethyl-carbamates are higher than those of cyano-substituted phenyl *N*-methyl-carbamates. 2-Nitro-3,5-dimethylphenyl *N*-methyl-carbamate shows higher insecticidal activity than 4-nitro-3,5-dimethylphenyl *N*-methyl-carbamate. Substituted 2-allylphenyl *N*-methyl-carbamates and substituted 3,5-dimethylphenyl *N*-methyl-carbamates have high insecticidal activities against the corn leaf aphid.

METABOLIC PATHWAY IN ANIMALS

Hydrolysis

The first metabolic study in insects, with ring-^{14}C-labelled carbaryl, was made in 1961[6] Considerable variation with species was observed. For instance, 1-naphthol was found only in German cockroach tissues, in which there were five other metabolites. By contrast, milkweed bug formed one metabolite, and houseflies three. No identification of metabolites other than 1-naphthol, were made.

Oxidation

The most important advances in our understanding of carbamate metabolism have come from Casida's laboratory. The metabolism of carbaryl-carbonyl-^{14}C, carbaryl-methyl-^{14}C and O-isopropoxyphenyl N-methyl-carbamate-carbonyl-^{14}C was investigated in the presence of NADPH by using rat liver microsome, and the fat body of cockroach and houseflies. Metabolites tentatively identified:were 1-naphthyl N-hydroxymethyl-carbamate, 4-hydroxy-1-naphthyl N-methyl-carbamate and 5-hydroxyl-1-naphthyl N-methyl-carbamate. At least two unidentified metabolites have the C—O—C(O)—N—C structure intact. Hydrolysis yielded 1-naphthol and at least two unidentified metabolites lacking the carbamyl group. These eight metabolites, five of which are carbamates, are formed by the liver microsomes and insects. Certain of these metabolites appear in the milk of a goat treated orally with carbaryl-carbonyl-^{14}C[7]. In subsequent experiments, ether-extractable carbaryl metabolites found in the urine of treated rabbits and formed by enzyme preparations from rat, mouse and rabbit liver were tentatively identified: 1-naphthyl N-hydroxymethyl-carbamate; 4-hydroxy-1-naphthyl methyl-carbamate; 5-hydroxy-1-naphthyl methyl-carbamate; 5,6-dihydro-5,6-dihydroxy-1-naphthyl methyl-carbamate; 1-hydroxy-5,6-dihydro-5,6-dihydroxynaphthalene; 1-naphthol. Additional unidentified metabolites were also present in ether and butanol extracts of the urine. Each of the ether-extractable metabolites formed by liver enzymes was of reduced biological activity compared with carbaryl. Optimum conditions were given for the metabolism of carbaryl by rat liver microsomes plus soluble fractions[8]. In combination with the above-mentioned results, Oonnithan and Casida[9] investigated the metabolism of 10 ^{14}C-labelled methyl- and dimethyl-carbamates by rat liver, in order to determine the nature of the rat liver enzymes involved in the metabolism reactions, the number of carbamate metabolites formed, the chemical nature of the metabolic products, the anticholinesterase activity of the metabolites relative to the original insecticide and the extent of carbamoylation of microsomal proteins by methyl- and dimethyl-carbamate, in the presence and absence of added co-factor. Each of the 33 methyl- and dimethyl-carbamate insecticide chemicals and related compounds studied was metabolized by the rat liver microsome–reduced nicotinamide–adenine dinucleotide phosphate (NADPH) system, producing one or more carbamate metabolites in each case. In this system, NADPH is required for each of the following types of enzymatic reactions, as demonstrated with the listed carbamates: N-demethylation (dimetilan, Matacil, Zectran and 1-naphthyl dimethyl-carbamate); conversion of N-methyl into N-formamide (Zectran) and into N-hydroxymethyl groups (Banol, Baygon, carbaryl, HRS-1422, Matacil, UC 10854 and Zectran); aromatic ring hydroxylation (Baygon and carbaryl) or formation of a dihydrodihydroxy derivative (carbaryl); O-dealkylation (Baygon); alkyl hydroxylation of aralkyl

165

substituent (UC 10854); sulphoxidation (Mesurol and Temik). Carbaryl is produced on N-demethylation of 1-naphthyl dimethyl-carbamate by the microsome–NADPH system, and on spontaneous or enzymatic hydrolysis of 1-naphthyl N-acetyl-N-methyl-carbamate. The microsome–NADPH system usually forms one or more anticholinesterase metabolites from methyl- and dimethyl-carbamate insecticide chemicals, and certain of these metabolites are more potent inhibitors than the carbamate from which they are derived. Although hydrolysis of the carbamate ester group is not a major reaction in this enzyme system, certain of the products formed in its presence are hydrolysed, spontaneously or by enzymatic action. Carbamoylation of microsomal proteins probably occurs with certain of the methyl-carbamates, their carbamate metabolites and metabolites of the dimethyl-carbamates[9].

Conjugate formation

The water-soluble conjugate, especially the urinary conjugate in the metabolism of carbaryl, had not been isolated and identified in the above-cited studies. However, Knaak et al.[10] re-examined the metabolism and succeeded in identifying the conjugates in urine by a chromatographic method. The metabolic fate of methyl-^{14}C, carbonyl-^{14}C and naphthyl-^{14}C carbaryl in the rat and guinea-pig was investigated. The overall recovery of the naphthyl, carbonyl and methyl label was, respectively, 95, 99 and 91 per cent of dose. Tissue residues (2 to 3 per cent of dose) were found only with methyl-labelled carbaryl. The metabolites identified were 4-(methylcarbamoyloxy)-1-naphthyl glucuronide, 1-naphthyl glucuronide, 4-(methyl-carbamoyloxy)-1-naphthyl sulphate, and 1-naphthyl sulphate. Evidence is presented for the possible direct conjugation of carbaryl with glucuronic acid to form 1-naphthyl methyl-carbamate N-glucuronide and 1-naphthyl methylimido-carbamate O-glucuronide. The assay of carbaryl, carbaryl derivatives, and metabolites in water by fluorimetry was investigated in conjunction with ^{14}C chromatographic studies and the method applied to the analysis of urine from men exposed to carbaryl dust. The only detectable metabolites present were 1-naphthyl glucuronide and sulphate. In later studies the metabolic fate of carbaryl in the pig, sheep, man and monkey was investigated. The overall recovery of the naphthyl-^{14}C and methyl-^{14}C label of carbaryl in the pig was, respectively, 85 and 71 per cent of dose, while in the sheep the recovery of the naphthyl and methyl label was, respectively, 74.8 and 67.8 per cent of dose. 1-Naphthyl methylimido-carbonate O-glucuronide and 4-(methyl-carbamoyloxy)-1-naphthyl glucuronide were the major metabolites excreted in the urine by the pig. In addition to these, the sheep excreted 4-(methyl-carbamoyloxy)-1-naphthyl sulphate, 1-naphthyl glucuronide and sulphate. The overall recovery of carbaryl equivalents in the urine of man by using the fluorimetric method (26 to 28 per cent) was lower than that obtained with the colorimetric method (37.8 per cent). The metabolites identified in urine were 4-(methyl-carbamoyloxy)-1-naphthyl glucuronide, 1-naphthyl glucuronide and sulphate. The monkey excreted carbaryl primarily as 1-naphthyl methylimido-carbonate O-glucuronide and 4-(methyl-carbamoyloxy)-1-naphthyl glucuronide[11]. These results show the same tendency as those with rat and guinea-pig.

In Japan, 3,4-dimethylphenyl N-methyl-carbamate (Meobal) is used to control various kinds of plant hoppers on the rice plant. The study on the metabolism of Meobal has been carried out to determine the extent of biodegradation and to clarify the metabolic pathways of the carbamate compound in white rat[12]. Up to now, the following results have been obtained. 3,4-Dimethylphenol, formed through hydrolysis of the original carbamate chemical, and its conjugation products, 3,4-dimethylphenyl sulphate and 3,4-dimethylphenyl glucuronide, were also demonstrated in the urine, but the amount of these three metabolites was less than five per cent of the total radioactivity in the urine. Relatively little of the radioactive metabolites from the carbamate compound appeared to be identical with those obtained from the urine of rats given 3,4-dimethylphenol, although 17 radioactive metabolites amounting to approximately 35 per cent of the total radioactivity in the urine have not been characterized yet. These facts might imply that 3,4-dimethylphenyl N-methyl-carbamate is rather resistant to hydrolysis in the animal body and that biodegradation of the carbamate compound proceeds mainly through oxidative pathways. Among these metabolites 3-methyl-4-carboxyphenyl N-methyl-carbamate is only weakly inhibitory on mouse brain cholinesterase *in vitro* (at 10^{-3} M, 19 per cent inhibition, while the original carbamate at 10^{-6} M inhibits 50 per cent of the enzyme activity). So oxidation leads ultimately to detoxification, although 3-methyl-4-hydroxymethylphenyl N-methyl-carbamate is as inhibitory as 3,4-dimethylphenyl N-methyl-carbamate.

METABOLISM IN PLANTS

Certain carbamate insecticides such as Isoran (1-isopropyl-3-methylpyrazalyl-5 NN-dimethylcarbamate) and 3-isopropyl phenyl N-methyl-carbamate have been shown to have systemic insecticidal properties. However, these compounds are highly species specific and have not come into general use as systemics. More recently, however, two exceptionally effective carbamate insecticides have been shown to have outstanding systemic properties, necessitating extensive investigations of their plant metabolism.

Temik [2-methyl-2-(methylthio)-propionaldehyde O-(methyl-carbamoyl)-oxime] contains the thioether moiety and was found in studies with ^{14}C-labelled radiotracers in cotton to undergo rapid oxidation to the sulphoxide and more slowly to the sulphone. The Temik sulphoxide is relatively stable in the plant environment and is the major active metabolite responsible for persistent systemic activity. It is slowly degraded to the Temik sulphoxide oxime, which is the principal degradative metabolite. The metabolism of Temik is therefore somewhat similar to disulphoton and phorate. The sulphoxide and sulphone oxidation products are considerably more active as anticholinesterases and it appears that this systemic carbamate is another example of the importance of both oxidative activation and the delaying factor in promoting prolonged systemic activity in the leaves of treated plants[13].

Furadan (2,2-dimethyl-2,3-dihydrobenzofuranyl-7-N-methyl-carbamate) is of quite different structure from Temik and has been found to undergo a much more elaborate metabolism in cotton leaves in work with ^{14}C-labelled products. The principal pathway of oxidative metabolism consists in hydroxylation at the benzyl carbon atom to give 3-hydroxy Furadan which is rapidly oxidized further to 3-keto Furadan. Hydrolysis of the N-methyl-carbamate derivatives also occurs and the resulting phenols are conjugated as glucosides. The oxidative products in Furadan metabolism retain high anticholinesterase and some degree of insecticidal activity. However, oxidation in this series also promotes hydrolytic instability and the 3-keto Furadan is hydrolysed about 170 times as rapidly as Furadan at pH 9.5[14].

Friedman and Lemin[15] studied the metabolism of ^{14}C-labelled Banol (6-chloro-3,4-xylenyl N-methyl-carbamate) in the bean. The principal metabolite is a glucoside of either 2- or 5-hydroxyl Banol. Studies with eight substituted phenyl methyl-carbamate and two substituted pyrazolyl dimethyl-carbamate insecticide chemicals indicate that the water-soluble metabolites formed from them, after injection into bean plants, result in part from hydroxylation of the carbamate on the N-methyl group, on the ring, or on a ring substituent, followed by conjugation of the hydroxylated carbamates, mainly as glycosides. These glycosides are quite persistent and, in many cases, yield anticholinesterase agents on hydrolysis by β-glucosidase. The aglycones derived from carbaryl, which include the N-hydroxymethyl, 4-hydroxy, 5-hydroxy and 5,6-dihydro-5,6-dihydroxy derivatives, are the same carbamate intermediates as involved in carbaryl metabolism by mammals and insects. N-Hydroxymethyl formation also occurs with Banol, Baygon and UC 10854. Hydroxylation of the tertiary carbon atom of the isopropyl group yields hydroxypropyl UC 10854 from UC 10854, and 2-hydroxyphenyl methyl-carbamate on O-depropylation of Baygon. Horseradish peroxidase degrades Matacil and Zectran while tyrosinase systems do not metabolize the four carbamates studied[16].

COMPARATIVE TOXICOLOGY

Enzymatic studies, metabolism and selective toxicities

During the past several years numbers have shown that a variety of organophosphorus, carbamate and organochlorine insecticides are activated (rendered more toxic) or detoxified by microsomal preparations from various insects. Many of these biotransformations, such as side chain and ring oxidation, epoxidation, hydroxylation, N- and O-dealkylation, reduction, hydrolysis and conjugation, are catalysed by microsomal enzyme requiring NADPH and oxygen.

In work on the metabolism of carbamate, evidence has been accumulated that in the microsomes from the liver of various mammals and organs of several insects there exists a carbon monoxide-binding pigment designated as cytochrome P-450[17, 18].

For example, newly emerged male and female flies are considerably more susceptible to Baygon than are older flies. This finding is in line with the occurrence of low levels of cytochrome P-450 at an early age, but it does not correlate favourably for all ages[17]. Green and Dorough[19] found that susceptibility to three carbamate insecticides was greatest in 1-day-old and 15-day-old houseflies and least in 5-day-old flies, but that neither variation in total cholinesterase activity nor its sensitivity to the carbamates was sufficient to explain the difference in mortality. However, the inhibition of cholinesterase *in vivo* did correlate with the observed toxicity of the carbamates. These results might also be interpreted along the line of reasoning suggested above, i.e. that greater susceptibility corresponds with lower titres of cytochrome P-450 in the very young and old flies

When piperonyl butoxide is applied topically, 76.5 per cent inhibition of cytochrome P-450 resulted as early as 4 h after treatment and 61 per cent after 24 h. When 5 µg Baygon per fly is applied either at 4 h or at 24 h after the synergist is applied, 100 per cent mortality of the flies resulted. This dose of Baygon is sub-lethal when applied alone, and the synergist is non-toxic even at higher doses. Some inhibition is still evident 48 h after treatment, and the corresponding mortality, although only 63 per cent, is nevertheless significant. The pattern was the same with other carbamates. Eventually the cytochrome P-450 reaches the level of the control, indicating either removal of the synergist by catabolic processes or synthesis *de novo* of cytochrome P-450, or both[17].

The insecticides DDT, aldrin, malathion and Baygon showed neither inductive nor inhibitory effects on cytochrome P-450 *in vivo* in resistant or susceptible houseflies. Repeated sub-lethal doses of Baygon applied at 24 h intervals to the Diazinon-resistant strain showed no increase in cytochrome P-450, but symptoms of poisoning were manifested after the third application[17, 20].

The toxicity of six carbamate insecticides, alone and synergized with several methylenedioxyphenyl synergists, has been evaluated against the housefly, honey bee and the German cockroach. The topical LD_{50} values of the carbamates are markedly affected by the age and sex of the housefly and cockroach, but the differences are almost completely abolished by synergism with piperonyl butoxide, sesamex and methylenedioxynaphthalene. The variations in the toxicity of the carbamates to the housefly and German cockroach are well correlated with the titre of soluble phenolases in the various life stages, sexes and in adults of different ages. However, the honey bee is extremely susceptible to these carbamate insecticides, and little synergism occurs with the methylenedioxyphenyl compounds. In the honey bee only a very low titre of phenolase can be demonstrated[21].

In combination with this result, Metcalf *et al.*[22] found that the insecticidal carbamates are synergized by a wide variety of methylenedioxyphenyl compounds. These act as inhibitors of phenolases, which detoxify the carbamates largely by ring hydroxylation. The active inhibitors appear to require a three-point attachment to the phenolase to orient the methylene carbon atom so that interaction with a nucleophilic group at the enzyme active site takes place. Tyrosinase, which is abundant in the housefly, has served as a model enzyme for study of the kinetics of this interaction. Soluble housefly tyrosinase has been highly purified and accepts insecticidal carbamates as substrates for hydroxylation. The susceptibility of individual carbamates to enzymatic detoxication is greatly influenced by the nature of the aryl ring. The methylenedioxynaphthalenes and piperonyl carbamates are exceptionally active carbamate synergists.

However, the work of Kuhr[18] on the role of tyrosinase and/or cytochrome P-450, suggests that they might play some role in the metabolism of methylcarbamate insecticides by the housefly. In this work, housefly microsomes plus NADPH were found to metabolize carbaryl to its 4-hydroxy, 5-hydroxy, and, probably, N-hydroxymethyl and 5,6-dihydrodihydroxy derivatives, and phenyl methyl-carbamate formed one major organosoluble metabolite. The metabolism of both carbamates by housefly microsomes was inhibited by carbon monoxide, and this inhibition was partially reversed by light. Tyrosinase present in housefly microsome preparations does not appear to be involved in the metabolism of either of these carbamates. A soluble tyrosinase prepared from adult houseflies does not degrade carbaryl, Baygon or phenyl methyl-carbamate.

Metabolism and insect resistance

The exact mechanism of carbamate resistance in the housefly is not clear. Earlier research suggests that a hydrolytic mechanism, i.e. altered aliesterase, may be responsible for carbamate resistance as it sometimes is for organophosphate resistance[23].

A more general theory of carbamate resistance is based on the well-known synergism of carbamate insecticides by piperonyl butoxide and related methyen-dioxyphenyl synergists. Compounds of this class inhibit certain oxidative reactions involved in insecticide detoxification and, since they are particularly effective as synergists against resistant strains of houseflies, it follows that oxidative mechanisms may be responsible for resistance. The occurrence of high activities of microsomal oxidases in carbamate-resistant houseflies, as reported by Tsukamoto and Casida[24], supports this theory.

Oppenoorth[25] found that a fifth chromosomal oxidative mechanism, which is blocked by antioxidant synergists, confers resistance to DDT and organophosphate insecticides in a strain he designates as Fc. This strain is resistant also to carbamates, presumably because of the same oxidative mechanism. Thus strain Fc with its fifth chromosomal resistance gene(s) may differ significantly in type of carbamate resistance from the strains previously developed in the Corvallis laboratory[26] in which second chromosomal genes are primarily involved. The studies are therefore designed to measure the relative contribution of the second and fifth chromosomes to carbamate resistance in the housefly. For this purpose, two resistant strains, Isolan-R and Fc, were crossed with a susceptible strain carrying visible recessive mutants on the second, third and fifth chromosomes. The inheritance of dominant resistance factors was then studied by assaying backcross populations from the cross. These results indicate that no single gene contributes to a high resistance to carbamate insecticides in the housefly. Furthermore, no single genetic factor is responsible for more than fivefold resistance to synergized carbamates. Therefore, it is apparent that when high resistance to carbamates occurs in the housefly, this is probably caused by the interaction of several genetic factors. If the results reported are representative of the species, a second chromosomal gene(s) is of major importance, but other genes contribute significantly to the total resistance[27].

REFERENCES

[1] R. D. O'Brien. In *Metabolic Inhibitors*. Ed. by O. M. Hochester and J. H. Quastel. Academic Press: New York (1963).
[2] F. W. Plapp and W. S. Bigley. *J. Econ. Ent.* **54**, 793 (1961).
[3] R. L. Metcalf and T. R. Fukuto. *J. Agr. Food Chem.* **13**, 220 (1965).
[4] T. R. Fukuto, M. A. H. Fahmy and R. L. Metcalf. *J. Agr. Food Chem.* **15**, 273 (1967).
[5] H. Kazano, K. Asakawa, T. Tanaka and K. Fukunaga. *Jap. J. Appl. Ent. Zool.* **12**, 202 (1968).
[6] M. E. Eldefrawi and W. M. Hoskins. *J. Econ. Ent.* **54**, 401 (1961).

[7] H. W. Dorough and J. E. Casida. *J. Agr. Food Chem.* **12**, 294 (1964).

[8] N. C. Leeling and J. E. Casida. *J. Agr. Food Chem.* **14**, 281 (1966).

[9] E. S. Oonnithan and J. E. Casida. *J. Agr. Food Chem.* **16**, 28 (1968).

[10] J. B. Knaak, J. Marilyn, W. Tallant, J. Bartley and J. L. Sullivan. *J. Agr. Food Chem.* **13**, 537 (1965).

[11] J. B. Knaak, M. J. Tallant, S. J. Kozbelt and J. L. Sullivan. *J. Agr. Food Chem.* **16**, 465 (1968).

[12] J. Miyamoto. *Biochemical Toxicology of Insecticides*, p 115. Ed. by R. D. O'Brien and I. Yammamoto. Academic Press: New York and London (1970).

[13] R. L. Metcalf, T. R. Fukuto, Crystal Collins, Kathlen Borck, Janet Burk, H. T. Reynolds and M. F. Osman. *J. Agr. Food Chem.* **14**, 579 (1966).

[14] R. L. Metcalf, T. R. Fukuto, Crystal Collins, Kathlen Borck, S. A. El-Aziz, R. Munoz and C. C. Cassill. *J. Agr. Food Chem.* **16**, 300 (1968).

[15] A. R. Friedman and A. J. Lemin. *J. Agr. Food Chem.* **15**, 642 (1967).

[16] R. J. Kuhr and J. E. Casida. *J. Agr. Food Chem.* **15**, 814 (1967).

[17] A. S. Perry. *Life Science* **9**, 335 (1970).

[18] R. J. Kuhr. *J. Agr. Food Chem.* **17**, 112 (1969).

[19] L. R. Green and H. W. Dorough. *J. Econ. Ent.* **61**, 88 (1968).

[20] B. Meeksongsee, B. R. S. Yang and F. E. Guthrie. *J. Econ. Ent.* **60**, 1469 (1967).

[21] S. A. El-Aziz, R. L. Metcalf and T. R. Fukuto. *J. Econ. Ent.* **62**, 318 (1969).

[22] R. L. Metcalf, T. R. Fukuto, C. Wilkinson, M. H. Fahmy, S. Abd El-Aziz and E. R. Metcalf. *J. Agr. Food Chem.* **14**, 555 (1966).

[23] F. W. Plapp Jr., G. A. Chapman and W. S. Bigley. *J. Econ. Ent.* **57**, 692 (1964).

[24] M. Tsukamoto and J. E. Casida. *Nature, Lond.* **213**, 49 (1967).

[25] F. J. Oppenoorth. *Entomol. Exp. Appl.* **10**, 75 (1967).

[26] F. W. Plapp Jr and R. F. Hoyer. *J. Econ. Ent.* **60**, 768 (1967).

[27] F. W. Plapp Jr. *J. Econ. Ent.* **63**, 138 (1970).

CARBARYL RESIDUES IN MILK AND MEAT OF DAIRY ANIMALS

H. Wyman Dorough

Department of Entomology, University of Kentucky,
Lexington, Kentucky 40506, USA

ABSTRACT

Cows fed on a diet containing 10, 30 or 100 p.p.m. [naphthyl-^{14}C] carbaryl for 14 days eliminated daily about 0.2 per cent of the consumed doses in the milk, 5–10 per cent in the faeces and 70–85 per cent in the urine. Average daily levels of [^{14}C] carbaryl equivalents in the milk for the three feeding levels were 0.02, 0.07 and 0.28 p.p.m. respectively. Residue levels in the tissues after 14 days of feeding the three levels of carbaryl were as follows: kidney, 0.10, 0.53, 1.00; liver, 0.03, 0.10, 0.41; lung, 0.02, 0.06, 0.21; muscle, 0.01, 0.03, 0.10; heart, 0.01, 0.04, 0.10; blood 0.01, 0.04, 0.14; fat, 0.0, 0.02, 0.02. The chemical nature of these residues in the milk and meat is discussed.

INTRODUCTION

The evaluation of the residual nature of carbaryl in cattle has been a major source of progress in defining the metabolic fate of carbamate insecticides. Even before the realization that oxidative and hydroxylative mechanisms played a significant role in the metabolism of carbaryl, some of the more complete fate studies with this carbamate were performed with cows (Gyrisco et al.[1]; Claborn et al.[2]; Whitehurst et al.[3]). Although the analytical methods used by these scientists were later reported to be inadequate for the detection of total carbaryl residues in meat and milk (Dorough[4]) they did establish that carbaryl was rapidly metabolized and excreted by dairy animals.

In 1964, a report on the metabolism of carbaryl indicated that the biochemistry of this carbamate, and probably carbamates in general, was a very complex subject (Dorough and Casida[5]). These authors demonstrated the presence of certain carbaryl metabolites in the milk of a treated goat that were neither carbaryl of 1-naphthol nor any product which could be converted into 1-naphthol by alkaline hydrolysis. Subsequent studies on the metabolism of carbaryl in dairy cows were instrumental in confirming the identity of some carbaryl metabolites and in suggesting the chemical nature of others isolated for the first time (Baron et al.[6,7]; Dorough[4]). Progress towards the complete elucidation of the metabolic fate of carbaryl in cows and other animals has recently been reviewed (Dorough[8]).

A report on a study still under way in our laboratory relative to the residues in milk and meat of cows fed carbaryl continuously in the diet for extended periods will serve as a quick review of carbaryl metabolism. In addition, the detection of certain new materials will be discussed, along with the effect of prolonged exposure of carbaryl on its metabolism in lactating animals.

GENERAL STUDY PLAN

A summary of the overall study is presented in *Table 1*. One Holstein cow was used at each of the feeding levels indicated. All animals were in a medium stage of lactation, and production was considered satisfactory for

Table 1. Study plan for [naphthyl-^{14}C]carbaryl cow feeding experiment

Dietary dose (p.p.m.)	0, 10, 30, 100
Treatment method	Gelatin capsule (one every 12 h)
Treatment schedule	14 days on 'cold' carbaryl followed by 14 days on [naphthyl-^{14}C]carbaryl
Sampling	Milk, urine, faeces: every 12 h. Tissues: 18 h after last dose
Sensitivity	0.005 p.p.m. [^{14}C]carbaryl equivalents

a commercial dairy. They were housed in metabolism stalls, which permitted separate and quantitative collection of urine and faeces. Non-radioactive carbaryl was administered to the animals for a two-week period before feeding of the ^{14}C-labelled carbamate began. Collection of samples for analysis began 12 h after the first [^{14}C]carbaryl treatment.

The 5 p.p.b. level of sensitivity for total [^{14}C]carbaryl equivalents was determined on the basis of the specific radioactivity of the parent compound, which was 1.2 mc/mmol, and the size of sample radioassayed. For milk, 0.5 g was routinely assayed, and 1 g dry weight of tissue was assayed. The sensitivity was increased when necessary by assaying larger samples. The basic procedures used for quantitation of residues and for their isolation and identification were similar to those described in a study involving aldicarb (Dorough et al.[9]).

ELIMINATION OF CARBARYL

As expected from the earlier studies on the metabolism of carbaryl in cows, there was very rapid elimination of the doses from the animals (*Figure 1*). It was evident that an equilibrium between 'intake' and 'output' of carbaryl was established in rather fast order. Generally, the percentage of the previously applied dose present in the excreta remained fairly consistent after three or fours days of feeding the radioactive compound.

Milk from cows fed 10, 30 or 100 p.p.m. carbaryl contained about 0.2 per cent of the consumed carbamate. There were no indications that the pattern of excretion was altered significantly by increasing the dose tenfold. It was noted that the residues in the milk of the cow fed 100 p.p.m. did not reach their maximum levels as quickly as they did in animals fed the two lower doses. However, this may have been caused by some biochemical difference in this particular animal since [^{14}C]carbaryl equivalents in the urine and faeces exhibited a similar excretion pattern.

174

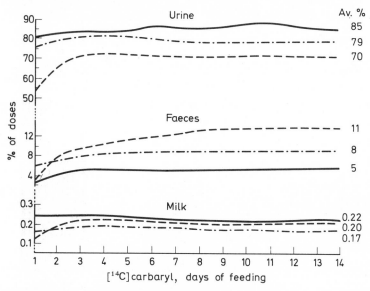

Figure 1. Elimination of [^{14}C]carbaryl equivalents in the urine, faeces and milk of cows on feeding with [^{14}C]carbaryl in the diet at : — 10 p.p.m.; — · — 30 p.p.m.; — — — 100 p.p.m.

Most of the administered carbaryl doses were eliminated from the body in the urine. From 70 to 85 per cent of the consumed carbamate was detected in the urine. There was a correlation between dose and percentage of dose excreted in the urine, with more complete elimination occurring as the dose decreased. The opposite pattern was indicated in the faeces, where 5 to 11 per cent of the doses was excreted. This type of excretion suggested that the metabolism of carbaryl may have been hindered somewhat by the larger levels of toxicant consumed. However, it is important to note that the total elimination of carbaryl equivalents exceeded 80 per cent of the administered doses regardless of the level fed to the animals.

[^{14}C]Carbaryl equivalents in the milk as p.p.m.

Having established that the percentage of the carbaryl doses eliminated in the milk remained at a fairly constant level during the 14-day study, it was expected that the same would hold true when the residues were converted into p.p.m. in the milk. Generally this was found to be the case (*Figure 2*). However, there was some day-to-day variation in milk production, which resulted in slight variations in the p.p.m. level observed in the milk. These minor variations were expected but were not considered too important since there was no indication that [^{14}C]carbaryl equivalents were increased as the time of feeding was extended.

Therefore our investigations showed that the level of total [^{14}C]carbaryl equivalents in the milk of cows on a continuous diet containing carbaryl was approximately 1/400 of that level in the diet. The non-accumulative nature of this carbamate in milk was likewise observed when aldicarb was fed to cows for 14 days (Dorough *et al.*[9]).

175

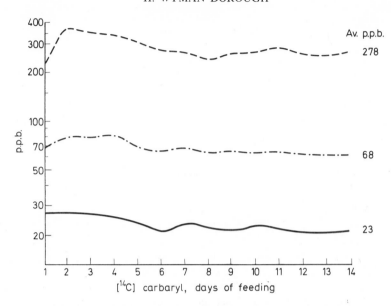

Figure 2. Total [^{14}C]carbaryl equivalents (p.p.b.) in the milk of cows on feeding with [^{14}C]-carbaryl in the diet at : — 10 p.p.m. ; — · — 30 p.p.m. ; — — — 100 p.p.m.

Extraction of carbaryl metabolites from milk

From a practical and toxicological viewpoint, the numbers defining the total carbaryl equivalents in milk have little significance. What is important, however, is the amount of those equivalents that were toxic or which should be considered toxic until proven otherwise. Generally, the latter would include any metabolite having the carbamate moiety still attached to the naphthyl ring and any other metabolites of unknown identity.

In the previous studies on the metabolism of radioactive carbaryl in dairy cows, the milk was extracted with organic solvent and the total residues in the organic extract, water phase and milk solids were quantitated. Only those metabolites appearing in the organic solvent phase have been subjected to rigorous testing to establish their identity. Such techniques were effective in identifying, or tentatively identifying, less than one-half of the total residues (Dorough[4]).

A major portion of our efforts in the current study was devoted to the development of an extraction procedure that would remove all residues from the water and solid phases of milk. Finally, a procedure that accomplished this goal was perfected ; a condensed outline version of the extraction procedure is shown in *Figure 3*. The outline shows that 50 ml of whole milk was used. This can be increased to 100 ml with only small increases of solvents required.

Acetone was added to the milk contained in a glass-stoppered, 250 ml Erlenmeyer flask and the contents were thoroughly shaken before addition of the acetonitrile. Reversing the order, or adding the two solvents together, coagulated the milk proteins so rapidly that residues were trapped in the

176

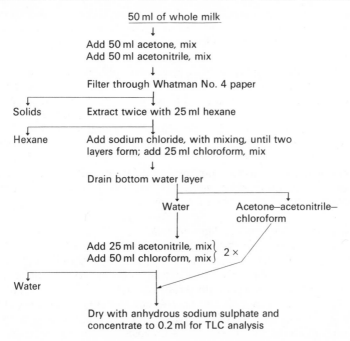

Figure 3. Outline of the procedure used for extracting [^{14}C]carbaryl equivalents from milk.

solids, and additional extractions with either acetone or acetonitrile were ineffective in their removal. The acetonitrile, after the acetone, coagulated the milk proteins without trapping the carbaryl residues and allowed the proteins to be removed by filtration. However, the flask and solids were thoroughly washed with acetonitrile. Analysis of 1 g of the dried milk solids by combustion techniques revealed that they were free of radioactive residues.

The filtrate was added to a separatory funnel and extracted with hexane to remove the fats and oils. After back-extracting the combined hexane with 20 ml of acetonitrile, the hexane was discarded. The acetonitrile was returned to the separatory funnel containing the milk extract.

Once all [^{14}C]carbaryl equivalents were removed from the milk solids, the most important step in this procedure was the removal of the water while retaining the residues in the organic solvent phase. This was done by adding sodium chloride to the extraction mixture, slowly with shaking, until two layers were formed. Chloroform (50 ml) was then added and the funnel shaken vigorously, and then the layers again were allowed to separate completely. Chloroform was necessary in this procedure because considerable water was present in the acetonitrile–acetone layer when chloroform was not used. Without the addition of the salt, the more polar metabolites were only partially extracted.

The water layer was extracted twice more with acetonitrile and chloroform and the water phase then discarded. No radioactive residue was detected in a 1 ml aliquot of the water, and only traces were evident when the entire water layer was concentrated and radioassayed directly. Thus all the carbaryl equivalents had been extracted from the milk and were present in an organic solvent.

The extract of the milk was then dried with anhydrous sodium sulphate and concentrated just to dryness on a rotary evaporator. Small washes of acetonitrile were used to transfer the residue to a 15 ml centrifuge tube. If the extract appeared to contain too much oily material for application to a thin-layer chromatogram, the acetonitrile was extracted with 2–4 ml of hexane. This step was usually necessitated by impure solvents rather than by oils from the milk.

Recent work has shown that the butterfat of milk is free of carbaryl metabolites. Therefore skim milk can be used without any changes in results and with less oil to be removed by the hexane washes.

Separation and isolation of residues in milk

A series of thin-layer-chromatographic (TLC) analyses, on Chromar 500 sheets, was used to separate and help identify the radioactive residues from the milk (*Figure 4*). The entire extract was applied to a chromatogram and developed two-dimensionally as shown in TLC No. 1. Radioautograms of the TLC revealed that six radioactive components were resolved by the solvent systems used. Each of the areas above the origin was isolated separately and analysed in several two-dimensional solvent systems. These

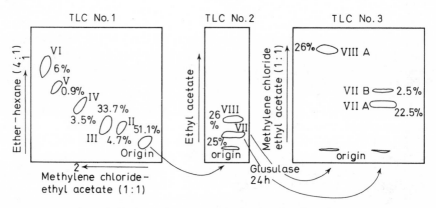

Figure 4. Drawings of thin-layer chromatograms showing the separation of metabolites of carbaryl, which were extracted from milk. (Chromar 500 sheets, Mallinckrodt Chemicals, St Louis, Mo., were used for all TLC analyses.) Percentages are with reference to the total radioactive residues in milk.

analyses demonstrated that each radioactive area, II–VI, was composed of a single material. Metabolites II–VI are those referred to in previous studies as the 'organo-solubles'. The radioactive materials remaining at the origin of TLC No. 1 were a combination of the 'water-solubles' and 'solids or unextractables' that were obtained with extraction procedures reported earlier (Dorough[4]).

178

The TLC No. 1 origin material was extracted with methanol and then applied to a new TLC and developed in ethyl acetate. When this was done, the radioactive material was resolved into two distinct areas (TLC No. 2, *Figure 4*). Since such polar metabolites of carbaryl and other carbamates have been shown to be conjugates of some type (Dorough[8]), metabolites VII and VIII were extracted from the TLC No. 2 and subjected to Glusulase enzyme. This enzyme contained both β-glucuronidase and sulphatase and therefore would cleave the metabolites if they were glucuronide or sulphate conjugates.

To determine if cleavage would occur, an aliquot of the methanol extract of either metabolite VII or VIII was added to a 25 ml Erlenmeyer flask and the solvent removed by evaporation. Citrate–phosphate buffer pH 5.0 (4 ml), and 0.5 ml of the Glusulase solution, as received (Endo Lab. Inc., Garden City, New York 11530), was added to the flask. A drop of toluene was added to retard microbial growth and the flasks were incubated, with shaking, at 37°C for 24 h.

After incubation the contents of the flask were transferred to a separatory funnel with water washes of the flask until the final volume was approximately 20 ml. Extraction of the radioactive products from the water was accomplished by using the procedure described for the extraction of milk.

The concentrated extract was applied to a TLC and developed in methylene chloride–ethyl acetate (1:1). Radioautographic analysis of the TLCs showed that metabolite VII yielded two aglycones, VII A and VII B, and that metabolite VIII yielded only one product, VIII A (TLC No. 3, *Figure 4*). Cleavage of metabolites VII and VIII by Glusulase enzyme was about 60 to 70 per cent during the 24 h period of incubation. Repeated isolation of the non-cleaved material and additional incubation with Glusulase enzyme showed that metabolites VII and VIII could be converted almost quantitatively into the aglycones shown in TLC No. 3.

Over 90 per cent of the applied radioactivity was routinely recovered from TLC No. 1 and No. 2. Therefore the metabolites shown on these TLCs were not unusually volatile, and no special precautions were required for good recovery and re-chromatography. However, metabolite III was often converted almost completely into metabolite IV. This conversion was kept to a minimum by using very pure solvents and maintaining metabolite III under slightly acid conditions whenever possible.

Poor recoveries of metabolites VII A and VIII A from TLC No. 3 were often encountered when attempts were made to isolate them for further study. This was primarily a function of volatility during the evaporation of solvents since direct counting of the radioactive areas of the TLC yielded recoveries exceeding 85 to 90 per cent of the applied materials.

Chemical nature of residues in milk

Once techniques for separating and isolating carbaryl metabolites from milk had been accomplished, each material was subjected to a variety of tests to determine its identity. The small concentrations of certain of the metabolites precluded detailed analysis of their chemical nature. When the same metabolite also was present in cow urine, but at much higher levels, that material was isolated and used for identification purposes. This was the case for metabolite II (and its hydrolytic product not detected in milk) and metabolites III and IV.

Table 2. Chemical nature of carbaryl metabolites in cow's milk and their average concentrations after feeding with carbaryl (100 p.p.m. in the diet for 14 days)

Metabolite No.	Chemical nature	Amount in milk (p.p.b.)	% of total
VI	Carbaryl	17	6
II	3,4-Dihydrodihydroxy-1-naphthyl methylcarbamate	13	5
III	5,6-Dihydrodihydroxy-1-naphthyl methylcarbamate	94	34
V	5-Hydroxy-1-naphthyl methyl-carbamate	3	1
IV	5,6-Dihydrodihydroxynaphthalene	9	3
VIII	1-Naphthyl sulphate	72	26
VII A	1-Methoxy-5-(methylcarbamoyloxy)-2-naphthyl sulphate	63	23
VII B	5-Methoxy-1,6-naphthalenediol	7	2

Results of the characterization studies of the metabolites in milk are shown in *Table 2*. A summary of the data supporting these findings is presented below.

Metabolite III—This product is considered first because it was the major metabolite of carbaryl in the milk and because its chemical characteristics were important in the identification of metabolite II. Moreover, it has been tentatively identified in a number of organisms in the past, and its identity after isolation from milk has been recently confirmed (Baron et al.[6,7]).

The bases on which our particular metabolite III from milk was identified as 5,6-dihydro-5,6-dihydroxy-1-naphthyl methylcarbamate were: (a) metabolite II co-chromatographed with an authentic sample synthesized by Union Carbide Chemists; (b) both the material from milk and the synthetic product could be dehydrated to form 5-hydroxy-1-naphthyl methylcarbamate; (c) mass spectra and infra-red spectra of metabolite II and the synthetic product were identical and supported the proposed structure.

Metabolite II—This metabolite and its hydrolytic product were found in rather large quantities in the urine. Therefore, these materials were isolated from the urine in sufficient quantity for mass spectral analysis. Since 3,4-dihydro-3,4-dihydroxy-1-naphthyl methylcarbamate has not been synthesized, identification of metabolite II as this product was based largely on its similarity to the 5,6-dihydrodihydroxy derivative of carbaryl. In addition to the fact that the mass spectral data were consistent with the proposed structure, metabolite II could be dehydrated to yield 4-hydroxy-1-naphthyl methylcarbamate. This reaction was comparable to that already mentioned in reference to metabolite III.

Metabolites V and VI—Each of these two materials was present at low levels in the milk, and the evidence for their structures was based primarily on co-chromatography with authentic samples. There was sufficient quantity of metabolite VI to establish that it yielded 1-naphthol upon hydrolysis, which further supported its identity as carbaryl.

Metabolite VIII—This metabolite was identified as 1-naphthyl sulphate. Before its incubation with Glusulase it co-chromatographed with a standard sample of 1-naphthyl sulphate (potassium salt). That this product exists interchangeably as a number of salts was pointed out by Paulson *et al.*[10]. These salts chromatograph differently on TLC and can lead to confusion about the identity of the material. This can be avoided by converting the compound into the sulphate by the addition of acid, or by converting it into a single salt by adding any one salt in excessive amounts. Glusulase enzyme cleavage of metabolite VIII yielded the aglycone, 1-naphthol (metabolite VIII A on TLC No. 3, *Figure 4*) in the same manner as the standard sample.

Metabolite VII—This material represents an entirely different type of carbaryl metabolite and one which has not been previously isolated. It is a carbamate and is formed by two types of conjugation, namely, sulphate conjugation and methylation. Data to support its identity as 1-methoxy-5-(methylcarbamoyloxy)-2-naphthyl sulphate are as follows: (a) It is a conjugate metabolite. This is based on the polar nature of the metabolite and the fact that Glusulase enzyme treatment yields two aglycones, metabolites VII A and VII B. About 99 per cent of metabolite VII is a conjugate of VII A. (b) It is a sulphate conjugate. Sulphatase hydrolysed twice as much as metabolite VII as did β-glucuronidase. By inhibiting the sulphatase activity in the glucuronidase preparation, the β-glucuronidase did not hydrolyse any of the conjugate metabolite. (c) Aglycone VII A is a ring-modified carbamate metabolite of carbaryl. If aglycone VII A was not a ring-modified derivative of carbaryl, alkaline hydrolysis would yield 1-naphthol. However, hydrolysis of VII A yielded a product that co-chromatographed with VII B. Mass spectral analysis of aglycone VII A showed a loss of methyl isocyanate, which also demonstrated that the ring was modified and, more important, showed that the metabolite was definitely a carbamate material. Other peaks of the mass spectrum suggested the presence of an hydroxyl group and a methoxy group. Mass spectral and i.r. data on 5-methoxy-6-hydroxy-1-naphthol methylcarbamate synthesized by Union Carbide chemists were identical with that of aglycone VII A.

Aglycone VII B is probably the hydrolytic product of VII A. However, the yield of VII B from the enzyme hydrolysis of metabolite VII is so small that detailed studies have not been possible. It is known that alkaline hydrolysis of VII A does yield a product that co-chromatographs with aglycone VII B. These data suggest the possibility that VII B is not present in milk as a conjugate but may form from aglycone VII A during the enzymatic cleavage of metabolite VII.

Residues in meat

The total [^{14}C]carbaryl equivalents in various tissues of cows fed with carbaryl for 14 days are shown in *Table 3*. The animals were slaughtered and the tissues taken approximately 18 h after the last treatment with the insecticide. Total residues in each sample were determined by combusting 1 g of dry tissue and collecting the radioactivity as ^{14}C-labelled carbon dioxide.

All of the tissues from cows fed with carbaryl at 30 and 100 p.p.m. contained detectable levels of residues. At the 10 p.p.m. feeding level, all of the tissues contained residues except the fat. A good correlation existed between

Table 3. Total [^{14}C]carbaryl equivalents in cow tissues after feeding with [naphthyl-^{14}C]carbaryl (10, 30 and 100 p.p.m. in the diet for 14 days)

Tissues	[^{14}C]carbaryl equivalents (p.p.b.)		
	10 p.p.m.	30 p.p.m.	100 p.p.m.
Kidney	0.095	0.531	1.003
Liver	0.033	0.100	0.411
Lung	0.020	0.064	0.207
Muscle	0.009	0.031	0.104
Heart	0.012	0.038	0.095
Fat	0.000	0.015	0.025
Blood	0.008	0.036	0.141

the level of pesticide fed and that which appeared in the tissues. Total [^{14}C]carbaryl equivalents in the muscle were 1/1000 of that level fed in the diet.

Although the total radioactive content of the tissues was quite low, attempts were made to determine the nature of the residues in all tissues except the fat. Tissue (25 g) was homogenized with 50 ml of water and then 100 ml of acetonitrile was introduced and blending continued. Again, the blender was stopped, 25 ml of acetone added and homogenization continued for about 1 min. The acetone aided protein coagulation and facilitated filtering. After being filtered off on Whatman No. 1 paper, the solids were extracted once more. The extracts were combined and analysis was continued by using a procedure similar to that described for milk. Unlike those in milk, however, some radioactive residues remained in the tissue solids

Table 4. Radioactive residues in cow tissues after feeding with [^{14}C]carbaryl (100 p.p.m. in the diet for 14 days)

Metabolites	% of total radioactivity in sample					
	Kidney	Liver	Lung	Muscle	Heart	Blood
Carbaryl (No. VI)	3.3	9.2	2.1	17.0	3.7	0
5,6-Dihydrodihydroxy carbaryl (No. III)	4.5	3.0	8.8	38.6	31.3	22.0
5,6-Dihydrodihydroxy naphthol	1.8	4.1	0	0	4.9	2.0
Naphthyl sulphate (No. VIII)	29.3	4.1	27.3	0	4.0	51.8
Water-soluble unknowns	43.2	32.9	47.5	30.6	41.8	7.1
Unextractable unknowns	17.9	46.7	14.3	13.8	14.3	17.1

after extraction and in the water phase after the addition of sodium chloride and partitioning with acetonitrile and chloroform. The concentration of these unknown materials and those residues that were identified are shown in *Table 4*.

Carbaryl was detected in all tissues except the blood. It accounted for 17 per cent of the [^{14}C]carbaryl equivalents in the muscle but constituted a lesser proportion of the total residues present in the other tissues.

The only other identified carbamate metabolite from the tissues was 5,6-dihydro-5,6-dihydroxy-1-naphthyl methylcarbamate. It was a major constituent of the residues in the muscle, heart and blood. Small quantities of the hydrolytic product of this metabolite were found in other tissues except the muscle and lungs.

Naphthyl sulphate was identified as 52 per cent of the [^{14}C]carbaryl equivalents in the blood. The same material accounted for about 30 per cent of the residues in the kidney and lung but was low in the liver and heart; none of this product was evident in the muscle tissue.

Metabolites of unknown identity, the water-solubles and unextractables, are currently being investigated with techniques described for the identification of the polar metabolites in milk.

ACKNOWLEDGEMENT

The data reported herein are the results of the combined efforts of Dr M. L. Saini, R. B. Davis and C. N. Thomas of our laboratory. We are particularly grateful to Dr W. J. Bartley (Union Carbide Corp., S. Charleston, W. Va, USA), for his cooperation and for providing metabolite standards and mass spectral data for this study. This work was supported by funds from Union Carbide Corp. (Chemicals and Plastics), U.S. Public Health Grant FD-00273 and from Regional Project S-73.

REFERENCES

[1] F. G. Gyrisco, D. J. Lisk, S. N. Fertig, E. W. Huddleston, F. H. Fox, R. F. Holland and G. W. Trimberger, *J. Agr. Food Chem.* **8**, 409 (1960).

[2] H. V. Claborn, R. H. Roberts, H. D. Mann, M. C. Bowman, M. C. Ivey, C. P. Weidenbach and R. D. Radleff, *J. Agr. Food Chem.* **11**, 74 (1963).

[3] W. E. Whitehurst, E. T. Bishop, F. E. Critchfield, F. G. Gyrisco, E. W. Huddleston, H. Arnold and D. J. Lisk, *J. Agr. Food Chem.* **11**, 167 (1963).

[4] H. W. Dorough, *J. Agr. Food Chem.* **15**, 261 (1967).

[5] H. W. Dorough and J. E. Casida, *J. Agr. Food Chem.* **12**, 294 (1964).

[6] R. L. Baron, N. J. Palmer, R. Ross, J. Doherty and W. C. Jacobson, *J. Ass. Offic. Anal. Chem.* **51**, 32 (1968).

[7] R. L. Baron, J. A. Sphon, J. T. Chen, E. Lustig, J. D. Doherty, E. A. Hansen and S. M. Kolbye, *J. Agr. Food Chem.* **17**, 883 (1969).

[8] H. W. Dorough, *J. Agr. Food Chem.* **18**, 1015 (1970).

[9] H. W. Dorough, R. B. Davis and G. W. Ivie, *J. Agr. Food Chem.* **18**, 135 (1970).

[10] G. D. Paulson, R. G. Zaylskie, M. S. Aehr, C. E. Portnoy and V. J. Feil, *J. Agr. Food Chem.* **18**, 110 (1970).

TOXICOLOGICAL CONSIDERATIONS OF METABOLISM OF CARBAMATE INSECTICIDES: METHOMYL AND CARBARYL

R. L. BARON

Environmental Protection Agency, Washington, D.C., U.S.A.

ABSTRACT

The ultimate goal in a toxicological consideration of contaminating substances is to evaluate their effect on man, including his ecosystem. In the absence of significant experimental conditions for man, the only alternative is the examination of data from animals and the assessment of their potential hazard to man. The metabolic fate of the contaminants in plants, experimental animals and man plays a significant role in this evaluation. This paper considers the role of metabolism in the toxicological consideration of two carbamate insecticides, carbaryl and methomyl.

Metabolism of methomyl in plants and rats apparently results in the rapid complete degradation of the molecule, yielding carbon dioxide, methylamine and acetonitrile as the major residual products. Small quantities of methomyl appear to be the only residue containing an intact carbamate skeleton. Evaluation of toxicological studies with rats and dogs has demonstrated a no-effect level of 100 p.p.m. Reproduction studies and other parameters have shown no unusual effects.

Experimental data on the fate of carbaryl in plants and animals have shown that the major carbamate residues in food appear to be polar conjugates of molecules which have undergone oxidative degradation. The significance to man of a toxicological effect reported to be elicited by carbaryl in certain species is examined in the light of the apparent lack of carbaryl residues in food and the metabolic fate of carbaryl in experimental animals and man.

The development and toxicological evaluation of anticholinesterase carbamate insecticides has been stimulated in recent years by their use as biodegradable agricultural insecticides potentially useful as substitutes for the more persistent chlorinated hydrocarbons. Esters of methyl- and dimethyl-carbamic acid have been used for many years, including their non-scientific use as a poison in certain African tribal customs. Development of carbamates as insecticides can be traced back to workers in Switzerland (Hans Gysin) and the United States (Robert Metcalf). The acute parasympathomimetic action resulting from inactivation of the enzyme acetylcholinesterase has been well documented and reviewed extensively. Many investigators have reported on the metabolic fate of various carbamates in plants, animals and other biological systems, and of the toxicological hazard to man associated with these compounds. This discussion will briefly and selectively examine two aspects in the toxicological consideration of carbamate insecticides: metabolism and the reproductive hazard.

In the report prepared for the Secretary of the U.S. Department of Health, Education and Welfare by the Secretary's Commission on Pesticides and their Relation to Environmental Health[1] it has been stated that 'Compounds suspected to affect DNA or to be converted enzymatically to effective compounds must be tested for their mutagenicity in higher organisms'. Certain methyl- and dimethyl-carbamate insecticides are included in the list of carbamates. These include: Bux, carbaryl, carbofuran, Carzol, Mobam and aldicarb. The Mrak report suggests a relationship between insecticidal carbamates and ethyl carbamate with regard to introducing chromosome breaks, cancer and teratogenic effects—probably through an N-hydroxylation reaction, other intermediates and free-radical formation. The N-methyl-carbamates currently used as insecticides have not been shown to be metabolized to N-hydroxy derivatives. Furthermore, in my opinion, the implication that a compound is mutagenic or can produce teratogenic effects by virtue of a proposed degradation intermediate based upon analogy with other compounds is untenable without supporting data.

The United States Government presently allows residues of 5-N-methyl-carbamate insecticides to be present in or on certain food crops. These compounds include aldicarb, carbaryl, carbofuran, methomyl and a mixture of two compounds commonly known as Bux. Additional temporary tolerances have been granted for formetanate, Baygon, and another mixture commonly known as Landrin. The metabolic fate of these compounds in insects, plants and mammals has been well documented in the literature.

With regard to the problems associated with food residues of carbamates, this discussion must distinguish between the metabolic fate of carbamates in plants and animals that constitute a part of the human diet from the comparative metabolic fate in experimental animals and man. Obviously, the metabolic fate of carbamates in and on edible tissues is of prime consideration in determining those materials actually in the food supply. Knowledge of comparative metabolism in mammalian species is also important. In the absence of relevant studies in man, that species which has the ability to alter the molecule in a manner most like man's must be chosen for study to evaluate the potential hazard to man. In many instances a considerable quantity of data exists on the toxicological effects of carbamates that have been granted tolerances in the U.S.A. These include life-time studies and reproduction studies, generally in rodents, shorter (two-year) studies in non-rodents, interaction studies, biochemical studies and many acute and subacute studies. When it has been shown that the residue in edible tissues is a metabolic product and the occurrence of the parent compound as a residue in the diet is of minor consideration, a question has to be raised about the significance of toxicological studies of the parent compound with regard to the potential danger to human health. A greater degree of relevance should be given to studies where the compound under investigation is the material actually consumed by man.

I would like to present a portion of the data presented to the United States Food and Drug Administration, as evidence of the lack of toxicological hazard of residues in food, as a result of the agricultural use of methomyl.

This discussion will, in part, point out, on the basis of the metabolic data, the relevance of studies where methomyl was examined for its toxicological hazard. A second part of this presentation, a review of the reproduction effects associated with carbaryl administration, will attempt to illustrate the problems which have thus far arisen with this compound. Problems which may in time be found to exist for the whole class of carbamate insecticides and which may or may not constitute a human hazard.

The data I am going to present are part of an unpublished presentation from E. I. Dupont de Nemours and Co. It includes portions of the studies on the metabolic fate of methomyl in corn, tobacco and cabbage, and preliminary experiments of the metabolic fate in rats. The methomyl results constitute a portion of the data required as a basis for granting a tolerance for use that results in residues in or on food. It is hoped that in the near future a full presentation of these data will be made by the investigators to a scientific journal for evaluation by the scientific community†.

METHOMYL

As seen in *Figure 1*, methomyl (S-methyl N-[(methylcarbamoyl)oxy]thio-acetimidate) (Lannate) has a structure very similar to another known oxime carbamate, aldicarb (Temik). The differences in these compounds are two

Methomyl (Lannate®)

$$CH_3-C=N-O-C(O)NHCH_3$$
$$S-CH_3$$

S-Methyl N-[(Methylcarbamoyl)oxy] thioacetimidate

Carbaryl (Sevin®)

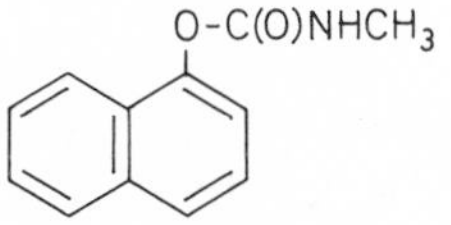

$$O-C(O)NHCH_3$$

1-Naphthylmethylcarbamate

Figure 1.

carbon atoms strategically placed in the molecule. The metabolism of aldicarb has been well documented. Briefly, it includes oxidation of the sulphur atom to form a sulphoxide, which is the toxic entity. This is slowly transformed into a less-toxic molecule before degradation by hydrolysis and other mechanisms. The degradation of methomyl, although the compound appears to be similar to aldicarb, is significantly different enough to be of extreme interest.

A diagrammatic view of the plant metabolism apparatus and trapping system is given in *Figure 2*. Modifications of the basic trapping system in these studies include: the use of several alkali or acid traps before an oxidation furnace, consisting of a quartz tube containing copper oxide to convert

† This presentation of data on the metabolic fate of methomyl does not reflect endorsement by the United States Government nor does this presentation constitute a review of the data as normally would occur when data are submitted for publication.

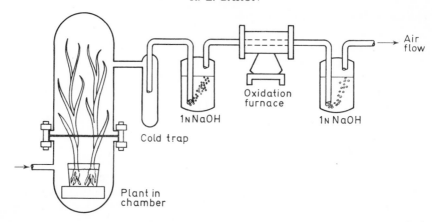

Figure 2. Diagram of plant metabolism apparatus and trapping system.

all organic materials which pass through the tube into carbon dioxide; the inclusion of two trapping trains, rather than one, to separate volatilizing materials coming from the ground level from those coming from the plant itself; a cold trap to collect materials not trapped in alkali or acid. Data in *Table 1* were obtained with tobacco when methomyl was administered to the plant by soil application. Tobacco was grown in the presence of 10 p.p.m. of methomyl dissolved in nutrient solution. It was found that between 20 and 25 per cent of the radioactivity was absorbed into the plant. The data are essentially similar for three replicated plants. It is obvious that quite a bit of material was trapped from the aerial and the root portions in trap 1, little was trapped in trap 2 and a considerable portion of material passed both traps, was oxidized to carbon dioxide and collected in the third trap. Materials that were trapped in the sodium hydroxide traps were shown to be carbon dioxide by complete precipitation as barium carbonate. Radioac-

Table 1. Volatilization of radioactivity from tobacco treated with methomyl

Portion of plant	Trap no.†	Radioactivity (μCi) Plant no. 1	Plant no. 2	Plant no. 3
Aerial	1	2.39	1.87	2.43
Aerial	2	0.53	0.32	0.48
Aerial	3	<u>4.98</u>	<u>3.52</u>	<u>4.81</u>
Aerial	Total	7.90	5.71	7.72
Root	1	1.37	1.39	2.11
Root	2	0.38	0.04	
Root	3	<u>0.62</u>	<u>0.39</u>	<u>1.25</u>
Root	Total	2.37	1.82	3.36
Radioactivity found in acid traps over the fourth 1-week period				
Aerial	acid	0.09	0.02	0.03
Root	acid	0.00	0.00	0.00

† Traps 1 and 2 were positioned between the plant chamber and the oxidation furnace. Trap 3 collected carbon dioxide from the oxidation furnace.

tivity data from the roots indicate that a significant amount of material is volatilized directly from the nutrient solution as carbon dioxide and is neutral in nature. There appears to be a small quantity of basic material, which was found in an acid trap from the aerial portion of the plant. *Table 2* shows a quantitative recovery of residues utilizing tobacco plants Nos 1 and 2. Approximately 75 per cent of the original ^{14}C treatment was unchanged in the growth medium. The plants absorbed 25 and 20 per cent respectively of the radioactivity in the nutrient solution. This was divided into two parts, the volatile component and the plant tissues. The volatile components, as

Table 2. Metabolic distribution of methomyl in tobacco

Fraction	Plant no. 1		Plant no. 2	
	μCi	% of original dose	μCi	% of original dose
Plant tissues				
Leaf extract	2.31	4.3	1.84	3.4
Leaf residue	0.80	1.5	0.78	1.4
Stem extract	0.08	0.1	0.08	0.1
Stem residue	0.08	0.1	0.09	0.2
Root extract	0.02	0.1	0.03	0.1
Root residue	0.04		0.05	
Volatile components†				
Acidic fraction	4.67	8.6	3.62	6.7
Neutral fraction	5.69	10.5	3.93	7.3
Condensate	0·09	0.2	0.29	0.5
Sub-total (dose absorbed by plant)	13.78	25.4	10.71	19.7
Growth medium residue				
Nutrient solution	37.92	70.0	41.67	77.0
Sand residue	0.30	0.6	0.35	0.7
Total recovery	52.00	96.0	52.73	97.4

† Acidic components: pre-furnace trap; neutral components: post-furnace trap; condensate: plant chamber wash.

noted in *Table 1*, were acidic and were trapped by sodium hydroxide or were neutral. The neutral material passed the sodium hydroxide traps to the combustion chamber. The condensate was material that was found on the inside of the walls of the plant chamber at the conclusion of the experiment. With tobacco, approximately the same quantity of acidic and neutral components was observed. The term 'plant tissue' includes a methanol extract of the leaves, the roots and the stems. Data are presented on the distribution of radioactivity in both the extract and the residue. It is obvious that the vast majority of the absorbed material is in the leaf. The material apparently passed into the roots, up the stems and into the leaf where it accumulated as a small residue.

The data in *Table 3* were obtained from a ^{14}C recovery study with corn. In this particular study, 5.44 μCi of methomyl per plant was placed in the growing whorl of a young corn plant. After ten days a methanol extraction of the roots and aerial portions was performed. It was found that 108 per cent

189

Table 3. Metabolic distribution of methomyl in corn

Fraction	μCi	% of recovered radioacitivity
Plant tissues		
Aerial portions—extract	1.537	26.1
Aerial portions—unextractable	1.120	19.0
Roots—extract	0.002	0.4
Roots—unextractable	0.019	
Volatile components†		
Acidic fraction	0.373	6.3
Neutral fraction	1.407	24.5
Cold trap	0.037	
Condensate	0.732	12.5
Soil contamination		
Soil extract	0.034	
Soil residue	0.624	11.2
	5.885	
	(108% recovery)	

† Acidic components: pre-furnace trap; neutral components: post-furnace trap; cold trap: between plant chamber and first trap; condensate: chamber wash.

of the original dose was recovered in this study. There was some soil accumulation, where materials apparently washed down to the soil. Volatile components in this study accounted for approximately 45 per cent of the recovered radioactivity. The neutral fraction was approximately four times the size of the acidic fraction. Approximately 45 per cent of the recovered radioactivity was found to be residues present in the aerial portion of the plant as methanol-extractable and non-extractable fractions. The methanol-extractable material consisted of 26 per cent of the radioactivity. In *Table 4*, data are presented from a study in which cabbage was treated with 4.42 μCi of methomyl and

Table 4. Metabolic distribution of methomyl in cabbage

Fraction	μCi	% of recovered radioactivity
Plant tissues		
Aerial portions—extract	2.293	54.4
Aerial portions—unextractable	0.933	22.1
Roots	0.035	0.8
Volatile components†		
Acidic fraction	0.343	8.1
Neutral fraction	0.323	7.9
Cold trap	0.011	
Condensate	0.195	2.1
Soil contamination		
Soil	0.087	2.1
	4.220	
	(96% recovery)	

† See *Table 3* for explanation.

harvested after seven days, and the aerial portions were extracted in methanol. Approximately 96 per cent of the original ^{14}C dose was accounted for in this study. The soil contained a very small quantity of radioactivity. Again volatile components included both an acidic and a neutral fraction. In this study with cabbage, in contrast to corn but similar to tobacco, the neutral and acidic fractions were comparable. Approximately 70 per cent of the plant residue was present as a methanol-extractable fraction.

Table 5. Countercurrent distribution of plant leaf extract

Tobacco	µCi	Recovered radioactivity (%)
Polar fraction	0.14	7.5
Methomyl oxime	0.003	0.2
Methomyl	1.53	82.3
Non-polar fraction	0.19	10.2
Total	1.86	
Corn		
Polar fraction	0.885	81.8
Methomyl oxime	0.015	1.4
Methomyl	0.061	5.6
Non-polar fraction	0.121	11.2
Total	1.082	
Cabbage		
Polar fraction	1.03	62.4
Methomyl oxime	0.02	1.2
Methomyl	0.11	6.7
Non-polar fraction	0.49	29.7
Total	1.65	

The methanol-extractable material from all experiments was further examined by countercurrent distribution, with a fractionation between benzene and water (Table 5). Radioactivity was found in four fractions: the first lower phases contained a polar fraction; a second fraction contained small quantities of a known metabolite of methomyl, the free oxime; another fraction accounted for methomyl itself; a fourth was designated as the non-polar fraction. The polar fraction was further examined with regard to cholinesterase inhibition and found to be non-inhibitory to bovine red blood cell acetylcholinesterase. Further studies with thin-layer-chromatographic techniques and mass-spectral analysis indicated that approximately 85 per cent of the methanol-extractable materials from tobacco was unchanged methomyl. A small fraction was found to be the oxime. Examination of the methanol extract of corn indicated the majority of the residue to be very polar material (82 per cent of the total residue) with a small amount of methomyl (6 per cent) and a non-polar component (11 per cent). Again the polar fraction was non-inhibitory toward cholinesterase. Examination of the methanol extract from cabbage indicated a predominantly polar fraction with a small quantity of methomyl and a substantial non-polar fraction. The polar fraction was not inhibitory towards cholinesterase. Recovery of radioactivity in the studies with the methanol extract of corn and cabbage was approximately 70 per cent of the material applied to the countercurrent

191

apparatus. It is significant to note the differences obtained in these particular studies in which corn and cabbage were both treated topically, resulting in residues of a very polar nature, from those with tobacco treated by nutrient solution uptake which resulted in a residue consisting primarily of methomyl.

A study utilizing tobacco traced the radioactivity after foliar application of methomyl (*Table 6*). These data indicate that methomyl, although taken

Table 6. Movement of radioactivity in the tobacco plant after foliar application of S-methyl[1-^{14}C]—N—[(methylcarbamoyl)oxy]thioacetimidate

Portion of plant	Radioactivity (µCi)			
	3 days after treatment		7 days after treatment	
	Extract	Residue	Extract	Residue
Growing tip	0.0	0.00	0.00	0.01
Leaves and stem above treated leaf	0.00	0.00	0.00	0.02
Treated leaf	1.53	0.04	0.75	0.13
Leaves and stem below treated leaf	0.00	0.00	0.00	0.02
Roots	0.00	0.00	0.00	0.02

† Only 0.01 µCi of radioactivity was obtained by washing the surface of the leaf seven days after treatment.

into the plant, did not appear to migrate to any great extent from the area of the treated leaf. Little if any radioactivity was found in the leaves and stem above or below the treated leaf. There was no indication of the nature of the radioactivity in the treated plant. Little if any radioactivity was found on the surface of the leaf seven days after treatment. In another experiment (*Table 7*) methomyl and its oxime were applied to a paper disc and examined for radioactive components in the trapping system. The data obtained with two sodium hydroxide traps and a combustion furnace indicate that a significant quantity of material volatilizes from methomyl and is trapped as a neutral or basic component. Approximately 22 per cent of the applied dose of methomyl was volatilized, with 90 per cent of the material being trapped as an extremely volatile component. Volatilization of the oxime accounted

Table 7. Radioactivity collected in alkali traps from air drawn over dry deposits of S-methyl thioacetimidates

From compound	Trap no.	Radioactivity collected	
		µCi	% of amount in traps
S-Methyl[1-^{14}C]—N—[(methylcarbamoyl)oxy]-thioacetimidate	1 NaOH	0.19	6.9
	2 NaOH	0.10	3.6
	3 Volatiles	2.47	89.5
S-Methyl[1-^{14}C]—N—hydroxythioacetimidate	1 NaOH	1.37	87.8
	2 NaOH	0.03	1.9
	3 Volatiles	0.16	10.3

for approximately 17 per cent of the applied dose and the majority of material was trapped as an acidic product in the first trap. These experiments were done over a two-week interval. The material trapped in the alkali solutions, as might be expected, was carbon dioxide. The volatile component was collected in a cold trap, examined by several techniques and shown to be acetonitrile.

The polar metabolites obtained in the corn and cabbage experiment, which in corn amounted to 82 per cent of the methanol extract and in cabbage to 62 per cent of the extract, were examined and found to be natural products (*Figure 3*) identified in part as glycollic acid, tartaric acid, various ^{14}C-labelled

Volatiles
C^*O_2 [^{14}C]Carbon dioxide
CH_3C^*N [^{14}C]Acetonitrile

Undegraded fraction
CH_3—$^*C(NO)$—$CO(NH)$—CH_3
            |
          SCH_3

Polar fraction
HO—CH_2—C^*OOH [^{14}C]Glycollic acid
HO—CH—COOH [^{14}C]Tartaric acid
      |
HO—CH—COOH

C^*—Sugars ^{14}C-labelled sugars
C^*—Amino acids ^{14}C-labelled amino acids

Non-polar fraction
C^*—Lipids ^{14}C-labelled lipids, which yield on alkaline saponification:

C_{16}, C_{18} and C_{20} fatty acids containing ^{14}C

Figure 3. Partial list of methomyl metabolites in corn and cabbage.

sugars and possibly some ^{14}C-labelled amino acids. The small quantities of the non-polar fraction, which in corn amounted to 11 per cent and in cabbage to approximately 30 per cent of the recovered radioactivity, were found to be ^{14}C-labelled lipids, which upon alkaline saponification yielded C_{16}, C_{18} and C_{20} fatty acids. Further examination of the fraction designated as methomyl again confirmed its presence.

Methomyl, unlike aldicarb, is active as the parent compound, which, if it does undergo oxidative attack to the *S*-oxide, results in a less toxic compound and is followed by extensive breakdown. The mechanism by which methomyl is degraded is one that, with regard to residues in foods, is an academic question. Accordingly, toxicological examination of the parent compound would apparently be sufficient to satisfy all requirements for the safety of the compound in regard to food residues unless some plant system is found that affects the metabolism of methomyl in a manner different from the systems thus far examined.

Toxicological examination of methomyl has been accomplished by long-term feeding studies in rats and dogs at levels up to 400 p.p.m.[2]. A no-effect level was estimated to be approximately 100 p.p.m. in both species. A three-generation rat reproduction study was also evaluated to show 100 p.p.m. to be a no-effect level. Potentiation studies with methomyl in combination with 18 other anticholinesterase compounds revealed effects only with carbaryl and ronnel. The effects were minimum with carbaryl but ronnel showed approximately fourfold acute toxic potentiation. Methomyl is a relatively toxic compound; its acute oral LD_{50} is 17 (14–20) mg/kg to male rats and 24 (22–25) mg/kg to female rats. Acute toxicity of the sulphoxide and sulphone analogues to male rats showed that these compounds were almost non-toxic with an oral LD_{50} of greater than 1000 mg/kg. This type of acute data was exemplified when methomyl was assayed against red blood cell cholinesterase. Methomyl showed a Ki of $2.0 \pm 0.2 \times 10^{-7}$ in comparison to $4.3 \pm 0.2 \times 10^{-6}$ for the sulphoxide, indicating the sulphoxide to be considerably less potent than methomyl. Methomyl was found to induce no demyelination hazard when examined in White Leghorn chickens. Feeding methomyl to a lactating cow at levels of 0.2 and 20 p.p.m. in the diet showed no adverse growth effects and no residues (less than 0.02 p.p.m.) in the milk, meat, fat, liver or kidney.

Table 8. Distribution of radioactivity after treatment of rats with
S-methyl[1-^{14}C]—N—[(methylcarbamoyl)oxy]thioacetimidate

	(1 day)		(3 day)		(3 day)	
	µCi	%O.T.†	µCi	%O.T.	µCi	%O.T.
External fractions						
carbon dioxide	0.94	15	1.50	23	1.03	17
neutral volatile metabolite	N.D.‡		N.D.		2.00	33
metabolites in urine	1.75	27	1.59	24	0.95	16
faeces	0.02	1	0.13	2	N.D.	
Body fractions						
blood	0.034		0.084		N.D.	
brain	0.003		0.003		N.D.	
fat	0.002		0.000		N.D.	
g.i. tract	0.167		0.122		N.D.	
heart	0.003		0.005		N.D.	
hide	0.105		0.169		N.D.	
kidneys	0.010		0.007		N.D.	
liver	0.042		0.035		N.D.	
lungs	0.005		0.004		N.D.	
muscle	0.004		0.003		N.D.	
spleen	0.003		0.003		N.D.	
testes	0.006		0.005		N.D.	
carcass	0.227		0.234		N.D.	
Body total	0.611	10	0.674	10		

† O.T. Original treatment
‡ N.D. Not determined.

The metabolic fate of methomyl in male rats was given a preliminary examination. A summary of the distribution data is presented in Table 8. For approximately eight days young adult male rats were fed with diets containing 200 p.p.m. of unlabelled methomyl. At the end of this period the animal was given orally 1.2 mg of methomyl (approximately 5 mg/kg) containing 6.5 µCi and examined over various intervals in a metabolism unit. The data collected after one day or three days were very similar: between 15 and 23 per cent of the original dose was eliminated as carbon dioxide; approximately 25 per cent of the original dose as metabolites in the urine;

about ten per cent of the original dose was retained in the body in various tissues. Recovery in these experiments was approximately 59 to 60 per cent of the original dose. Another experiment utilized a combustion furnace and a trapping system in a manner similar to the plant metabolism studies, and an additional 30 per cent of the original dose was recovered in this manner. These data account for approximately 90 per cent of the administered dose and indicate the rapid removal of methomyl from the animal body. An examination was made of the neutral volatile metabolite found in the third study. The radioactive peak from a liquid nitrogen trap was examined by mass spectrometry and again found to be acetonitrile. Examination of the metabolites in urine indicated that they were primarily very polar components with less than 10 per cent unchanged methomyl.

CARBARYL

A request for a tolerance for carbaryl in or on raw agricultural commodities was originally submitted to the United States Food and Drug Administration in 1958. At the time of this original request, referring to residues on certain selected agricultural crops, it was suggested that 'the toxicity and mechanism of action of the insecticide, Sevin, are now sufficiently well understood, and that the chronic toxicity is low enough, so that commercial use in agriculture would be safe . . .'. Since this submission extensive toxicological and chemical data have been collected. The metabolic fate of carbaryl in animals has been studied in many species of animals including the chicken, goat, cow, dog, guinea pig, monkey, pig, rabbit, rats, sheep and man[3]. Carbaryl does not accumulate in the animal body. It is rapidly metabolized through two primary mechanisms, hydrolysis and oxidation, with the resulting polar metabolites being conjugated and readily voided and excreted. Qualitatively, carbaryl is cleaved through hydrolysis to form 1-naphthol and methylcarbamic acid. Oxidation results in ring hydroxylation to produce 4-hydroxycarbaryl, 5-hydroxycarbaryl and 5,6-dihydro-5,6-dihydroxycarbaryl (all of which have been reported primarily as water-soluble conjugates). In man, the primary metabolites in urine have been demonstrated to be conjugates of 4-hydroxy-carbaryl and 1-naphthol. Chromatographic profiles of metabolites in urine from other experimental animals indicate that several species metabolize carbaryl in a manner qualitatively similar to man[4, 5]. At the present time there are insufficient data to enable a selection of a single animal species that will degrade carbaryl in a manner both qualitatively and quantitatively similar to man. In further research it is vital to resolve the question of comparative metabolism to define that animal species or strain which will detoxify carbaryl and all carbamates in a manner closest to that described for man[6]. Only then can data from animal studies be extrapolated with measurable assurances to evaluate potential hazards to man.

The metabolic fate of carbaryl in plants has also been extensively studied. The half-life of carbaryl on a leaf surface has been estimated to be approximately three to four days. Carbaryl, which appears almost entirely on the leaf surface, has been found to be unaffected by photo-oxidation processes. The 'market basket surveys' made by the FDA show that no carbaryl residues were consumed in the average diet in 1968[7]. A small fraction of the residue deposit penetrates plant tissues, where it undergoes biotransformation to its primary metabolites including hydroxymethylcarbaryl, 7-hydroxycarbaryl and 4-hydroxycarbaryl; to a lesser extent 5-hydroxycarbaryl, 1-naphthol and 5,6-dihydro-5,6-dihydroxycarbaryl are also produced. These metabolites are conjugated to form water-soluble glycosides. The formation of the oxidized carbaryl metabolites appears to be the rate-limiting step, since the primary metabolites are not found free but only as conjugates in plant tissues. It is significant that the primary metabolite in plant systems, the hydroxymethylcarbaryl, is apparently a very minor metabolite in animal systems.

In general, sensitive methods of routine analyses must be available to determine the major metabolites of carbamates in food.

The single most important toxicological problem at this time relating to the safety of the use of carbaryl and possibly other carbamates is the possibility of a hazard to reproduction.

A considerable number of species respond to the reproductive (and potential teratogenic) stimulus of carbaryl[1, 8-26], while several appear to be resistant[19, 26]. The ultimate problem is: does carbaryl in good agricultural and economic practice represent a hazard to reproduction in man? Other questions raised include: should we be interested in the reproductive potential of carbaryl *per se* where it has been demonstrated by plant and animal metabolism studies that carbaryl is not a significant residue in food? Are there constant differences in metabolism between resistant and susceptible species or strains? What are the qualitative and quantitative relationships in the metabolism of carbamates and pesticides in general in experimental animals with regard to man? For carbaryl, where the toxicological evaluation of the parent compound with regard to a potential reproductive effect has resulted in questioning its use, it becomes more apparent that the total metabolic picture must be examined and used as an indicator to guide the selection of suitable species for further, more definitive, toxicological studies. Sullivan and his co-workers[27, 28] are attempting to select such a species based upon metabolic similarity to man. The realization that both the quantitative and qualitative aspects of the metabolic fate of a compound in an experimental animal are similar to that found in man is a first step in adequately choosing an animal species which will generate data that can be extrapolated to man. The ultimate goal in any toxicological evaluation is to determine the significance of the effects of a compound on experimental animals in relation to the effects which might occur in man. Thus, the qualitative and quantitative determination of the metabolic fate of the compound in animals and man is primary consideration in choosing the best animal species for study.

In summary, the metabolic fate in plants, experimental animals and man is one of the primary considerations in the evaluation of the toxicological hazards of carbamates arising from good agricultural and economic use. The metabolic data on the degradation of methomyl in plants suggest that the toxicological studies thus far performed with the parent compound are most relevant, as apparently methomyl is the only chemical entity which exists as a carbamate residue in food. In contrast, metabolic studies in plants and animals indicate that carbaryl is not the significant residue in food.

Therefore toxicological studies with carbaryl are of limited value in evaluating the hazard to man associated with food residues. Some well-defined studies are currently under way with metabolites of carbaryl and other insecticidal carbarmates to determine if a hazard to man exists as a result of the small quantities of metabolites expected to occur as residues in food. Additional studies are also under way to define that species of experimental animal from which data can be extrapolated to man. It must be re-emphasized that in evaluating the toxicological potential of carbamates to man the role of metabolism is of primary consideration.

REFERENCES

[1] E. M. Mrak, *Report of the Secretary's Commission on Pesticides and Relationship to Environmental Health.* U.S. Department of Health, Education and Welfare (1969).

[2] E. I. Dupont de Nemours & Co. Unpublished Report. (1968).

[3] H. W. Dorough, *J. Agr. Food Chem.* **18**, 1015 (1970).

[4] J. B. Knaak, M. J. Tallant, W. T. Bartley and L. J. Sullivan, *J. Agr. Food Chem.* **16**, 465 (1965).

[5] J. B. Knaak and L. J. Sullivan, *J. Agr. Food Chem.* **15**, 1125 (1967).

[6] R. J. Kuhr, *J. Agr. Food Chem.* **18**, 1023 (1970).

[7] R. E. Duggan and G. Q. Lipscomb, *Pest. Monitoring J.* **2**, 153 (1969).

[8] FAO/WHO: FAO/PL 1967/M/11/1 WHO/FOOD ADD./68–30 (1968).

[9] T. F. X. Collins, W. H. Hansen and H. V. Keeler. *Tox. Appl. Pharmacol.* In press (1971).

[10] V. I. Vashakidze, *Soobshch. Akad, Nauk. Gruz. S.S.R.* **39**(2), 471 (1965). (Cited in *Chem. Abstr.* **64**, 2689h, 1966).

[11] V. I. Vashakidze, N. S. Shavladge and I. S. Guineriya, *Sb. Tr. Nauck.-Issled. Inst. Gig. Tr. Profzabol., Tiflis,* **10**, 205 (1966). (Cited in *Chem. Abstr.* **68**, 113580m, 1968).

[12] V. I. Vashakidze, *Soobshch. Akad, Nauk, Gruz, S.S.R.* **48**(1), 219 (1967). (Cited in *Chem^i Abstr.* **68**, 28750x, 1968).

[13] M. N. Rybakova, *Hygiene and Sanitation,* **31**, 402 (1966).

[14] M. N. Rybakova, *Vop. Pitan.* **26**, 9 (1967).

[15] A. I. Shtenberg and M. N. Rybakova. *Fd. Cosmet. Tox.* **6**, 461 (1968).

[16] N. V. Orlova and E. P. Zhalbe, *Vop. Pitan.* **27**, 49 (1968). (Cited in *Chem. Abstr.* **70**, 46402f, 1969).

[17] H. E. Smalley, J. M. Curtis and F. L. Earl, *Tox. Appl. Pharmacol.* **13**, 393 (1968).

[18] W. J. Dougherty, L. Golberg and F. Coulston, Oral Presentation to Society of Toxicology: 8–11 March, 1971).

[19] J. F. Robens, *Tox. Appl. Pharmacol.* **15**, 152 (1969).

[20] M. Gharidi, D. A. Greenwood and W. Binss, *Tox. Appl. Pharmacol.* **10**, 393 (1967).

[21] J. B. DeWitt and C. M. Menzie, Unpublished Report by Bureau of Sport Fisheries and Wildlife, U.S. Department of Interior (1961).

[22] M. Gharidi and D. A. Greenwood, *Tox. Appl. Pharmacol.* **8**, 342 (1966).

[23] K. S. Khera, *Tox. Appl. Pharmacol.* **8**, 345 (1966).

[24] A. I. Olefir and V. Kh. Vinogradova, *Vrach. Delo.* **11**, 103 (1968). (Cited in *Chem. Abstr.* **70**, 19205n 1969).

[25] J. P. Marliac, *Fed. Proc.* **23**, 105 (1964).

[26] H. E. Smalley, P. J. O'Hara, C. H. Bridges and R. D. Radeliff, *Tox. Appl. Pharmacol.* **14**, 409 (1969).

[27] L. J. Sullivan, B. H. Chin and C. P. Carpenter, Unpublished Report (1970).

[28] B. H. Chin and L. J. Sullivan, Oral Presentation to Society of Toxicology: 8–11 March, 1971).

THE FORMATION AND IMPORTANCE OF CARBAMATE INSECTICIDE METABOLITES AS TERMINAL RESIDUES

R. J. KUHR

Department of Entomology, New York State Agricultural Experiment Station, Geneva, New York 14456, USA

ABSTRACT

The formation of carbamate insecticide metabolites in a plant or animal is primarily dependent on the hydrolytic, oxidative and conjugative potential of the organism. Hydrolysis appears to be a more significant metabolic mechanism in mammals than it is in insects, which lends a degree of selectivity to certain carbamates. The extent of oxidation is generally higher in plants and insects, while conjugation of hydrolytic and oxidative metabolites is involved in the metabolism of almost all of the insecticidal carbamates in any living system. In animals, and probably plants, a mixed-function oxidase(s) serves as the catalyst for most of the oxidations producing essentially the same series of metabolites in a variety of plants and animals. In some cases, metabolites can be equally or more toxic than the applied carbamate, but these products are usually present in minor amounts. Most important are the sulphoxidation products of aldicarb and the 4-dimethylamino analogues of Zectran and aminocarb. Data on the toxicity of carbamate metabolite conjugates are very limited.

INTRODUCTION

Before any chemical can be registered for use as an insecticide in the USA, voluminous experimental data must be acquired with respect to its chemistry, toxicology, metabolism, effectiveness and residue evaluation procedures. As analytical methods for residue determination and metabolic pathway elucidation improve, and as public concern over pollution increases, the amount of data, and expense, needed to satisfy government regulations also increases. It has recently been estimated that the average cost of developing a new pesticide from the laboratory bench to the field is over $4 million[1].

Regardless of the economics involved, a variety of conditions and demands must be satisfied by a candidate insecticide. It must, of course, be toxic to insects; but preferably it should have some degree of selectivity, particularly against beneficial insects. The chemical as it is applied, and the metabolites formed, must be non-toxic to non-target organisms, particularly man and wildlife. It and any toxic metabolite should not persist in the environment, although they must persist long enough to give effective control. The candidate should be amenable to formulation and application and stable when mixed with other pesticides and diluents. It must be inexpensive to produce in large quantities so that its intended use is economically feasible. The chemical and its metabolites, in many cases, must be non-phytotoxic. Finally, a precise residue analysis method must be developed to allow determination of at least 1 p.p.m. of the candidate chemical.

After considering the above information, it is sometimes surprising that any insecticide becomes registered. However, several companies screen thousands of chemicals each year as potential insect control agents. The early era of synthetic insecticides was dominated by the organochlorine compounds, notably DDT. The environmental persistence of these compounds has led, in some cases, to restrictions on their use. The discovery of the more 'biodegradable' organophosphorus and carbamate insecticides has replaced, and will probably continue to replace, the organochlorines.

Of course, some of the problems associated with insecticide use could be overcome through the use of alternative control methods presently being investigated. The use of attractants, repellents, sterility, hormones, microbial pathogens, predators and parasites has met with some success. However, until these methods are refined and proved effective in the control of our major insect pests, insecticides will be needed. Thus it is imperative that efforts toward finding safer and more effective insecticides continue.

In this regard, certain of the carbamate insecticides appear to have a good future. Evidence to date indicates that, as a group, they are generally non-persistent in the environment and are relatively low in mammalian toxicity, with some exceptions. They are effective against a wide range of insects, but also exhibit selectivity, both among arthropods and between insects and mammals. Information on the metabolism of carbamates is abundant and continues to increase. These studies are necessary to insure that carbamates and their metabolites pose no threat to the survival of non-target organisms or to our total environment. This paper will briefly summarize the status of knowledge on carbamate metabolism and discuss further investigations that are needed. Other review articles have recently appeared and should be consulted for a complete picture of carbamate metabolism[2-8].

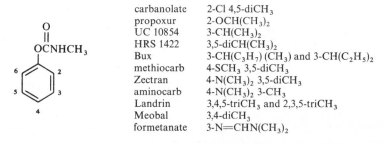

carbanolate	2-Cl 4,5-diCH$_3$
propoxur	2-OCH(CH$_3$)$_2$
UC 10854	3-CH(CH$_3$)$_2$
HRS 1422	3,5-diCH(CH$_3$)$_2$
Bux	3-CH(C$_3$H$_7$) (CH$_3$) and 3-CH(C$_2$H$_5$)$_2$
methiocarb	4-SCH$_3$ 3,5-diCH$_3$
Zectran	4-N(CH$_3$)$_2$ 3,5-diCH$_3$
aminocarb	4-N(CH$_3$)$_2$ 3-CH$_3$
Landrin	3,4,5-triCH$_3$ and 2,3,5-triCH$_3$
Meobal	3,4-diCH$_3$
formetanate	3-N=CHN(CH$_3$)$_2$

Figure 1. Structures of substituted phenyl methylcarbamate insecticide chemicals

The structures of carbamate insecticides derived from phenols are given in *Figure 1* and other carbamate structures are given in *Figure 2.* They will be referred to throughout the text by their common names.

200

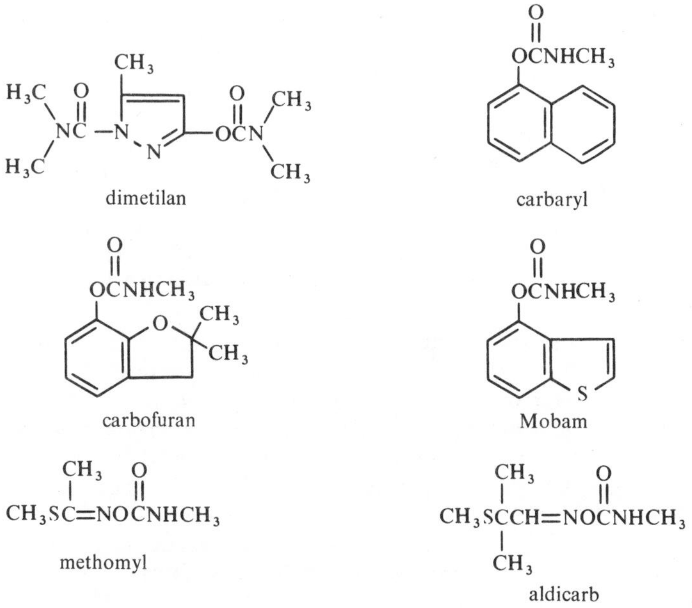

Figure 2. Structures of various methyl- and dimethylcarbamate insecticide chemicals

METABOLISM OF CARBAMATES IN MAMMALS, PLANTS AND INSECTS

A combination of hydrolysis, oxidation and conjugation govern the biological fate of a carbamate insecticide. In some species, hydrolysis or oxidation predominates, but both of these mechanisms are usually followed by conjugation. Rates of metabolism also vary with species, but generally the more efficient degradation, circulation and excretion systems present in mammals and insects result in a faster rate compared to plants[2]. Often, the metabolites formed in plants, mammals and insects are identical, although the conjugating moieties may differ. Whereas plants tend to accumulate metabolites, insects and mammals usually excrete them.

Hydrolysis

Initial carbamate degration studies concentrated on hydrolysis as the major metabolic mechanism. Later it was discovered that oxidation and conjugation probably play a greater role in metabolism, and hydrolysis was almost forgotten. However, it is important to consider carefully all of these degradation modes with each new carbamate insecticide and with each new test organism.

The majority of carbamates investigated are esters of methylcarbamic acid with various phenols and aliphatic oximes. These compounds are subject to hydrolysis as shown overleaf.

The methylcarbamic acid is believed to be biologically unstable, and breaks down to carbon dioxide and methylamine. Presumably the latter

201

$$\underset{R—OCNH—CH_3}{\overset{O}{\overset{\|}{}}} \longrightarrow ROH + \underset{HOCNH—CH_3}{\overset{O}{\overset{\|}{}}}$$

$$\longrightarrow CO_2 + H_2O + CH_3NH_2$$

partially degrades to carbon dioxide also. The fate of these hydrolysis products has received some attention. Usually the phenols are conjugated and the oximes are either conjugated or metabolized further as discussed below.

A number of experiments have shown that mammals and insects treated with *carbonyl-* or *methyl-*[14]C-labelled carbamates expire a certain percentage of the administered radioactivity as $^{14}CO_2$. Since most of the administered sodium [^{14}C]carbonate is rapidly expired from certain mammals[9, 10] and insects[11] as $^{14}CO_2$, the trapping of $^{14}CO_2$ released by an animal treated with a [*carbonyl-*[14]C]carbamate has been used to determine the amount of hydrolysis of the carbamate. However, 60 per cent of the ^{14}C from the sodium carbonate injected into bean plants is recovered as insoluble residues, probably due to incorporation of the $^{14}CO_2$ into natural plant constituents[12]. Incorporation of a low percentage of $^{14}CO_2$, resulting from carbamate hydrolysis, into natural animal products has been demonstrated[3, 10, 13]. [^{14}C]Methylamine also releases $^{14}CO_2$ after administration to rats[9] and bean plants[12], but probably not in houseflies[11]. However, most of the radioactivity is recovered as water-soluble materials or insoluble residues, both of which may represent natural products. In one instance, methylamine has been identified as a metabolite of carbanolate in rat urine[14]. Another possibility is that methyl isocyanate, an unstable precursor of methylcarbamic acid, transmethylcarbamoylates proteins or other natural products[9, 14, 15].

Hydrolysis appears to be more important in the degradation of carbamate insecticides in mammals than it is in plants or insects. Indeed this difference is partially responsible for the selective action of carbamates. Carbaryl is readily hydrolysed in the rat[9, 16, 17], guinea pig[17], sheep[18] and dog[19], but not in the monkey or pig[18]. Evidence also exists for hydrolysis of carbaryl in dairy cows[3] and rabbits[20]. The chemical structure of a carbamate can influence its hydrolysis rate. Thus in rats[9] one-fourth of the injected dose of carbaryl is hydrolysed compared with one-third for propoxur and three-fourths for isolan and Zectran. The latter is also extensively hydrolysed in dogs[21] and mice[22].

Other carbamates very susceptible to hydrolysis are Bux and Mobam. Approximately 65 per cent of the administered dose of each compound metabolizes via hydrolysis in the rat[23, 24]. Substantial hydrolysis of Mobam and Mobam sulphoxide also occurs in cows and goats[25]. Carbofuran and derivatives are hydrolysed in rats[26], mice[27] and cows[10]. About half of the administered ^{14}C from carbonyl-labelled carbanolate is expired from rats as $^{14}CO_2$[9, 14]. When rats were put under stress, the rate of carbanolate hydrolysis increased significantly but the degradation rate of methylamine to carbon dioxide was not changed[14]. Two carbamates fairly resistant to mammalian hydrolysis are Landrin, about 35 per cent in mice[28], and Meobal, about 30 per cent, probably much less, in rats[29]. However, extensive hydrolysis of Meobal oxidative metabolites occurs in the rat.

The oxime carbamates are also hydrolytically cleaved in mammals. In 24 h, a large percentage of orally administered [carbonyl-^{14}C]aldicarb is released from rats as [14]CO_2[30]. However, part of the carbon dioxide is from aldicarb sulphoxide and other oxidative metabolites[30, 31]. A number of the aldicarb products formed in dairy cows result from hydrolysis of parent compound and/or oxidative metabolites[32, 33]. Limited published information suggests that methomyl is rapidly hydrolysed in the rat[24].

Detoxication of carbamates by hydrolysis may not be as important in insects as it is in mammals. When nine methyl- and carbonyl-^{14}C-labelled carbamates were applied topically to houseflies, the only insecticides that yielded considerable [14]CO_2 were methiocarb (20–23 per cent) and carbanolate (15–20 per cent)[34]. Although the major metabolic pathway of carbaryl in the German cockroach is hydrolysis[35], this appears to be a minor pathway in American cockroaches[36] and cabbage loopers[37], and intermediate in boll weevils[38, 39], bollworms[38], cotton leaf worms[40], houseflies and rice weevils[39]. Houseflies detoxify propoxur[11] and Landrin[28] almost exclusively by oxidation and conjugation. Evidence indicates some hydrolysis of carbofuran in flies[26] and salt marsh caterpillars[27], of dimetilan in German cockroaches[41] and of aldicarb and its sulphoxide in houseflies[42], boll weevils, tobacco budworms and bollworms[43].

The carbamate ester bond appears to be quite stable in plants. Very little 1-naphthol, free or as a conjugate, is recovered from bean plants after injection or topical application of carbaryl[12, 44, 45]. Cotton plants seem to hydrolyse more carbaryl than do bean plants, but hydrolysis is probably not the major pathway[46]. A small amount of hydrolysis of carbofuran and its 3-hydroxy and 3-keto analogues takes place in bean[47] and cotton plants[27]. Carbanolate[12, 48] and Landrin[28] are not significantly hydrolysed in bean plants. The oxime carbamate, aldicarb, and particularly its sulphoxide, are prone to hydrolytic cleavage in cotton plants[42, 49–51]. In fact, the formation of the sulphoxide and subsequent hydrolysis of this material appears to be of prime importance in the metabolism of aldicarb in cotton[49]. Formetanate is slowly metabolized in orange seedlings with some hydrolysis evident, both of the parent compound and metabolites[52]. The only plant in which hydrolysis was found to be the major metabolic pathway is broccoli, where Zectran is extensively converted into its phenol, which is subsequently degraded[53]. Limited information suggests that methomyl is transformed rapidly in plants to small fragments, acetonitrile, carbon dioxide and methylamine, all of which are probably incorporated into natural plant components[24]. The sulphoxide and sulphone of methomyl apparently are not formed.

Thus it is evident that hydrolysis must be considered when investigating the fate of a carbamate insecticide. As pointed out briefly above, not only the parent compound but oxidative metabolites which still possess the carbamate moiety are subject to hydrolysis. In fact, with some compounds such as aldicarb, Meobal and carbofuran, hydrolysis of the oxidative metabolites is much more important than hydrolysis of the parent compound.

Not too much work has been done to characterize the enzymes responsible for carbamate hydrolysis. Although cholinesterases and aliesterases apparently decarbamylate certain carbamates, it is unlikely that these enzymes could be responsible for the large amount of hydrolysis that occurs with some compounds. Plasma albumin has been shown to hydrolyse certain carbamates[54, 55], whereas the hydrolysis of p-nitrophenyl methylcarbamate is not catalysed by human plasma cholinesterase or arylesterase, chymotrypsin, trypsin, pepsin, papain, lipase or egg albumin[55]. Relatively non-specific esterases have been proposed as the responsible agent for carbamate hydrolysis in insects[56, 57] and this may be true for mammals and plants as well. However, non-enzymic factors could catalyse hydrolysis, particularly in plants. Hydrolytic products may also be detected as a result of drastic analysis procedures or because of the innate instability of intermediate metabolites.

Oxidation

Over the past ten years, the importance of oxidation of carbamate insecticides as a metabolic mechanism has been fully realized. Much of this work involved the use of systems in vitro, which generally limit hydrolysis and conjugation and allow isolation of the oxidation products. Important reactions include hydroxylation, epoxidation, N-dealkylation, O-dealkylation and sulphoxidation. Hydroxylation may take place on the carbamate or ring N-methyl groups, on the aromatic ring or on ring substituents, especially at a benzylic carbon atom. Many of the oxidative metabolites from a particular carbamate formed in mammals, insects and plants are identical.

Hydroxylation of carbaryl in the 4- and 5-positions of the aromatic ring occurs in a number of insects[7, 36, 37, 58–60], plants[12, 44–46] and mammals[17, 18, 20, 36, 61–63], and recently it was shown that hydroxylation also takes place in the 7-position in bean plants[45]. In fact, 7-hydroxycarbaryl may have been a metabolite in a number of other systems but was not properly identified since it chromatographs with hydroxymethylcarbaryl in the commonly used chromatography procedure[45]. The phenyl ring of propoxur is hydroxylated in the 5-position in insects[11, 64], mammals[63] and probably plants[12]. Landrin-2,3,5 and Landrin-3,4,5 form their 4-hydroxy and 2-hydroxy analogues respectively, in mammal and insect enzyme systems[28]. Some of these metabolites are illustrated in Figure 3A.

Benzylic carbon hydroxylation is of prime importance in the metabolism of carbofuran. The resulting 3-hydroxy analogue is found in plants[27, 47], insects[26, 27] and mammals[10, 26, 27]. Further oxidation results in the formation of 3-keto carbofuran. Ring methyl groups of Landrin are hydroxylated in vivo in houseflies and bean plants, and in mice the oxidation continues to the benzoic acid derivatives[28]. Hydroxymethyl and benzoic acid derivatives of Meobal are metabolites in white rats[29]. In each case, either the hydroxymethyl or benzoic acid metabolite may be conjugated or hydrolysed with subsequent conjugation. Thus the potential number of metabolites is much larger than it is for some of the simpler aryl methylcarbamates. Enzymatic hydroxylation does not seem to be sterically hindered, as evidence by attack on the isopropyl group of UC 10854[12, 63] and the 1-methylbutyl group of Bux[24]. A few of these hydroxy derivatives are shown in Figure 3B.

In a similar manner, the tertiary carbon atom of the isopropoxy group of propoxur is hydroxylated in houseflies[11, 59, 64], rat liver microsomes[62, 63]

CARBAMATE INSECTICIDE METABOLITES AS TERMINAL RESIDUES

A. *Ring Hydroxylation*

7-hydroxy
carbaryl

5-hydroxy
propoxur

4-hydroxy
Landrin

B. *Benzylic Carbon Hydroxylation*

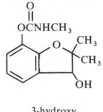

3-hydroxy
carbofuran

3-hydroxymethyl
Meobal

1-methyl-1-hydroxybutyl
Bux

C. *Propoxyl Hydroxylation and Decomposition*

propoxur → unstable → O-depropyl propoxur + acetone

$+ (CH_3)_2C{=}O$

D. *Carbamate N-Methyl Hydroxylation*

hydroxymethyl
carbanolate

hydroxymethyl
UC10854

hydroxymethyl
Zectran

E. *N-Dealkylation*

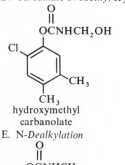

methylamino
aminocarb

demethyl
formetanate

methylamido
dimetilan

Figure 3. Examples of carbamate insecticide metabolites formed by hydroxylation

205

and bean plants[12]. However, an unstable compound [o-(1-hydroxy-2-propoxy)phenyl methylcarbamate] results, which rapidly decomposes to acetone and the respective phenol[11, 65], the latter being the recovered metabolite (*Figure 3C*).

All of the methyl- and dimethylcarbamates have one potential oxidative site in common, namely, the carbamate N-methyl group. Plants metabolize carbanolate[12], carbaryl[12, 44, 45], carbofuran[47], Landrin[28], propoxur[12] and UC 10854[12] to their respective hydroxymethyl derivatives (*Figure 3D*). Mammalian enzymes catalyse carbamate N-methyl hydroxylation of aminocarb[62, 63], Bux[24], carbanolate[62, 63], carbaryl[20, 36, 61–63], carbofuran[10, 26, 27], HRS 1422[63], propoxur[62, 63], UC 10854[63] and Zectran[62, 63]. With the exception of Bux and UC 10854, all of these insecticides form hydroxymethyl derivatives in insects as well[7, 11, 26–28, 36–38, 41, 54, 55, 60, 66, 67]. Dimetilan, and some other dimethylcarbamates, are hydroxylated on one of the carbamate N-methyl groups by mammalian enzymes[68, 69] and insects[41]. In some cases, the hydroxymethyl analogues are relatively unstable and it is possible that they are not detected as metabolites because of this. Very few of the demethyl derivatives (N-dealkylation) have been isolated; either they are not formed, possibly because of conjugation of the hydroxymethyl intermediate, or they are unstable. The oxime carbamates may be less susceptible to this type of degradation.

Hydroxylation of ring N-methyl groups appears to be an analogous reaction, but the hydroxymethyl derivatives are not usually isolated. Instead, formamido derivatives are. Thus the p-dimethylamino group of aminocarb and Zectran is demethylated, presumably through the hydroxymethyl form (unstable) and the formamido form in plants[12, 70], insects[59, 64, 66] and mammals[62, 63] as shown:

$$R-N\begin{array}{c}CH_3\\ \diagdown\\CH_3\end{array} \longrightarrow \left[R-N\begin{array}{c}CH_2OH\\ \diagdown\\CH_3\end{array}\right] \longrightarrow R-N\begin{array}{c}CHO\\ \diagdown\\CH_3\end{array} \longrightarrow R-N\begin{array}{c}H\\ \diagdown\\CH_3\end{array}$$

The same reaction may then proceed on the other N-methyl group. More removed N-dealkylation occurs with formetanate in orange seedlings[52] and rats[71] and with dimetilan in insects[41] and rats[62, 63] (*Figure 3E*).

Oxidation of the sulphur atom occurs with methiocarb in bean plants[70], in rat liver microsomes[62, 63] and by housefly enzymes[59]. Mammals treated with Mobam excrete 4-benzothienyl sulphate-1-oxide in the urine, but it is not apparent whether sulphoxidation takes place before hydrolysis of Mobam. Probably the most important reaction of aldicarb in insects[42, 43], plants[42, 49–51, 72] and mammals[30–33] involves sulphoxidation to the sulphoxide, and less to the sulphone. Some of these metabolites are shown in *Figure 4A*.

Limited evidence suggests that carbaryl undergoes epoxidation as an intermediate in the formation of its metabolite, 5,6-dihydro-5,6-dihydroxycarbaryl (*Figure 4B*). This metabolite is then subject to degradation and

CARBAMATE INSECTICIDE METABOLITES AS TERMINAL RESIDUES

A. *Sulphoxidation*

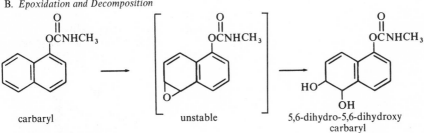

methiocarb sulphone

aldicarb sulphoxide

Mobam sulphate-1-oxide

B. *Epoxidation and Decomposition*

carbaryl   unstable   5,6-dihydro-5,6-dihydroxy carbaryl

C. *Conjugation of Primary Metabolites*

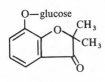

glucoside of
3-keto carbofuran phenol

glucuronide of
Mobam phenol

sulphate of
4-hydroxy carbaryl

D. *Postulated Conjugation of Original Carbamates*

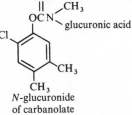

N-glucuronide
of carbanolate

O-glucuronide
of carbaryl

N-glucoside
of formetanate

E. *UV Irradiation Products*

C-8353
phenol

C-8353
aldehyde

C-8353
cyclic product

Figure 4. Examples of carbamate insecticide metabolites formed by oxidation, conjugation and photodegradation

207

may convert into the 5-hydroxy metabolite. These are well-known products of carbaryl in mammals[20, 61-63, 73], plants[12, 44, 45] and insects[7, 36-38, 58, 60].

The primary enzyme system(s) responsible for the catalysis of insecticide oxidations in mammals and insects is a mixed-function oxidase(s) (mfo) requiring NADPH and oxygen[7, 8, 74-79]. In mammals, the primary location of the mfo system is in the liver, whereas in insects the fat body and/or gut appear to be the main sites of metabolism. Studies with mammalian liver *in vitro* usually involve a discrete centrifugal fraction, the microsomes, which contains cytochrome *P*-450. Microsomal sediments from whole insects or insect tissues are less discrete, but cytochrome *P*-450 has been found in these fractions as well as in tissue homogenates. This cytochrome, together with the mfo system, forms an active-oxygen complex, which is believed to be the attacking species in many oxidations. The action of this system is inhibited by a variety of insecticide synergists and by carbon monoxide. The level of mfo activity varies with respect to species, age, sex, diet and history of exposure to other chemicals.

In plants, much less is known about the oxidative enzymes, principally because procedures *in vitro* have not been developed. Recent studies with plant tissues and subcellular fractions from these tissues have demonstrated hydroxylation[80], *N*-dealkylation[81], epoxidation[82, 83] and the 'NIH shift'[84]. Aldrin epoxidase activity in pea root homogenates appears to be present in the 'soluble' fraction rather than the 'microsome' fraction and does not require NADPH[82]. On the other hand, bean root fractions oxidize aldrin to its epoxide and diol in a manner characteristic of an mfo system[83]. A microsomal preparation from cotton hypocotyl extracts that *N*-demethylates substituted 3-(phenyl)-1-methylureas has many of the characteristics of a typical animal mixed-function oxidase[81]. However, oxidation of carbamates by plants *in vitro* has not yet been accomplished.

As with hydrolysis, investigators should be mindful of the fact that some recovered oxidation products may result from the analytical procedures used to isolate metabolites. It is also likely, particularly with the sulphur-containing carbamates, that a certain amount of non-enzymic oxidation may take place both *in vivo* and *in vitro*.

Conjugation

For lipophilic toxicants to be eliminated from an insect or mammal they must be converted into a more water-soluble form. This conversion is achieved through hydrolysis and oxidation, followed by conjugation with sugars, uronic acids, phosphoric acid, sulphuric acid and amino acids. Similar transformations take place in plants, but the resulting conjugates are stored rather than excreted. This important aspect of carbamate metabolism has received little attention to date. Perhaps part of the reason is the fact that conjugation is generally not a factor until after primary metabolism of the carbamate, i.e. hydrolysis and oxidation. Also, the water-soluble nature of these products makes isolation and identification more difficult. In most cases the water-soluble materials are hydrolysed with acids or an array of enzymes to release the organosoluble insecticide residue, which can be identified. This procedure, particularly with acid, tells little about the conjugating moiety, or indeed, if conjugation, as opposed to 'binding' or 'multihydroxylation', or incomplete extraction has taken place. In addition, acid conditions may alter the carbamate portion of the conjugate.

Cleavage of water-soluble conjugates with β-glucosidase, β-glucuronidase, aryl sulphatase, glusulase, acid phosphatase and alkaline phosphatase, prepared from various sources, has been demonstrated in many of the above-listed metabolism studies. However, it is important to realize that many of these enzyme preparations contain minor amounts of other hydrolases. For example, β-glucuronidase preparations from *Helix pomatia* hydrolyse ethereal sulphates, glucosides, glucuronides and phosphates; bovine β-glucuronidase hydrolyses glucuronides and glucosides[85]. Other glucuronidase preparations also contain a combination of hydrolytic enzymes[86]. Almond emulsion preparations of β-glucosidase probably contain a number of glycosidases, as well as glucuronidase, and β-glucosidase can cleave glycosides other than β-glucose conjugates[12]. Screening of some readily available carbohydrases indicated that carbaryl conjugates from bean plants could be partially hydrolysed (30–50 per cent) by maltase and pectinase preparations and effectively hydrolysed (50–80 per cent) by cellulase and glusulase, but not (less than five per cent) by amylase, amyloglucosidase, hemicellulase and invertase[87]. Most of these enzymes were crude preparations so that it is not known which hydrolase or combination of hydrolases was responsible for conjugate cleavage.

In some cases the identity of the conjugates has been confirmed (*Figure 4C*). The glucoside of 3-keto-carbofuran phenol from cotton plants and insects has been characterized by mass spectrometry and infra-red analysis[27]. Sulphate and β-glucuronide conjugates of Mobam phenol were isolated from the rat and identified by gel filtration, liquid ion-exchange, paper and gas–liquid chromatography[23]. Sulphate and β-glucuronide conjugates of carbaryl metabolites isolated from chicken urine were identified by acylation, ultra-violet and infra-red analysis, and mass spectrometry[88].

Additional evidence for the nature of conjugates has been obtained through the use of synthesis *in vitro*. Mammalian liver homogenates and microsomal preparations fortified with uridine diphosphoglucuronic acid (UDPGA) and NADPH, in the presence of carbaryl, form glucuronides of 1-naphthol and 4-hydroxycarbaryl[17]. Rat liver microsome plus soluble fractions have been incubated with carbaryl metabolites in the presence of glucuronide (UDPGA), glutathione or sulphate-conjugating systems[20]. Little or no glutathione conjugates were formed, but conjugation did occur in the UDPGA and sulphate systems.

Recently, a conjugating system has been shown to be active in rat liver microsomes when fortified with UDPGA and NADPH (necessary for oxidation but not conjugation)[89]. In fact, the rate of overall metabolism seems to be dependent on the rate of conjugation. Synergists that block mfo activity also inhibit the conjugating system. Tobacco hornworm tissue homogenates fortified with UDPGA do not form 1-naphthol conjugates, but, in the presence of uridine diphosphoglucose, a glucoside is produced. Organs other than the liver may be involved in glucuronide formation. For example, rat small intestine will hydrolyse carbaryl and conjugate the released 1-naphthol[90].

These limited studies, plus knowledge of plant and animal biochemistry, suggest that certain oxidative and hydrolytic metabolites of carbamates are conjugated as β-glucuronides in mammals and as β-glucosides or other glycosides in plants and insects. Sulphates seem more likely to occur in mammals whereas phosphates may be more common in insects. Plants may not form either. All are capable of amino acid conjugation. However, differences in conjugation rates may be important. For example, ring-hydroxymethyl derivatives of Landrin are oxidized to the acid analogues before conjugation in rats, whereas houseflies and bean plants presumably conjugate the hydroxymethyl compound before further oxidation can take place[28].

Perhaps the most important, and potentially hazardous, conjugation involves direct conjugation of the parent carbamate (*Figure 4D*). There is evidence for the formation of an *O*- and *N*-glucuronide of carbaryl in several mammals[17, 18] and possibly in chickens[88]. Rats appear to form an *N*-glucuronide of carbanolate[14]. Direct conjugation of formetanate may occur in plants[52] and animals[71], and conjugation of carbaryl with sugars has been implied from studies with bean plants[12]. Recent findings indicate that carbaryl and its metabolites form pi complexes with certain flavonoid plant pigments[91]. These complexes, which can be decomposed with acid, may represent a significant portion of the water-soluble products recovered from plants treated with carbaryl. However, it is not known if these materials result from extraction procedures or if such binding occurs *in vivo*.

In almost all investigations that employ radiolabelled carbamates, a certain percentage of the radiotracer is not recovered, i.e. is unextractable or insoluble. As discussed earlier, when the label is ^{14}C in the carbamic acid portion, the resulting degradation products are expired and/or incorporated into normal biochemical pathways. However, unextractable products from carbamates labelled in the phenolic portion are more difficult to explain. In broccoli, 18 per cent of the applied Zectran ^{14}C is incorporated into lignin, probably as catechol derivatives formed after hydrolysis of Zectran[53]. It was suggested that lignin incorporation may serve as a permanent storage facility for toxic materials. Radioactivity from [1-^{14}C]naphthol injected into bean plants is rapidly incorporated into insoluble residues[12]. However, the amount of insoluble radioactivity in bean plants injected with carbaryl labelled in the ring or carbamate portion is almost the same, suggesting that some of these unextractable materials may still possess the carbamate moiety[12, 44]. On a long-term basis it appears that water-soluble metabolites are converted into insoluble products, which may represent 75 per cent of the injected carbaryl[44]. It is also possible that intact carbamates and/or their hydroxymethyl analogues carbamolate proteins, forming relatively stable carbamoyl–protein bonds, which would result in insolubility[63]. Finally, a certain portion of these insolubles may only arise because of inefficient homogenization and/or extraction procedures.

METABOLISM OF CARBAMATES IN HUMANS AND VARIOUS OTHER ANIMALS

The metabolic fate of carbaryl in humans is similar to that discussed for other mammals. After oral ingestion by men of 2 mg/kg of this insecticide, the 4-hydroxy and 1-naphthyl glucuronide and 1-naphthyl sulphate were present in the urine during the first 24 h[18]. After three days no metabolites could be found. Autopsy of a man who had ingested a fatal dose of carbaryl revealed the presence of one metabolite in the stomach, three in the intestines, four in the liver and kidney, and five in the urine, with carbaryl present in all these organs[92]. Metabolites of propoxur in urine from humans include the parent phenol and its glucuronide conjugate[93].

Human liver homogenates catalyse the formation of methiocarb sulphone (the sulphoxide was not detected), the hydroxylation of carbaryl in the 4- and 5-positions, the dealkylation of the ring dimethylamino groups of aminocarb and Zectran, and the hydroxylation of the carbamate N-methyl group of aminocarb, carbaryl and Zectran[94]. Comparative studies between rat and human liver homogenates demonstrated some differences, notably the formation of more metabolites by human liver. Cell cultures derived from normal human embryonic lung tissue have been used to examine carbaryl metabolism[95]. A monolayer of 3–4 million cells completely metabolizes 10 p.p.m. of carbaryl in three days. The major metabolite recovered is the hydrolysis product of 4-hydroxycarbaryl. Other metabolites postulated are N-glucuronides of 4-hydroxy- and 5,6-dihydro-5,6-dihydroxycarbaryl. Introduction of piperonyl butoxide into the culture medium does not effect carbaryl metabolism. The procedure offers a potential tool for preliminary investigation of pesticide metabolism.

The degradation of carbamates in animals other than mammals has not been extensively investigated. Chickens treated with carbaryl excrete at least 15 metabolites in urine[88]. Those identified include 1-naphthol and its sulphate and glucuronic acid conjugates, the sulphate conjugates of 4- and 5-hydroxycarbaryl, and other conjugates of 5,6-dihydroxycarbaryl and its phenol, 1,5-naphthalenediol, 4- and 5-hydroxycarbaryl, and two of carbaryl itself. Perhaps most interesting is the partial identification of the dihydroxy derivative of carbaryl, which has not been characterized in any previous carbaryl studies. A metabolite of aldicarb formed in laying hens, the hydroxymethyl analogue of aldicarb sulphone, has not been reported as a mammalian metabolite of this insecticide[3].

Carbaryl is predominantly hydrolysed in the cattle tick, but oxidative metabolites are also produced[96]. Although no 4-hydroxycarbaryl was identified, evidence indicates attack on the 5-position and on the hydroxymethyl group and formation of the 5,6-dihydro-5,6-dihydroxy derivative. Interestingly, these metabolites were present as water-soluble products that were cleaved by acid but not by glusulase. Preliminary data reveal that grey garden slugs oxidize carbaryl to products identical with those isolated from mammals[97].

DEGRADATION OF CARBAMATES BY SOIL AND LIGHT

The biodegradable nature of many of the carbamate insecticides suggests that they would be relatively non-persistent in most soils. Since few of the aryl methylcarbamates are used as systemics, published information on their fate in soils is limited. The predominant isomer of Bux is rapidly hydrolysed in soil with a half-life of approximately one week[24]. Granular formulation extends the half-life to three weeks and there is little translocation of insecticide or metabolites. The only metabolite identified was m-(1-methyl 1-hydroxybutyl)phenyl methylcarbamate.

Thirty days after applying methomyl to the soil, 50–75 per cent of the material had dissipated. In laboratory studies it took 42 days for soil to degrade half of the applied dose to unextractable materials (15 per cent) and volatile materials[24]. Aldicarb mixed with soil at a rate of 2 mg/100 g of soil and placed in the field was almost gone after one week, transforming into ten metabolites, three of which have not been found in plant studies[50]. The major breakdown product is aldicarb sulphoxide. After eight weeks, 86 per cent of the metabolites was lost by volatilization and translocation. Broadcast application of this insecticide results in rapid dissipation with 22 per cent of the dose left in the top six inches of soil, mostly as the sulphoxide and sulphone, after two months[72]. When aldicarb was mixed with three soil types (20 p.p.m.) and held in sealed bottles in the dark, its half-life ranged from nine to twelve days[51]. In three months, over 95 per cent of the aldicarb had metabolized, mostly to its sulphoxide. This metabolite is very stable in the soil and is not hydrolysed to its oxime. A large percentage of the applied dose was not extractable from the soil samples. Application to potting soils open to the atmosphere resulted in a more rapid rate of degradation.

Insecticides applied to the soil or plant surfaces are often exposed to sunlight and thus subject to photodecomposition. Ethanol or hexane solutions of five methylcarbamate insecticides irradiated with sunlight or ultra-violet light for 3 h all form decomposition products that inhibit human plasma cholinesterase[98]. Propoxur appears quite stable to light, while carbaryl only forms one inhibitory material unless subjected to intense u.v. irradiation. However, solid carbaryl or a 50 per cent w.p. formulation degrades to only one inhibitor even under prolonged exposure to intense ultra-violet light. Products other than cholinesterase inhibitors were not identified in these studies. Other work shows that formulated carbaryl slowly degrades to several unidentified materials after exposure to u.v. light or sunlight[99]. Isolan (1-isopropyl-3-methyl-5-pyrazolyl dimethylcarbamate) and pyrolan (1-phenyl-3-methyl-5-pyrazolyl dimethylcarbamate) yield several unidentified products when exposed to ultra-violet light on paper[100].

When eight methylcarbamates were placed on silica-gel plates, no degradation products formed under fluorescent light or long-wavelength ultra-violet light[70]. However, every insecticide except carbaryl produced two or more products when exposed to short-wavelength u.v. light. Modifications of the 4-dimethylamino group of aminocarb and Zectran account for most of their degradation products[101], while methiocarb forms its sulphoxide and sulphone plus four other materials[70]. On bean leaves, propoxur and UC 10854 form few, if any, breakdown products and they are rapidly lost from the plant surface. On the other hand, methiocarb is much more residual with a surface half-life of more than three days. Carbaryl, carbanolate and HRS 1422 are also persistent and few degradation products appear on leaf surfaces. In these studies no attempt was made to determine the amount of penetration of parent compound or metabolites into the leaves. A recent report shows that carbaryl does partially penetrate plant leaves, where it is subject to hydrolysis, oxidation and conjugation[45]. In sixteen days, 70 per cent of the applied dose was lost from the leaf surfaces.

Crystalline carbofuran subjected to two days of sunlight is converted into its 3-hydroxy derivative[27]. After two and one-half weeks, three other products become evident, one of which is probably carbofuran phenol. Thin-layer plates containing carbofuran exposed to fluorescent light also yield the 3-hydroxy compound. However, further oxidation to the 3-keto analogue does not occur after two weeks of exposure. Landrin is not hydrolysed on bean foliage held in sunlight and the parent compound is not present after four days[28]. Hydroxylation products involving attack on the ring-methyl and N-methyl groups are the major products formed.

Although many of the u.v. products separated in these studies are unidentified, those that have been characterized are identical with the oxidation products formed in living systems. However, this may not always be the case. Ultra-violet irradiation of Ciba's 2-(1,3-dioxolane-2-yl)phenyl methyl-carbamate (C-8353) in methanol results in almost complete conversion into a cyclic derivative whereas photolysis in water yields the parent phenol and a benzaldehyde derivative[102] (*Figure 4E*). Whether all these conversions take place in living systems is not known.

TOXICITY OF CARBAMATE METABOLITES

To evaluate the safety of a pesticide, not only must metabolites be identified, but the toxicity of these metabolites must also be evaluated. Then, if necessary, residue procedures can be developed which detect toxic metabolites as well as parent toxicant. This is particularly true when pesticides are applied to plants and soils where residues come in contact with, or are ingested by, man and other animals. In many cases, the level of metabolite is extremely small compared with the applied chemical, but care should be taken before these levels are called insignificant.

In general, hydrolysis of the carbamate ester bond results in detoxication. As illustrated above, the carbamate moiety rapidly decomposes to carbon dioxide and methylamine, while the phenolic portion, generally non-toxic *per se*, is conjugated and excreted. Unlike the organophosphorus insecticides, oxidation of carbamates rarely enhances the toxicity with respect to the parent compound. However, this does occur on occasion, which emphasizes the importance of toxicological studies of metabolites. The potential hazard

Table 1. Toxicity of carbaryl and some of its metabolites

	LD_{50} (mg/kg)		7-day no-effect level (mg/kg) Rat[45]	Molar I_{50} bovine anticholinesterase[3]
	Rat acute oral[45]	Mouse i.p.[36, 104]		
Carbaryl	270	29–42	125–250	5×10^{-8}
4-Hydroxycarbaryl	1190	74	>1000	4×10^{-7}
5-Hydroxycarbaryl	297	56	>1000	$4 \cdot 6 \times 10^{-8}$
7-Hydroxycarbaryl	4760		>1000	
Hydroxymethylcarbaryl	>5000	630–780	250–500	$1 \cdot 4 \times 10^{-5}$
1-Naphthol	2590		500–1000	1×10^{-3}

of conjugates of oxidative metabolites or, particularly, of unchanged carbamates and of products designated in studies as insoluble residues should be considered.

Considerable attention has been given to the toxic nature of metabolites of carbaryl, the most widely used methylcarbamate insecticide. Much of this data appears in *Table 1* with appropriate references. Many of the known metabolites, with the exception of 5-hydroxycarbaryl, are much less toxic to rats on an acute oral basis and are less potent cholinesterase inhibitors. Mouse intraperitoneal injection indicates a relatively high toxicity of the 4- and 5-hydroxy compounds, but it is less than that of carbaryl. All of the metabolites, including the ring-hydroxy analogues, are less detrimental than carbaryl in short-term feeding studies. The 'no-ill effect' level for hydroxymethylcarbaryl after 90 day feeding studies is approximately equivalent to carbaryl[45]. Another metabolite, 5,6-dihydro-5,6-dihydroxycarbaryl, is only one-fifth as potent an anticholinesterase agent as carbaryl[73]. All metabolites are less toxic to houseflies[20]. In one study carbaryl water-soluble metabolites recovered from bean plants were fed to rats[44]. Within 96 h. approximately 96 per cent of the total dose was excreted in the urine and faeces.

Table 2. Toxicity of Zectran and some of its metabolites[101]

	Cholinesterase pI_{50}		Mouse LD_{50} (mg/kg)	
	Human plasma	Fly head	i.p.	Dermal
Zectran	6.0	8.1	4.2	107
Methylformamido Zectran	5.0	6.9	23	1000
Methylamino Zectran	6.7	7.8	1.4	8
Formamido Zectran	5.5	6.8	18	1000
Amino Zectran	5.8	7.5	1.6	7

The biological activity of metabolites of Zectran and aminocarb resulting from attack on the dimethylamino constituent has been examined[101]. The data in *Table 2* are only for Zectran but aminocarb values are similar, although less toxic in each instance. Formamido derivatives are less potent cholinesterase inhibitors and less toxic to mice than are the parent or the amino derivatives. Mouse toxicity of the methylamino and amino analogues is greater than it is for Zectran, particularly on dermal application. The carbamate hydroxymethyl metabolites of Zectran and aminocarb are considerably less toxic than the original insecticides[103]. All of these analogues possess reduced activity toward houseflies compared with that of the parent insecticides. Thus residue methods for these two carbamates should detect the dimethylamino degradation products. Demethylation of the formetanate dimethylamino group, not attached directly to the ring, leads to less potent human plasma and housefly cholinesterase inhibitors[71]. None of the dimethylamino-modified dimetilan metabolites recovered from American cockroaches is more toxic to houseflies than dimetilan itself[41].

Oxidative and hydrolytic metabolites of propoxur formed in houseflies are all less toxic to this insect. The 3-hydroxy, 3-keto, hydroxymethyl and

3-keto-hydroxymethyl metabolites of carbofuran have less insecticidal action against houseflies and mosquitoes than does carbofuran[27]. Fly head cholinesterase inhibition is also lower with the metabolites. A conjugate of 3-hydroxycarbofuran has human plasma anticholinesterase activity with an I_{50} value of 3.6×10^{-6} M for fly head cholinesterase compared with 1.4×10^{-6} M for the unconjugated metabolite and 2.5×10^{-7} M for carbofuran. This indicates that conjugated metabolites with the carbamate portion intact may still possess toxic potential, especially if they are not rapidly excreted. Anticholinesterase activity of carbofuran, 3-hydroxycarbofuran and 3-keto carbofuran were reported to be higher in another study[26].

In studies involving the synthesis of a wide variety of potential carbamate metabolites, the anticholinesterase activity and male mouse intraperitoneal toxicity of many of these compounds was determined[103, 104]. The carbamate hydroxymethyl analogues of propoxur, UC 10854, HRS 1422, Landrin, aminocarb, Zectran and carbanolate are all generally less toxic, and usually much less toxic, than their parents. Ring-hydroxylated products of carbaryl, propoxur, UC 10854, HRS 1422 and Zectran are often more potent anticholinesterase agents, but have reduced toxicity to mice, with the exception of 4-hydroxy HRS 1422. Hydroxylation of the isopropyl group of UC 10854 does not alter its biological activity. The differences between cholinesterase activity and toxicity are probably related to the susceptibility of the aryl hydroxy position to conjugation in the mouse. However, conjugation of 4-hydroxy HRS 1422 may be sterically hindered.

One of the primary metabolites of aldicarb, the sulphoxide, is probably responsible for its long-lasting systemic properties and toxicity. As shown in *Table 3*, aldicarb sulphoxide is a more potent anticholinesterase agent than aldicarb itself. The sulphone also retains considerable anticholinesterase activity. On the other hand, the hydrolysis products are ineffective inhibitors. The alcohol, acid and amide metabolites formed from aldicarb sulphoxide and sulphone are relatively non-toxic, based on rat acute oral results[49].

Table 3. Toxicity of aldicarb and some of its metabolites

	LD$_{50}$ (mg/kg)	Cholinesterase molar I$_{50}$		
	Rat acute oral[105, 107]	Plasma[106]	Blood cells[43, 106]	Fly head[42, 43, 106, 107]
Aldicarb	1	5×10^{-6}	$1.2–1.8 \times 10^{-5}$	$1.0–8.4 \times 10^{-5}$
Aldicarb sulphoxide	1	5×10^{-7}	$8 –8.1 \times 10^{-7}$	$0.8–1.1 \times 10^{-6}$
Aldicarb sulphone	10	1×10^{-5}	$1.3–4.9 \times 10^{-5}$	$2.5–5.0 \times 10^{-6}$
Aldicarb oxime				$>1.0 \times 10^{-3}$

Aldicarb is one of the most toxic carbamate insecticides, having an acute oral LD$_{50}$ to rats of approximately 1 mg/kg and a dermal LD$_{50}$ to rabbits of 5 mg/kg[105]. The sulphoxide is equally toxic to the rat, but the sulphone is only one-tenth as toxic as aldicarb. After an oral dose of 0.33 mg/kg to rats, plasma, red blood cell and brain cholinesterase activity is depressed almost equally by aldicarb or aldicarb sulphoxide. However, aldicarb-treated rats recovered from inhibitions 2 h before the sulphoxide-treated rats. Intraperitoneal injection of this dose of aldicarb sulphoxide causes severe symptoms and sometimes death[31]. Rats fed daily doses of cow's milk containing aldicarb metabolites regularly excreted about 90 per cent of the administered dose in the urine[32]. Five days after treatment ceased, 96 per cent of the total milk metabolites had been excreted from the rats without significant additional degradation. One product was present in the rat urine that had not been detected in the cow's milk.

Topical application of the sulphoxide and sulphone of aldicarb to insects generally results in a lower toxicity for the oxidized analogues, although they are more effective cholinesterase inhibitors *in vitro* (*Table 3*). However, as suggested by many, the decreased lipid solubility of the sulphoxidation products compared with aldicarb probably slows their penetration through the insect cuticle. The toxicity of these products applied to flies via baits or injection is not greatly different[106]. Certain lepidopterous larvae are very tolerant to relatively large concentrations of aldicarb, even after injection[43]. The predominant metabolic products formed are toxic compounds, particularly aldicarb sulphoxide. Cholinesterase activity *in vitro* of larval homogenates does not appear to be inhibited by aldicarb, aldicarb sulphoxide or aldicarb sulphone. Methiocarb sulphoxidation reduces both insect toxicity and cholinesterase inhibition[34].

Thus it is apparent that certain carbamate metabolites can possess equal or greater toxic properties than do the original esters. Residue methods for carbamate detection often depend on an organosoluble extraction, which does not remove the water-soluble and insoluble products. These materials are often the predominant metabolites, although most of them are probably non-toxic. The large number of minor, unidentified products that are anticholinesterase agents found in several studies should receive additional attention.

Carbamates, other than aryl methylcarbamates, have been developed as herbicides and fungicides. One compound, dichlormate (3,4-dichlorobenzyl methylcarbamate), is quite similar in structure to the insecticidal carbamates. Metabolism studies with bean plants[108] and rats[109] indicate that its degradation is similar to that of the insecticides. Bean plants hydrolyse the herbicide to its benzyl alcohol, which is conjugated or oxidized to its benzoic acid, the latter also subject to conjugation. Hydroxylation occurs on the carbamate *N*-methyl group and probably on the ring in the 2-position. The metholyl derivative is conjugated, demethylated or hydrolysed. In the rat, hydrolysis, oxidation and conjugation are also involved. No ring-hydroxy or hydroxymethyl derivatives were identified, however. An additional metabolite, not found in beans, 3,4-dichlorohippuric acid, offers an interesting deviation from carbamate insecticide metabolites.

CONCLUSIONS

It is hoped that the preceding discussion will give the reader an appreciation for the important roles hydrolysis, oxidation and conjugation play in the biochemical transformation of a carbamate insecticide chemical. These metabolic mechanisms appear to be present in most plants and animals and their efficiency contributes appreciably to the selectivity and biodegradability of insecticidal carbamates. Non-enzymic mechanisms, such as photoalteration, and exposure to wind, heat, humidity and rainfall, may also contribute to degradation, particularly when the insecticide is applied to plants or soils.

In most instances the metabolites identified thus far are less toxic than their parent compounds, but there are exceptions. However, a large number of metabolites have not been fully characterized and their potential hazard as residues remains undetermined. Often these unknowns are minor products, but whether or not they are 'significant' is open to question. Generally, hydrolysis results in detoxication, but oxidation, particularly sulphoxidation, may increase toxicity. Conjugation in animals facilitates excretion of toxic materials whereas in plants conjugates are stored for a considerable length of time. Limited information implies that ingestion of animal or plant conjugates by mammals leads to rapid elimination of the intact conjugates. However, considerably more study is needed to ensure that these water-soluble products, especially those retaining the carbamate moiety, represent safe residues.

Studies with mammals and insects *in vitro* have established the importance of cytochrome *P*-450 and mixed-function oxidases in the oxidative metabolism of carbamates. Further work is needed to solubilize and fully characterize this enzyme system. Only recently have plant systems *in vitro* been successfully employed in insecticide metabolism studies, and these endeavours should be expanded. More attention should also be given to the mechanisms involved in conjugation, especially as they relate to species selectivity, insect resistance and mode of action of synergists. These studies should be expedited by new techniques for isolating and characterizing conjugated carbamate metabolites. Some of these procedures may have to be incorporated into the present residue analysis methods, which often detect only the original carbamate and/or its phenol.

The majority of carbamate metabolism studies with plants are performed under laboratory conditions. However, a few investigations indicate that the same metabolic mechanisms are of prime importance under field conditions, although a large portion of the applied material is lost and never penetrates the plant. In mammals, metabolic pathways are frequently determined after application of one rather large dose and it may be that more studies should be based on a steady dietary intake at low levels. Such studies are valuable in assessing whether potential hazardous metabolites discovered in the laboratory are real hazards under normal exposure.

Based on our present state of knowledge, methylcarbamate esters represent a relatively safe class of insecticide chemicals. They are rapidly metabolized in mammals and man, and do not appear to be stored in any tissue. Nor are they persistent in the environment to any great extent. Their metabolites, although not all known, are not likely to pose serious hazards. Where toxicity has been demonstrated, residue procedures should be revised, if necessary, to include these materials. Metabolism studies not only assist in evaluating the safety of commercial and experimental carbamates, but they also are valuable in the development of new, safer and more effective carbamates. For example, acylation of the carbamate *N*-methyl group often results in a compound that retains insect toxicity but reduces mammalian toxicity[110-112]. This increased selectivity is apparently due to the mammal's hydrolysis of the acylmethylcarbamate to its phenol whereas the insect forms the active methylcarbamate[113].

Although the chemistry, toxicology and metabolsim of carbamates is important in their development and safe use, more work should be done on the finished product. Method, time and rate of application, formulation and equipment modifications can greatly enhance or reduce a compound's effectiveness. Techniques such as low-volume and ultra-low volume spraying could significantly reduce exposure to non-target species. A combination of these field studies and laboratory investigations would ensure maximum distribution of the toxicant in the micro-environment of the insect with minimum distribution in the macro-environment of man and other non-target organisms.

ACKNOWLEDGEMENT

Approved by the Director of the New York State Agricultural Experiment Station as Journal Paper No. 1864, dated 12 February 1971.

REFERENCES

[1] R. von Rumker, H. R. Guest and W. M. Upholt, *BioSci.* **20**, 1004 (1970).
[2] J. E. Casida and L. Lykken, *Ann. Rev. Plant Physiol.* **20**, 607 (1969).
[3] H. W. Dorough, *J. Agr. Food Chem.* **18**, 1015 (1970).
[4] T. R. Fukuto and R. L. Metcalf, *Ann. N.Y. Acad. Sci.* **160**, 97 (1969).
[5] R. J. Kuhr, *J. Sci. Food Agr. Suppl.*, p 44 (1968).
[6] R. J. Kuhr, *Meded. Rijksfac. Landbouww. Gent.* **33**, 647 (1968).
[7] R. J. Kuhr, *J. Agr. Food Chem.* **18**, 1023 (1970).
[8] L. Lykken and J. E. Casida, *Canad. Med. Ass. J.* **100**, 145 (1969).
[9] J. G. Krishna and J. E. Casida, *J. Agr. Food Chem.* **14**, 98 (1966).
[10] G. W. Ivie and H. W. Dorough, *J. Agr. Food Chem.* **16**, 849 (1968).
[11] S. P. Shrivastava, M. Tsukamoto and J. E. Casida, *J. Econ. Ent.* **62**, 483 (1969)
[12] R. J. Kuhr and J. E. Casida, *J. Agr. Food Chem.* **15**, 814 (1967).
[13] R. L. Baron, *J. Ass. Offic. Anal. Chem.* **51**, 1046 (1968).
[14] R. L. Baron and J. D. Doherty, *J. Agr. Food Chem.* **15**, 830 (1967).
[15] J. E. Casida, *Ann. Rev. Entomol.* **8**, 39 (1963).
[16] A. Hassan, S. M. A. D. Zayed and F. M. Abdel-Hamid, *Biochem. Pharmacol.*, **15**, 2045 (1966).
[17] J. B. Knaak, M. J. Tallant, W. J. Bartley and L. J. Sullivan, *J. Agr. Food Chem.* **13**, 537 (1965).
[18] J. B. Knaak, M. J. Tallant, S. J. Kozbelt and L. J. Sullivan, *J. Agr. Food Chem.* **16**, 465 (1968).
[19] J. B. Knaak and L. J. Sullivan, *J. Agr. Food Chem.* **15**, 1125 (1967).
[20] N. C. Leeling and J. E. Casida, *J. Agr. Food Chem.* **14**, 281 (1966).
[21] E. Williams, R. W. Meikle and C. T. Redemann, *J. Agr. Food Chem.* **12**, 457 (1964).
[22] R. P. Miskus, T. L. Andrews and M. Look, *J. Agr. Food Chem.* **17**, 842 (1969).
[23] J. D. Robbins, J. E. Bakke and V. J. Feil, *J. Agr. Food Chem.* **17**, 236 (1969).
[24] K. R. Hill, *J. Ass. Offic. Anal. Chem.* **53**, 987 (1970).
[25] J. D. Robbins, J. E. Bakke and V. J. Feil, *J. Agr. Food Chem.* **18**, 130 (1970).
[26] H. W. Dorough, *J. Agr. Food Chem.* **16**, 319 (1968).
[27] R. L. Metcalf, T. R. Fukuto, C. Collins, K. Borck, S. Abd El-Aziz, R. Munoz and C. C. Cassil, *J. Agr. Food Chem.* **16**, 300 (1968).
[28] M. Slade and J. E. Casida, *J. Agr. Food Chem.* **18**, 467 (1970).
[29] J. Miyamoto, K. Yamamoto and T. Matsumato, *Agr. Biol. Chem.* **33**, 1060 (1969).
[30] N. R. Andrawes, H. W. Dorough and D. A. Lindquist, *J. Econ. Ent.* **60**, 979 (1967).
[31] J. B. Knaak, M. T. Tallant and L. J. Sullivan, *J. Agr. Food Chem.* **14**, 573 (1966).
[32] H. W. Dorough and G. W. Ivie, *J. Agr. Food Chem.* **16**, 460 (1968).

[33] H. W. Dorough, R. B. Davis and G. W. Ivie, *J. Agr. Food Chem.* **18**, 135 (1970).

[34] R. L. Metcalf, M. F. Osman and T. R. Fukuto, *J. Econ. Ent.* **60**, 445 (1967).

[35] T.-Y. Ku and J. L. Bishop, *J. Econ. Ent.* **60**, 1328 (1967).

[36] H. W. Dorough and J. E. Casida, *J. Agr. Food Chem.* **12**, 294 (1964).

[37] R. J. Kuhr, *J. Econ. Ent.* In press (1971).

[38] N. R. Andrawes and H. W. Dorough, *J. Econ. Ent.* **60**, 453 (1967).

[39] H. B. Camp and B. W. Arthur, *J. Econ. Ent.* **60**, 803 (1967).

[40] S. M. A. D. Zayed, A. Hassan and T. M. Hussein, *Biochem. Pharmacol.* **15**, 2057 (1966).

[41] M. Y. Zubairi and J. E. Casida, *J. Econ. Ent.* **58**, 403 (1965).

[42] R. L. Metcalf, T. R. Fukuto, C. Collins, K. Borck, J. Burk, H. T. Reynolds and M. F. Osman, *J. Agr. Food Chem.* **14**, 579 (1966).

[43] D. L. Bull, D. A. Lindquist and J. R. Coppedge, *J. Agr. Food Chem.* **15**, 610 (1967).

[44] H. W. Dorough and O. G. Wiggins, *J. Econ. Ent.* **62**, 49 (1969).

[45] O. G. Wiggins, M. H. J. Weiden, C. S. Weil and C. P. Carpenter. Paper presented at *VII International Congress of Plant Protection, Paris* (September 1970).

[46] I. Y. Mostafa, A. Hassan and S. M. A. D. Zayed, *Z. Naturforsch.* **216**, 1060 (1966).

[47] H. W. Dorough, *Bull. Environ. Contam. Toxicol.* **3**, 164 (1968).

[48] A. R. Friedman and A. J. Lemin, *J. Agr. Food Chem.* **15**, 642 (1967).

[49] W. J. Bartley, N. R. Andrawes, E. L. Chancey, W. P. Bagley and H. W. Spurr, *J. Agr. Food Chem.* **18**, 446 (1970).

[50] D. L. Bull, *J. Econ. Ent.* **61**, 1598 (1968).

[51] J. R. Coppedge, D. A. Lindquist, D. L. Bull and H. W. Dorough, *J. Agr. Food Chem.* **15**, 902 (1967).

[52] C. O. Knowles and A. K. Sen Gupta, *J. Econ. Ent.* **63**, 615 (1970).

[53] E. Williams, R. W. Meikle and C. T. Redemann, *J. Agr. Food Chem.* **12**, 453 (1964).

[54] J. E. Casida and K.-B. Augustinsson, *Biochim. Biophys. Acta*, **36**, 411 (1959).

[55] J. E. Casida, K.-B. Augustinsson and G. Jonsson, *J. Econ. Ent.* **53**, 205 (1960).

[56] H. T. Gordon and M. E. Eldefrawi, *J. Econ. Ent.* **53**, 1004 (1960).

[57] R. L. Metcalf, T. R. Fukuto and M. Y. Winton, *J. Econ. Ent.* **53**, 828 (1960).

[58] G. M. Price and R. J. Kuhr, *Biochem. J.* **112**, 133 (1969).

[59] M. Tsukamoto and J. E. Casida, *Nature, Lond.* **213**, 49 (1967).

[60] R. J. Kuhr, *J. Agr. Food Chem.* **17**, 112 (1969).

[61] H. W. Dorough, *J. Agr. Food Chem.* **15**, 261 (1967).

[62] E. S. Oonnithan and J. E. Casida, *Bull. Environ. Contam. Toxicol.* **1**, 59 (1966).

[63] E. S. Oonnithan and J. E. Casida, *J. Agr. Food Chem.* **16**, 28 (1968).

[64] M. Tsukamoto and J. E. Casida, *J. Econ. Ent.* **60**, 617 (1967).

[65] J. E. Casida, S. P. Shrivastava and E. G. Esaac, *J. Econ. Ent.* **61**, 1339 (1968).

[66] M. Tsukamoto, S. P. Shrivastava and J. E. Casida, *J. Econ. Ent.* **61**, 50 (1968).

[67] E. G. Gemrich, *J. Agr. Food Chem.* **15**, 617 (1967).

[68] E. Hodgson and J. E. Casida, *Biochim. Biophys. Acta*, **42**, 184 (1960).

[69] E. Hodgson and J. E. Casida, *Biochem. Pharmacol.* **8**, 179 (1961).

[70] A. M. Abdel-Wahab, R. J. Kuhr and J. E. Casida, *J. Agr. Food Chem.* **14**, 290 (1966).

[71] A. K. Sen Gupta and C. O. Knowles, *J. Econ. Ent.* **63**, 10 (1970).

[72] R. F. Skrentny and J. A. Ellis, *Pestic. Sci.* **1**, 45 (1970).

[73] R. L. Baron, J. A. Sphon, J. T. Chen, E. Lustig, J. D. Doherty, E. A. Hansen and S. M. Kolbye, *J. Agr. Food Chem.* **17**, 883 (1969).

[74] E. Hodgson Ed. *Enzymatic Oxidations of Toxicants*, North Carolina State University at Raleigh, N.C. (1968).

[75] E. Hodgson and F. W. Plapp, Jr., *J. Agr. Food Chem.* **18**, 1048 (1970).

[76] L. C. Terriere, *Ann. Rev. Entomol.* **13**, 75 (1968).

[77] H. B. Matthews and J. E. Casida, *Life Sci.* **9**, 989 (1970).

[78] R. D. O'Brien. In *Insecticides, Action and Metabolism*, Academic Press: New York (1967).

[79] J. R. Gillette, A. H. Conney, G. J. Cosmides, R. W. Estabrook, J. R. Fouts and G. J. Mannering. Eds. *Microsomes and Drug Oxidations*, Academic Press: New York (1969).

[80] P. F. T. Vaughan and V. S. Butt, *Biochem. J.* **111**, 32 (1969).

[81] D. S. Frear, H. R. Swanson and F. S. Tanaka, *Phytochem.* **8**, 2157 (1969).

[82] F. P. Lichtenstein and J. R. Corbett, *J. Agr. Food Chem.* **17**, 589 (1969).

[83] S. J. Yu, U. Kiigemagi and L. C. Terriere, *J. Agr. Food Chem.* **19**, 5 (1971).

[84] D. W. Russell, E. E. Conn, A. Sutter and H. Grisebach, *Biochim. Biophys. Acta*, **170**, 210 (1968).

[85] A. Binning, F. J. Darby, M. P. Heenan and J. N. Smith, *Biochem. J.* **103**, 42 (1967).

86 G. J. Dutton. Ed. *Glucuronic Acid.* Academic Press: New York (1966).
87 M. H. J. Weiden. Personal communication.
88 G. D. Paulson, R. G. Zaylskie, M. V. Zher, C. E. Portnoy and V. J. Feil, *J. Agr. Food Chem.* **18**, 110 (1970).
89 H. M. Mehendale and H. W. Dorough. In *Insecticides,* edited by A. S. Tahori, pp 15–28. Gordon and Breach: New York, London, Paris (1971).
90 J. C. Pekas and G. D. Paulson, *Science,* **170**, 77 (1970).
91 R. O. Mumma. Personal communication.
92 A. Farago, *Arch. Toxikol.* **24**, 309 (1969).
93 J. A. Dawson, D. F. Heath, J. A. Rose, E. M. Thain and J. B. Ward, *Bull. World Hlth Org.* **30**, 127 (1964).
94 A. Strother, *Biochem. Pharmacol.* **19**, 2525 (1970).
95 R. L. Baron and R. K. Locke, *Bull. Environ. Contam. Toxicol.* **5**, 287 (1970).
96 J. R. Bend, G. M. Holder, E. Protos and A. J. Ryan, *Austral. J. Biol. Sci.* **23**, 361 (1970).
97 F. D. Judge and R. J. Kuhr, *J. Econ. Ent.* In press (1971).
98 D. G. Crosby, E. Leitis and W. L. Winterlin, *J. Agr. Food Chem.* **13**, 204 (1965).
99 K. Okada, K. Nomura and S. Yamamoto, *Nippon Nageikagaku Kaishi,* **35**, 739 (1961).
100 L. C. Mitchell, *J. Ass. Offic. Agr. Chem.* **44**, 643 (1961).
101 A. M. Abdel-Wahab and J. E. Casida, *J. Agr. Food Chem.* **15**, 479 (1967).
102 B. E. Pape, M. F. Para and M. J. Zabik, *J. Agr. Food Chem.* **18**, 490 (1970).
103 M. H. Balba, M. S. Singer, M. Slade and J. E. Casida, *J. Agr. Food Chem.* **16**, 821 (1968).
104 M. H. Balba and J. E. Casida, *J. Agr. Food Chem.* **16**, 561 (1968).
105 M. H. J. Weiden, H. H. Moorefield and L. K. Payne, *J. Econ. Ent.* **58**, 154 (1965).
106 M. H. J. Weiden, *J. Sci. Food Agr. Suppl.,* p 19 (1968).
107 L. K. Payne, Jr, H. A. Stansbury, Jr and M. H. J. Weiden, *J. Agr. Food Chem.* **14**, 356 (1966).
108 N. R. Andrawes and R. A. Herrett. Paper presented at the *158th National American Chemical Society Meeting* (8 September 1969).
109 J. B. Knaak and L. J. Sullivan, *J. Agr. Food Chem.* **16**, 454 (1968).
110 D. K. Lewis, *Nature, Lond.* **213**, 205 (1967).
111 J. Fraser, I. R. Harrison and S. B. Wakerley, *J. Sci. Food Agr. Suppl.,* p 8 (1968).
112 R. P. Miskus, M. Look, T. L. Andrews and R. L. Lyon, *J. Agr. Food Chem.* **16**, 605 (1968).
113 R. P. Miskus, T. L. Andrews and M. Look, *J. Agr. Food Chem.* **17**, 842 (1969).

METABOLISM OF SUBSTITUTED PHENYLCARBAMATE INSECTICIDES IN MAMMALS

Junshi Miyamoto and Kazuo Fukunaga

The Institute of Physical and Chemical Research, Saitama, Japan

ABSTRACT

Orally administered 3,4-dimethylphenyl *N*-methylcarbamate or Meobal, labelled with ^{14}C at the 4-methyl group, was easily absorbed from the gastrointestinal tract of male Wistar rats and distributed into the tissues. Elimination of the radioactivity was rapid and substantially complete: during 48 h approximately 92 per cent and 5 per cent of the total radioactivity was excreted into urine and faeces respectively. The content of the intact Meobal in the urine was negligible. Major degradation products were identified as 3-methyl-4-carboxyphenyl *N*-methylcarbamate, its *N*-hydroxymethyl analogue and its component phenol. Direct evidence was obtained for oxidation of alkyl side chains *in vitro*. Much less of the hydrolysis product of the original carbamate, 3,4-dimethylphenol and its conjugates, was demonstrated in the urine. From these results 3,4-dimethylphenyl *N*-methylcarbamate is presumed to undergo biodegradation through oxidative pathways. Major metabolites were tested for their biological activity, among which 3-methyl-4-hydroxymethylphenyl *N*-methylcarbamate was similarly active to Meobal. Residues of Meobal in harvested rice grains determined by gas chromatography were on average 0.11 p.p.m. two weeks after application, which was far less than the permissible level of the compound calculated from the results of 90 consecutive days feeding to rats.

Metabolic studies on carbamate insecticides have been extensively carried out[1] and from the results it has gradually been made clear that biodegradation of *N*-methylcarbamates proceeds primarily through two pathways. One is hydrolytic cleavage of the ester linkage or carbamic acid by esterases, liberating component phenol or enol derivatives. By this reaction the carbonyl carbon atom of the molecule is converted into carbon dioxide. Terminal methylamine is also oxidized to carbon dioxide, and according to Hassan *et al.*[2] it is catalysed successively by several types of oxidizing enzymes. Carbon dioxide is presumably formed from *N*-hydroxymethyl analogues of *N*-methylcarbamates. Carbonyl carbon is usually more easily oxidized to carbon dioxide than is *N*-methyl carbon. Generally production of carbon dioxide from the carbamates takes place more in mammals than in insects.

Another degradation pathway is oxidative. Carbamate compounds undergo various types of oxidation reactions, dependent upon their chemical structures: for example, hydroxylation of ring structure, oxidation of *N*-alkyl or *O*-alkyl groups, alkyl side chain oxidation and sulphur oxidation. The

221

Table 1. Annual usage of carbamate insecticides in Japan

Compounds	Amount used annually (tons)				
	1966	1967	1968	1969	1970
1-Naphthyl N-methylcarbamate (carbaryl)	630	1030	1020	1120	ca. 1000
3,4-Dimethylphenyl N-methylcarbamate (Meobal)	—	220	630	880	ca. 730
3-Methylphenyl N-methylcarbamate	—	1	100	420	ca. 500
2-sec.-Butylphenyl N-methylcarbamate	—	—	—	ca. 10	ca. 330
2-Isopropylphenyl N-methylcarbamate	100	210	170	200	ca. 200
2-Chlorophenyl N-methylcarbamate	—	2	150	180	ca. 180
3,5-Dimethylphenyl N-methylcarbamate	—	—	—	4	ca. 4
Total	730	1460	2070	2810	ca. 2940

carbamate ester linkage remains intact during the oxidation reactions. Most of these oxidation reactions are confirmed or presumed to be catalysed by the so-called mixed function oxidase present in microsome fractions of mammalian liver or insect abdomen.

The carbamate insecticide dealt with in some detail here is also metabolized in the animal body by these two pathways.

In Japan some 3000 tons of carbamate insecticides are being used annually for the control of various species of plant hoppers and leaf hoppers in the paddy fields, as shown in *Table 1*. This carbamate compound with the structure of 3,4-dimethylphenyl *N*-methylcarbamate, or Meobal, accounts for approximately one-quarter of the total amount used annually. Meobal is moderately toxic to warm-blooded animals, as indicated in *Table 2*.

Table 2. Acute toxicity of Meobal in mammals

Animal species	Sex	Route	LD_{50}(mg/kg)
Mouse	Male	Oral	60
Mouse	Male	Dermal	> 2500
Mouse	Male	Inhalation	> 541[†]
Rat	Male	Oral	380
Rat	Female	Oral	290
Rabbit	Male	Oral	> 200
Dog	Male, female	Oral	*ca.* 100
Monkey	Male	Oral	> 100

[†] mg/m^3

Symptoms of poisoning are characteristic of stimulation of autonomic nervous systems resulting from inhibition of cholinesterases, such as tremor, myosis and salivation. They appear shortly after administration of the compound, but disappear also quite rapidly. Cholinesterase of blood or brain inhibited by the compound rapidly recovers to the normal activity.

To study the extent of biodegradation and to clarify the metabolic pathways of Meobal in mammals, 3,4-[^{14}C]dimethylphenyl *N*-methylcarbamate labelled at the 4-methyl group[3] was administered orally to male Wistar rats at a rate of 50 mg/kg body weight.

The content of total ^{14}C as well as intact Meobal in several tissues and blood was found to reach a maximum 15 min after treatment, as is shown in *Figure 1*, but it decreased rapidly thereafter and after 4 h only negligible amounts of the original carbamate were present in these tissues and blood[4].

Most of the radioactivity was excreted into urine[4]: approximately 90 per cent was recovered in 24 h, and during 48 h 91.5 per cent and 4.9 per cent of the administered radioactivity were obtained in urine and faeces respectively. No radioactive carbon dioxide was expired.

Radioactive metabolites were separated in 48 h pooled urine by acidic ether extraction, silica gel or DEAE-cellulose column chromatography, followed by preparative thin-layer chromatography, as described in detail elsewhere[4]. The metabolites were identified by co-chromatography with the

223

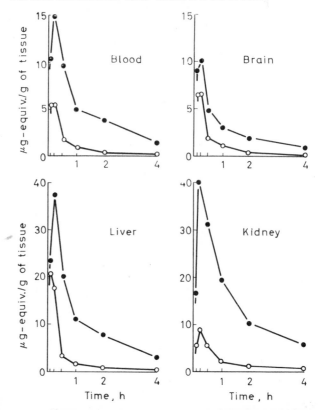

Figure 1. Content of total ^{14}C(●) and 3,4-dimethylphenyl *N*-methylcarbamate(o) in rat tissues and blood after oral administration of 50 mg of radioactive Meobal/kg.

authentic compound, as well as by careful examination of their infra-red and nuclear-magnetic-resonance spectra.

Urine contained only traces of intact Meobal and the most abundant metabolite proved to be 3-methyl-4-carboxyphenyl *N*-methylcarbamate (*Table 3*). *N*-Hydroxymethyl analogues of the 4-carboxy carbamate and their component 3-methyl-4-carboxyphenol were also identified. These three oxidation products accounted for about half of the total metabolites in the urine. 3-Hydroxymethyl-4-methyl analogue of the original compound and glucuronide conjugate of the hydroxymethylphenyl carbamate and its component phenol were also present in the urine.

The above-mentioned 3-hydroxymethyl-4-methyl phenol and 3-methyl-4-carboxyphenol may not be derived from 3,4-dimethylphenol, for these oxidized phenols were not detected in the urine from rats given free 3,4-dimethylphenol orally[4]. These oxidized phenols seem to be formed by hydrolysis of the corresponding oxidized carbamate compounds, once formed.

Direct hydrolysis products of Meobal, free 3,4-dimethylphenol and its conjugation products, accounted for less than 20 per cent of the metabolites in the urine.

Table 3. Radioactive metabolites of Meobal in rat urine

Compound identified		% of urinary radioactivity
(1) Intact Meobal		0.2
(2) Hydrolysis products		
3,4-dimethylphenol		0.6
3,4-dimethylphenylsulphate		3.5
3,4-dimethylphenylglucuronide		0.8
unidentified compounds (4)	at most	10
(3) Oxidation products		
3-hydroxymethyl-4-methylphenyl N-methylcarbamate		2.2
3-hydroxymethyl-4-methylphenyl N-methylcarbamate glucuronide		8.2
3-hydroxymethyl-4-methylphenol glucuronide and/or 3-methyl-4-hydroxymethyl isomer		4.0
3-methyl-4-carboxyphenyl N-methylcarbamate		30.1
3-methyl-4-carboxyphenyl N-hydroxy-methylcarbamate		4.9
3-methyl-4-carboxyphenol		10.1
3-methyl-4-carboxyphenol glucuronide	*ca.*	1
unidentified compounds (at least 13)	*ca.*	25

The oxidative conversion of Meobal was tested *in vitro* with rat liver preparations[4]. As indicated in *Table 4*, rat liver lysosome-free supernatant or microsomes were capable of oxidizing the ring-substituted methyl group of Meobal, and the NADPH-generating system, namely NADP, glucose 6-phosphate plus glucose 6-phosphate–NADP oxidoreductase, gave best results as a coenzyme for this conversion reaction. Major oxidation products *in vitro* were separated from 150 ml of the incubation mixture. They co-chromatographed with the authentic sample of 3-methyl-4-hydroxymethyl-phenyl *N*-methylcarbamate, but their infra-red and nuclear-magnetic-resonance spectra were a little different from those of the synthesized compound. By careful comparison of their spectra it was concluded[4] that the hydroxymethyl analogues obtained *in vitro* were a mixture of 3-hydroxy-methyl-4-methylphenyl *N*-methylcarbamate and 3-methyl-4-hydroxymethyl isomer.

Although in the above experiment *in vitro* only a trace amount of 3-methyl-4-carboxyphenyl *N*-methylcarbamate was detected, the oxidation of the 4-hydroxymethyl group to a 4-carboxy group was demonstrated *in vitro* by using rat liver microsome-free supernatant fraction fortified with NAD[4].

Thus direct, unequivocal evidence has been obtained for alkyl side chain oxidation of carbamate compounds in mammals *in vitro* and *in vivo*. From these results it was concluded that in mammals major portions of Meobal are metabolized oxidatively and that hydrolytic pathways are of minor importance. The suggested metabolic pathways for Meobal in rats are shown in *Figure 2*.

225

I

Table 4. Degradation of 3,4-dimethylphenyl *N*-methylcarbamate by rat liver preparations *in vitro*

	Degradation of added carbamate (%)	Formation of 3-hydroxymethyl and 4-hydroxy-methyl analogues (%)
(1) Localization		
Liver homogenate	48.1	40.5
Liver nucleus	5.0	4.7
Liver mitochondria	2.6	2.3
Liver lysosome	0.4	0.0
Liver lysosome-free supernatant	54.8	47.5
Liver microsome	40.8	35.5
Liver microsome-free supernatant	1.1	0.8
Kidney homogenate	2.7	2.1
(2) Coenzyme requirement by liver microsome		
No coenzyme	0.3	0.2
NAD plus NADP (each 6 μmol)	2.3	1.1
NADH (6 μmol)	9.1	7.1
NADPH (6 μmol)	34.3	28.8
NADP (6 μmol), glucose 6-phosphate (6 μmol) plus glucose 6-phosphate-NADP oxidoreductase (3.5 i.u.)	65.7	58.6

The results are the mean value of three replicated trials, and expressed as percentages of the carbamate initially added. The incubation mixture in Experiment 1 contained in 2 ml 4 μmol of radioactive 3,4-dimethylphenyl *N*-methylcarbamate, 20 μmol of niacin, 10 μmol of magnesium chloride, 4 μmol of NADP, 40 μmol of glucose 6-phosphate, 2.8 i.u. of glucose 6-phosphate-NADP oxidoreductase, 66.7 μmol of tris buffer, pH 7.2, and enzyme preparation (0.13 g-equiv. of the tissue. Incubated at 37.5°C for 1.5 h.

In Experiment 2, the reaction mixture contained in 3 ml 6 μmol of radioactive 3,4-dimethylphenyl *N*-methylcarbamate, 30 μmol of niacin, 15 μmol of magnesium chloride, 100 μmol of tris buffer, pH 7.2, coenzyme at the specified concentration and 0.14 g-equiv. of rat liver microsome fraction. Incubated at 37.5°C for 1 h in air.

These biodegradation pathways are consistent with those of Landrin, a mixture of 3,4,5-trimethylphenyl *N*-methylcarbamate and 2,3,5-trimethyl isomer reported recently by Slade and Casida[5]. From enzymatic experiments and experiments *in vivo* in mice, they also suggested that side chain oxidations are major pathways of the carbamate compounds.

Some of the metabolites of carbamate compounds are known to retain biological activity equivalent to or even more potent than the original carbamate. Therefore biological activity of some of the metabolites of Meobal was examined. *Table 5* summarizes the results. 3-Methyl-4-hydroxymethyl-phenyl *N*-methylcarbamate was similarly active, whereas the 4-carboxy analogue had a very poor biological activity. 3-Hydroxymethyl-4-methyl-phenyl *N*-methylcarbamate is possibly of low activity, although this compound has not yet been tested, as 3-hydroxymethylphenyl *N*-methylcarbamate

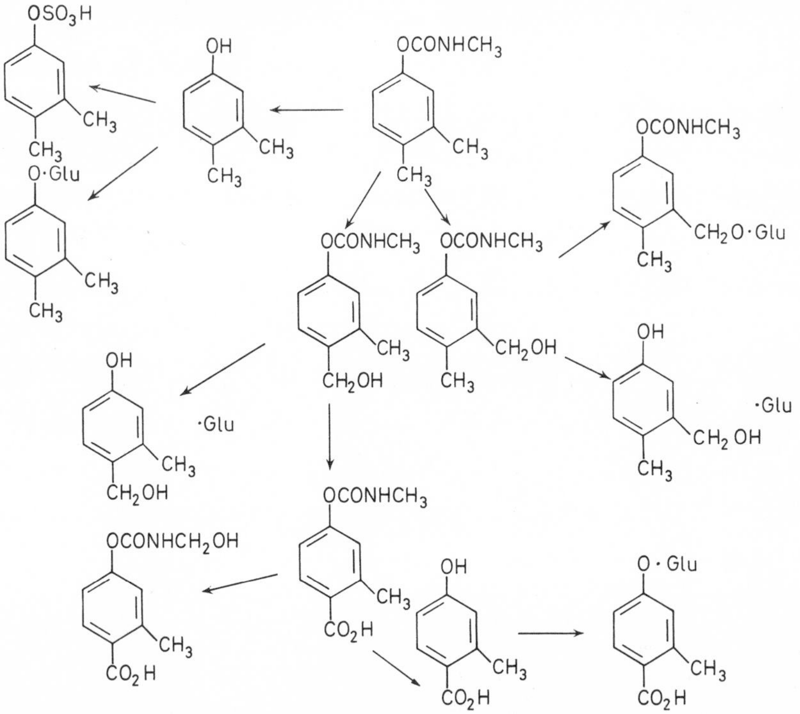

Figure 2. Metabolic pathways of 3,4-dimethylphenyl *N*-methylcarbamate in the rat. Glu, glucuronide conjugate.

had far weaker efficacy against plant hoppers than 3-methylphenyl *N*-methylcarbamate.

One point should be made about the residue of Meobal in rice grains and its toxicological implications. A microanalytical method for Meobal residue in rice grains has been elaborated[6, 7], in which the carbamate compound, after separation by column chromatography, was simultaneously hydrolysed and condensed with 2,4-dinitrofluorobenzene under alkaline conditions. The resultant *N*-methyl-2,4-dinitroaniline was determined by electron-capture gas chromatography. Two weeks after application of Meobal dust formulation, rice grains contained on an average 0.11 p.p.m. of Meobal, and 30–50 days after double applications, following the usual spraying programme in Japan, the residual amount decreased to 0.014 p.p.m.[8]. If 500 g of rice containing 0.11 p.p.m. of Meobal are taken daily, the amount of Meobal ingested would be 0.06 mg/man. On the other hand the no-effect level of the compound after 90 consecutive days feeding to rats proved to be 900 p.p.m. in the diet or 64 mg/kg per day[9]. Calculated with a safety factor of 2 000, the acceptable daily intake for man would be 1.6 mg/day. Therefore the maximum amount of Meobal to be ingested daily is much smaller than this acceptable daily intake. Therefore if it is assumed that rice grains do contain only small amounts of toxic metabolites of Meobal, this carbamate

227

Table 5. Biological activity of some metabolites of Meobal

Compound	Cholinesterase inhibition (IN_{50}, M)	Toxicity to mice, intravenous LD_{50} (mg/kg)	Insecticidal activity against plant hoppers
Meobal	9.6×10^{-6}	35	⧺
3-Hydroxymethyl-4-methylphenyl N-methylcarbamate	(weak)	(weak)	(weak)
3-Methyl-4-hydroxymethylphenyl N-methylcarbamate	9.6×10^{-6}	35	⧺ ~ ⧻
3-Methyl-4-carboxyphenyl N-methyl-carbamate	$> 10^{-3}$†	weak	± ~ +

† 30% inhibition at 10^{-3} M.

228

insecticide can be used without any potential danger of residual toxicity to humans.

REFERENCES

[1] H. W. Dorough, *J. Agr. Food Chem.* **18**, 1015 (1970).
[2] A. Hassan, S. M. A. D. Zayed and F. M. Abdel-Hamid, *Biochem. Pharmacol.* **15**, 2045 (1966).
[3] M. Hazue and K. Miyake, *Botyu-Kagaku* (*Scientific Pest Control*), **34**, 120 (1969).
[4] J. Miyamoto, K. Yamamoto and T. Matsumoto, *Agr. Biol. Chem.* **33**, 1060 (1969).
[5] M. Slade and J. E. Casida, *J. Agr. Food Chem.* **18**, 467 (1970).
[6] S. Sumida, M. Takagi and J. Miyamoto, *Agr. Biol. Chem.* **34**, 1576 (1970).
[7] S. Sumida, M. Takagi and J. Miyamoto, *Botyu-Kagaku* (*Scientific Pest Control*), **35**, 72 (1970).
[8] J. Miyamoto, Unpublished work (1970).
[9] T. Kadota, Unpublished work (1968).

THE CHEMISTRY AND METABOLISM OF
TERMINAL RESIDUES OF FUNGICIDES

TERMINAL RESIDUES OF DITHIOCARBAMATE FUNGICIDES

H. M. Dekhuijzen, J. W. Vonk and A. Kaars Sijpesteijn

Institute for Organic Chemistry T.N.O., Utrecht, Holland

ABSTRACT

In studies on terminal residues of dithiocarbamate fungicides two groups have to be distinguished; (1) dimethyldithiocarbamates (like thiram); (2) ethylenebisdithiocarbamates, such as nabam, zineb and maneb. The fates of these two groups are completely different. In group 1, (a) dimethyldithiocarbamate (DDC) ions are converted enzymatically in plants into: DDC-β-glucoside, L-DDC-alanine and non-enzymatically into thiazolidine-2-thione-4-carboxylic acid. (b) In micro-organisms such as fungi and bacteria DDC-α-aminobutyric acid is formed. (c) In animals, tetraethyliuram disulphide (Antabuse), and presumably also thiram, is converted into the glucuronic acid conjugate.

In group 2 nabam decomposes rapidly in water into ethylenethiourea (ETU) and ethylenebisisothiocyanate sulphide. ETU is taken up by plants and appears to be broken down only very slowly into 2-imidazoline. Conjugate formation of nabam has not been found. Micro-organisms are able to break down ETU in soil only very slowly.

In the field of pesticides research there has been an expansion of activities as compared with the activities of few years ago, when the emphasis of research was on the development of new chemicals with selective biological effects. This is still of utmost importance, but in recent years interest has also been aroused in the metabolic fate of pesticides, such as fungicides, in different organisms. This topic is not only of interest to those research workers who are striving to reduce the risks of terminal residues but also for anyone interested in the biological action of the compound.

In this paper we will deal with the metabolism of dithiocarbamate fungicides. In any study on residues of these it is appropriate to distinguish clearly between two groups of compounds, which although related show very different chemical properties[13, 20].

Group 1. Dialkyldithiocarbamates and their oxidation products, the thiuram disulphides. The sodium salt of dimethyl dithiocarbamate, sodium–DDC, $(CH_3)_2N$—C—S—Na, is often used in laboratory studies, but the iron
$$\overset{\|}{S}$$
salt (ferbam) and zinc salt (ziram) find practical application. The oxidation product, tetramethylthiuram disulphide:

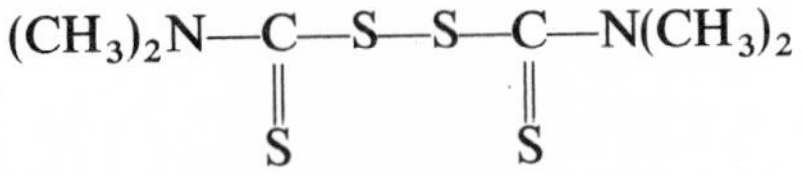

$$(CH_3)_2N-\underset{\underset{S}{\|}}{C}-S-S-\underset{\underset{S}{\|}}{C}-N(CH_3)_2$$

is also used as an agricultural fungicide.

Group 2 comprises the ethylenebisdithiocarbamates:

$$-S-\underset{\underset{S}{\|}}{C}-\underset{\underset{H}{|}}{N}-CH_2-CH_2-\underset{\underset{H}{|}}{N}-\underset{\underset{S}{\|}}{C}-S-$$

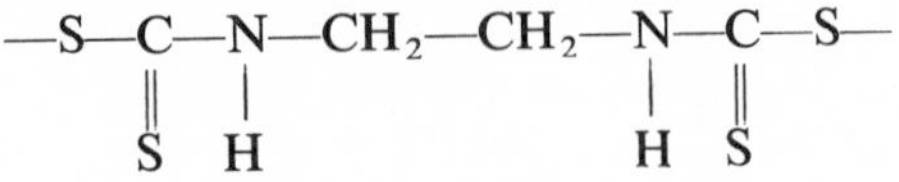

The sodium salt or nabam is only used for experimental purposes but the zinc and manganese salts find practical application (zineb, maneb).

These two general types of dithiocarbamate fungicides have entirely different chemical properties, their mode of fungicidal action is different and their pattern of breakdown differs.

DIALKYLDITHIOCARBAMATES

We will first briefly deal with the dialkyldithiocarbamates because the metabolism of this group has been studied extensively; it was followed more recently by a study of the fate of ethylenebisdithiocarbamates in plants at our Institute[2, 10, 24]. Thiram can easily be reduced to dimethyldithiocarbamate. At low pH dimethyldithiocarbamic acid is formed and this breaks down to dimethylamine and carbon disulphide[20].

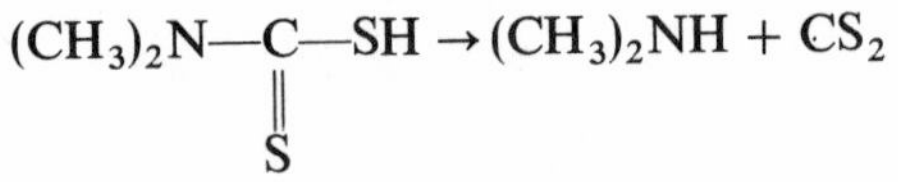

$$(CH_3)_2N-\underset{\underset{S}{\|}}{C}-SH \rightarrow (CH_3)_2NH + CS_2$$

Metabolism in plants

When taken up by plants, DDC ions are rapidly converted into three fungitoxic conjugates:

DDC–β-glucoside, $(CH_3)_2N-\underset{\underset{S}{\|}}{C}-S-\overset{\overset{\displaystyle O}{|}}{CH}-(CHOH)_3\overset{|}{CH}-CH_2OH$[7, 10, 11]

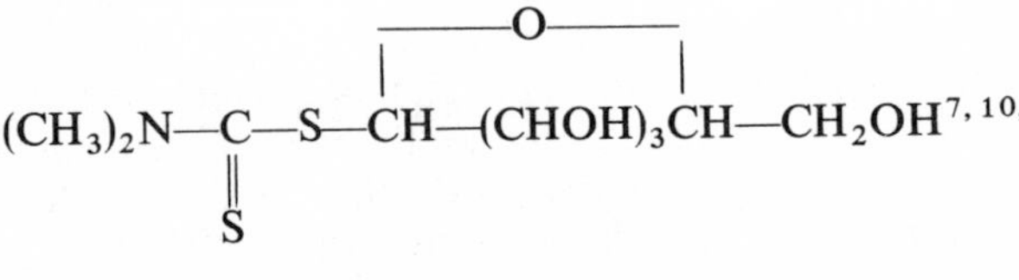

DDC–alanine, $(CH_3)_2N-\underset{\underset{S}{\|}}{C}-S-CH_2-\underset{\underset{NH_2}{|}}{\overset{\overset{H}{|}}{C}}-COOH$ (L-isomer)

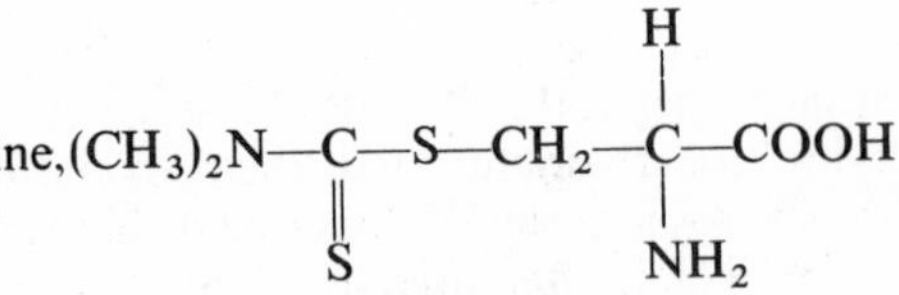

and an unknown fungitoxic compound, presumably also a conjugate[2, 7, 12]. DDC–alanine is converted non-enzymatically into thiazolidine-2-thione-4-carboxylic acid (TTCA)[2, 10]. Most of these reactions are interconvertible. Thiram undergoes exactly the same reactions, after reduction to DDC ions.

Massaux applied ^{35}S-labelled thiram to begonia and cucumber leaves and detected the same fungitoxic compounds[14]. No other compounds were found. Hylin and Chin[3], however, studied the fate of ^{35}S- and ^{14}C-labelled dimethyldithiocarbamate after application to *Carica papaya* and found, apart from DDC–glucoside, DDC–alanine, carbon disulphide and dimethylamine, four unidentified compounds.

Demethylation, which often occurs with non-natural compounds, does not take place as far as we know with DDC–alanine or DDC–glucoside. Demethylation is only known to occur with an experimental dimethyldithiocarbamate, carboxymethyldithiocarbamate[2].

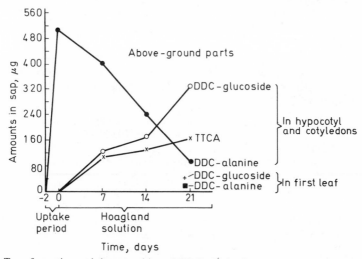

N-methylrhodanine

From consideration of these data we started a quantitative study of transformation and decomposition of DDC–alanine in cucumber seedlings after an uptake period of two days. DDC–alanine and DDC–glucoside can be separated by paper chromatography and are easily detected by growing a test fungus on paper. The size of the inhibition zone on the chromatograms

Figure 1. Transformation and decomposition of DDC–alanine in cucumber seedlings after an uptake for two days of 100 p.p.m. of DDC–alanine[2].

235

Table 1. Balance sheet for DDC–alanine

Days after uptake	Loss of DDC–alanine (% of the amount present after the uptake period)	DDC–alanine recovered (%)
7	69	47
14	76	41
21	90	25

can be used to determine the amount of the conversion products on the chromatograms[2]. DDC–alanine decreases slowly during 3 weeks, whereas the amounts of DDC–glucoside and of non-fungitoxic TTCA increase (*Figure 1*).

From this picture a balance sheet can be made (*Table 1*) showing the amount taken up by the plant and the amount present in the plant after various periods[2].

The results in *Table 1* raise the crucial question: what happened to the other, non-recovered part of DDC–alanine?

Partly it may have been decomposed into volatile carbon disulphide or hydrogen sulphide and unknown decomposition products. However, it is worthwhile to mention also another possibility. In our studies we investigated only those compounds that can be extracted with ethanol. The non-alcohol-soluble fraction, which contains proteins, has not been investigated. From work of Hylin and Chin[3] it is known that an appreciable portion of ^{35}S-labelled dimethyldithiocarbamate was recovered in the sulphur amino acids. Therefore it is conceivable that part of DDC–alanine or its breakdown products have been incorporated into the proteins of the alcohol-insoluble fraction. Moreover, Thorn and Richardson[21] showed complex-formation between dithiocarbamate, copper ions and protein. Therefore we cannot rule out the possibility that part of the non-recovered DDC is incorporated as breakdown product or as such into proteins of the alcohol-insoluble fraction. This problem can be solved only by using radioactively labelled dithio-carbamates.

Fate of thiram and sodium-DDC after application to leaves.—So far we studied the fate of sodium-DDC after uptake by the roots. When sprayed on the leaves sodium-DDC is taken up and converted into the three known conversion products.

Table 2. Concentration of conversion products in sap of mature leaves 4 days after spraying the leaves with sodium-DDC (1 000 p.p.m.)

	DDC–alanine (p.p.m.)	DDC–glucoside (p.p.m.)
Cucumber	50	94
Sugar beet	0	97
Cabbage	20	198
Broad beans	55	153
Tomato	27	130
Pea	17	400
Apple	0	30
Tobacco	14	7

Table 2 shows that the concentration of the conversion products in plants differs from one species to another; very much lower values are always found than in root application. It is striking that, as in root application, more DDC–glucoside than DDC–alanine is formed.

Thiram is used in agriculture and is taken up as such or as DDC ions by leaves of different plant species and converted into the known products. The concentration of DDC–alanine in cucumber leaves is about one-third of the concentration after a sodium-DDC spray (*Table 3*).

Table 3. Concentration and amount of conversion products in sap of mature leaves 4 days after spraying with thiram (1 000 p.p.m.)

	DDC–alanine		DDC–glucoside	
	p.p.m.	µg/g fresh wt	p.p.m.	µg/g fresh wt
Cucumber	15	12	0	0
Tobacco	5	4	7	6
Apple	0	0	0	0

For the small tobacco plants which we used this means that each leaf contained only about 20 µg of DDC–alanine four days after application of thiram. Twelve days after application neither DDC–alanine nor DDC–glucoside could be detected in sap of the tobacco leaves. From these experiments it appears that free DDC–alanine or DDC–glucoside after leaf application of thiram does not cause an important residue problem.

Metabolism by micro-organisms

It is interesting that by the influence of micro-organisms such as fungi and bacteria sodium-DDC is not converted into DDC–alanine but into DDC–α-aminobutyric acid

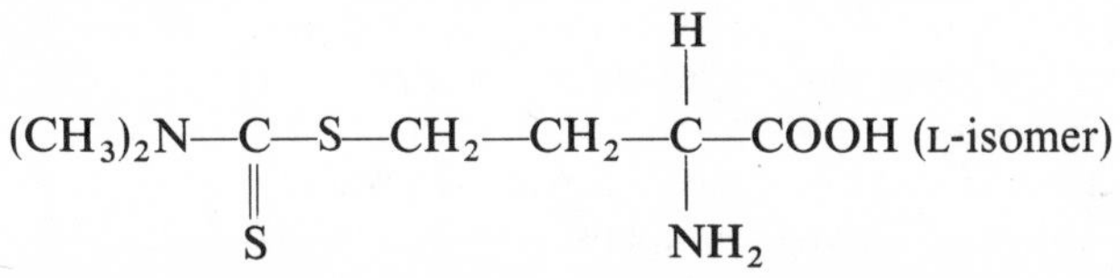

$$(CH_3)_2N-\underset{\underset{S}{\|}}{C}-S-CH_2-CH_2-\underset{\underset{NH_2}{|}}{\overset{\overset{H}{|}}{C}}-COOH \text{ (L-isomer)}$$

and its corresponding keto acid[4, 5, 6, 10]. No DDC-glucoside is formed.

Metabolism in animals

Most studies have been made with tetraethylthiuram disulphide or Antabuse, a drug for treatment of chronic alcoholism. This compound is broken down mainly to carbon disulphide and diethylamine. Partly it is converted into the glucuronic acid conjugate of diethyldithiocarbamic acid[9, 17]. This compound is excreted in the urine.

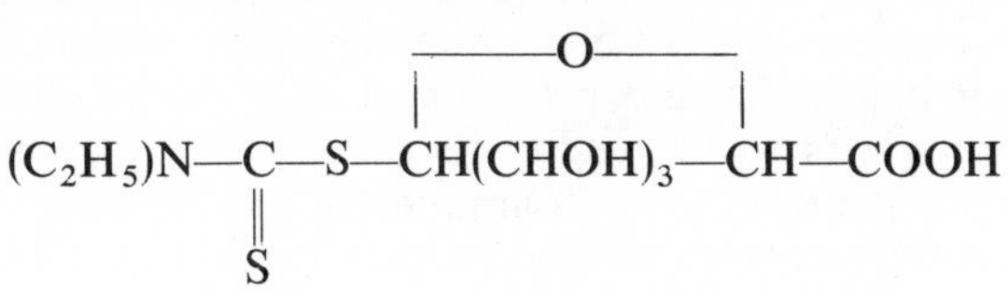

$$(C_2H_5)N-\underset{\underset{S}{\|}}{C}-S-\overset{\overset{O}{\overbrace{\qquad\qquad}}}{CH(CHOH)_3-CH}-COOH$$

237

From these results it is clear that although the fates of DDC in man, micro-organisms and higher plants differ from each other, they have in common a conjugation with naturally occurring metabolites. An interesting feature of these coupling reactions is that in plants foreign compounds are often transformed into glucosides, whereas in many animals glucuronides are formed.

The fate of ethylenebisdithiocarbamates differs completely from the fate of dialkyldithiocarbamates.

ETHYLENEBISDITHIOCARBAMATES

In an acid environment nabam decomposes to ethylenediamine and carbon disulphide. In neutral solution nabam decomposes mainly to ethylenethiourea (ETU) and ethylenethiuram monosulphide (ETM). ETM, moreover, is very slowly transformed into ETU[20]. Other compounds which may arise from aqueous nabam solutions are elementary sulphur, carbonyl sulphide[15], ($O = C = S$) and hydrogen sulphide.

It should be mentioned that recently doubts have arisen about the structure of ETM. Newer investigations with chemically pure ETM and determination of the molecular weight by mass spectrometry showed two hydrogen atoms less in the molecule than originally had been accepted. These investigations are in favour of one of the alternative structures originally considered by Thorn, ethylene bisisothiocyanate sulphide (EBS)[16].

Decomposition products of nabam can easily be separated by chromatography on cellulose thin-layer plates in propanol–water (85:15). Non-fungitoxic compounds with C=S groups such as ETU can be detected with colour reactions. Fungitoxic decomposition products such as EBS can be detected by spraying a dense conidial suspension on the plates. After 2 days at 24°C the zones are visible as inhibition zones. It appeared that nabam in water decomposed rapidly into ETU and EBS. EBS, the main fungitoxic decomposition product is slightly more fungitoxic than nabam[22, 24]. Next, Vonk studied the fate of nabam in cucumber seedlings[22, 24]. The seedlings were placed for two days in a 100 p.p.m. nabam solution and a thin-layer chromatogram was made of sap pressed from the above-ground parts. It appeared that sap contained no fungitoxic compounds (no EBS), but only ETU (30–50 p.p.m.). Most probably ETU has already been formed by decomposition of nabam in the aqueous solution before uptake by the roots. This result is consistent with results obtained by Sato and Tomizawa[18], who presented evidence for the presence of ETU in plants after zineb treatment. ETU appears to be readily taken up from aqueous solutions. *Figure 3* shows you the fate of this compound in cucumber plants after the uptake period. The concentration in expressed sap falls rapidly. However, the total amount did not decrease rapidly. This means that ETU is diluted in sap because of growth.

The fate of ETU has also been studied by Vonk, after feeding 500 p.p.m. ETU for five days to cucumber seedlings[22, 24]. Chromatograms of sap of above-ground parts contained, apart from ETU, another spot which reacted positively with nitroprusside reagent but negatively with iodine–sodium azide, indicating the absence of the C=S group. From chromatographic data and paper electrophoresis with a synthetic product the compound has recently been identified as 2-imidazoline[23] (*Figure 2*).

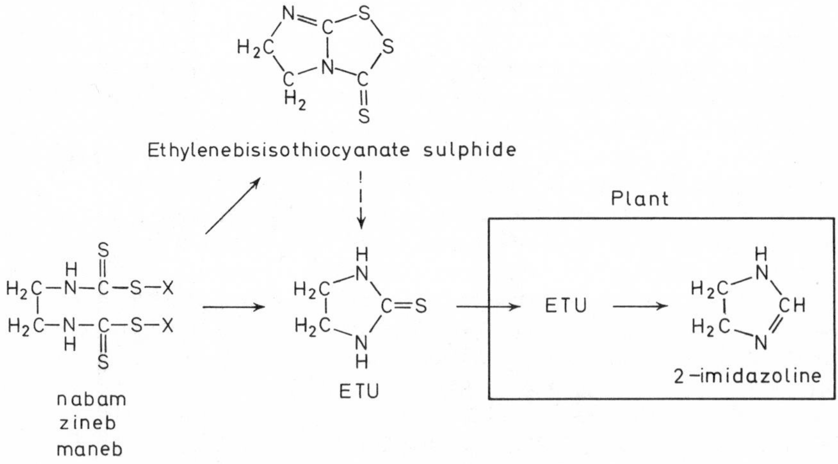

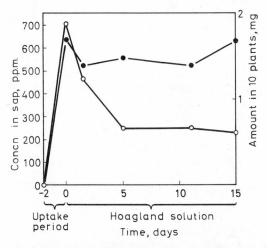

Figure 2. Scheme of transformation of ethylenebisdithiocarbamates [22–24].

Figure 3. Stability of ethylenethiourea (ETU) in cucumber seedlings after root treatment for two days with 300 p.p.m. of ETU. ○ Concentration in sap of seedlings; ●, total amount of ETU in ten seedlings[24].

239

The mechanism of conversion of ETU into 2-imidazoline is still obscure. The compound is formed in plant sap to which ETU has been added, and even in denatured sap, but not in water or phosphate buffer. It thus seems that certain plant constituents catalyse this non-enzymatic reaction. The compound is rather unstable in alkaline solutions. The removal of sulphur from cyclic thiourea derivatives by living organisms is surprising, since substitution of sulphur by oxygen is far more common, for instance, with thiouracil[25].

It must, however, be emphasized that ETU is only broken down very slowly. Plants were treated by root application with 500 p.p.m. of ETU. After five days sap contained 700 p.p.m. of ETU and only 10–20 p.p.m. of 2-imidazoline[23].

ETU could also be detected in plants after root treatment with zineb or maneb[24]. Cucumber seedlings placed for 2 days with the roots in 1 000 p.p.m. suspension of zineb or maneb contained about 300 p.p.m. ETU in the sap. In this case, however, no 2-imidazoline could be detected. Obviously the amount of ETU and thus of 2-imidazoline in the plant is so low after treatment with bisdithiocarbamates that 2-imidazoline escapes detection. It must be stressed here that in the FAO report on the evaluation of some pesticide residues in food (FAO/PL: 1967/MII/1, WHO/Food add./68.30, Rome 1968), 2-imidazoline and ETU were mentioned as intermediate degradation products of mancozeb applied to plants. No further details were given, however. Our work suggests that with mancozeb, too, 2-imidazoline was formed with ETU as an intermediate. At present, ETU must be considered as the most important terminal residue of bisdithiocarbamates such as nabam, zineb and maneb. It is very stable in plants but also in soil (pH 6)[8]. On incubation in soil the concentration of ETU declined only very slowly (Vonk, unpublished).

The known goitrogenic activity of ethylenebisdithiocarbamates[1] may stress the importance of a study on the fate of these compounds and ETU in animals. However, it must also be noted that after leaf application of zineb or maneb, with our method ETU could not be detected in sap from the leaves. Moreover, even if some ETU would be present in the plants after several leaf applications, we must consider the fact that ETU is highly soluble in water and not in fat. For this reason we do not expect a serious accumulation in fat of animals as occurs with DDT.

Summarizing, we can say that the breakdown of dialkyldithiocarbamates and ethylenebisdithiocarbamates runs along completely different lines. Whereas dialkyldithiocarbamates are subject to conjugate formation similar conjugates could not be detected with ethylenebisdithiocarbamates.

Finally I would like to make a general remark about studies on the fate of pesticides. Modern isotope techniques are useful to obtain a complete balance sheet of the pesticide. Conversion products or breakdown products which do not show up in colour reactions or bioassays can be detected when using radioactive labelled pesticides.

However, a warning is needed here. First, radioactive chemicals are often not as pure as indicated on the label. Secondly, often only those plant fractions soluble in organic solvents are examined for radioactivity, whereas the insoluble fractions, which often contain radioactivity, are not subjected to further studies. This must be regretted, not only by those studying the risks of residues but also by anyone who is interested in the mode of action of pesticides. In the fungicide field we rarely see an attempt to obtain a complete balance sheet. More often the study involves not more than a few paper-chromatographic or thin-layer results of a fraction soluble in an organic solvent.

Because of the emphasis laid upon us nowadays to decrease the hazards of unknown terminal residues we cannot be content until we can give a complete balance sheet of the pesticide.

REFERENCES

[1] R. Blackwell Smith, J. K. Finnegan, P. S. Larson, P. F. Sahyoun, M. L. Dreyfuss and H. B. Haag. *J. Pharmac. Exp. Ther.* **109**, 159 (1953).

[2] H. M. Dekhuijzen, *Neth. J. Plant Path.* **70**, suppl. 1, 1 (1964).

[3] J. W. Hylin and B. H. Chin. *Abstracts of the 6th Internat. Congress of Plant Protection*, 614 (1967).

[4] A. Kaars Sijpesteijn, H. M. Dekhuijzen, J. Kaslander, C. W. Pluijgers and G. J. M. van der Kerk. *Meded. Landbouw., Gent.* **28**, 597 (1963).

[5] A. Kaars Sijpesteijn and J. Kaslander. *Outlook on Agriculture*, **4**, 119 (1964).

[6] A. Kaars Sijpesteijn, J. Kaslander and G. J. M. van der Kerk. *Biochim. Biophys. Acta*, **62**, 587 (1962).

[7] A. Kaars Sijpesteijn and G. J. M. van der Kerk. *Ann. Rev. Phytopath*, **3**, 127 (1965).

[8] A. Kaars Sijpesteijn and J. W. Vonk. *Meded. Landbouw., Gent*, **35**, 799 (1970).

[9] J. Kaslander, *Biochim. Biophys. Acta*, **71**, 730 (1963).

[10] J. Kaslander, 'Metabolic fate of dithiocarbamates', *Dissertation*, Utrecht University (1966).

[11] J. Kaslander, A. Kaars Sijpesteijn and G. J. M. van der Kerk. *Biochim. Biophys. Acta*, **52**, 396 (1961).

[12] J. Kaslander, A. Kaars Sijpesteijn and G. J. M. van der Kerk. *Biochim. Biophys. Acta*, **60**, 417 (1962).

[13] G. J. M. van der Kerk. *Meded. Landbouw., Gent*, **21**, 305 (1965).

[14] F. Massaux, *Meded. Landbouw., Gent*, **28**, 590 (1963).

[15] W. Moje, D. E. Munnecke and L. T. Richardson. *Nature, Lond.*, **202**, 831 (1964).

[16] C. W. Pluijgers, J. W. Vonk and G. D. Thorn, *Tetrahedron Letters*, **18**, 317 (1971).

[17] R. C. Robbins and J. Kastellic. *J. Agr. Food. Chem.*, **9**, 256 (1961).

[18] T. Sato and C. Tomizawa. *Bull. Nat. Agr. Sci. Sect. C.*, **12**, 181 (1960).

[19] G. D. Thorn. *Canad. J. Chem.* **38**, 2349 (1960).

[20] G. D. Thorn and R. A. Ludwig. In *The Dithiocarbamates and Related Compounds*. Elsevier: Amsterdam (1962).

[21] G. D. Thorn and L. T. Richardson. *Canad. J. Bot.* **40**, 22 (1962).

[22] J. W. Vonk. *Meded. Landbouw., Gent*, **36**, 109 (1971).

[23] J. W. Vonk and A. Kaars Sijpesteijn. *Pesticide Biochem. Physiol.* In press (1970).

[24] J. W. Vonk and A. Kaars Sijpesteijn. *Ann. Appl. Biol.* **65**, 489 (1970).

[25] R. T. Williams. *Detoxification Mechanisms*. Chapman and Hall: London (1959).

THE METABOLIC FATE OF DITHANE M-45*
(COORDINATION PRODUCT OF ZINC ION AND MANGANOUS ETHYLENEBISDITHIOCARBAMATE)

W. R. Lyman

Rohm and Haas Co., Philadelphia, Pa 19105, USA

ABSTRACT

The degradation and metabolism of Dithane M-45 in water, in plants and in animals has been reviewed in this report. It is shown that degradation proceeds through a series of intermediate substances to yield metallic cations (Mn^{2+} and Zn^{2+}), inorganic materials (elemental sulphur, thiosulphate ion, sulphate ion etc.) and organic materials leading ultimately to ethylenediamine, which in turn is further metabolized to compounds which enter the general metabolic pool of plants and animals, and are converted into natural substances. It is of special significance that the degradation of Dithane M-45 apparently follows similar pathways in the animal system and in plants, and that the various intermediate compounds identified in each biological system are about the same. Chronic feeding studies on rats and dogs with Dithane M-45 have therefore obviously involved an evaluation of the toxicity of the metabolites as well as the parent compound. These chronic studies, including reproductive studies, reveal no unusual or unexpected effects from Dithane M-45. New residue analytical methods have been developed which determine: (1) total residues containing an ethylenediamine moiety (except ethylene thiourea) with a sensitivity of 0.05 p.p.m. as Dithane M-45; (2) ethylene thiourea specifically with a sensitivity of 0.01–0.05 p.p.m. These methods have been applied to Dithane M-45-treated potatoes from commercial growers and to milk and cow tissues from cows fed with various levels of Dithane M-45 residues, as they occur on leafy crops treated with the fungicide. From the information presented, it is concluded that total Dithane M-45 residues in potatoes will not exceed 1.0 p.p.m. and that ethylene thiourea is negligible as a result of current commercial usage of Dithane M-45 on potato plants to control fungus disease. It is further concluded that the feeding of potatoes or potato products to cattle does not lead to detectable residues from Dithane M-45 in milk or in edible tissues. Presently available information indicates that Dithane M-45 will not be persistent in the environment.

INTRODUCTION

Dithane M-45 is the most recent commercial development among the ethylenebisdithiocarbamate fungicides. Zineb and maneb are closely related products that have been in use as agricultural fungicides for many years.

---

* In some areas the generic name 'mancozeb' has been applied to this product.

Dithane M-45 has been a commercial product since 1962 and is used extensively as a fungicide on various fruits and vegetables throughout the world, now in greater volume in most use areas than either zineb or maneb.

Toxicological[1] and residue[2] studies have been conducted on this composition and separate crop tolerances have been established for it in the USA[3], and Canada and a few other countries. It is described chemically[3] as the coordination product of zinc ion and manganous ethylenebisdithiocarbamate containing 20 per cent manganese, 2.5 per cent zinc and 77.5 per cent ethylenebisdithiocarbamate. The structure may be represented by the formula shown in *Figure 1*[4].

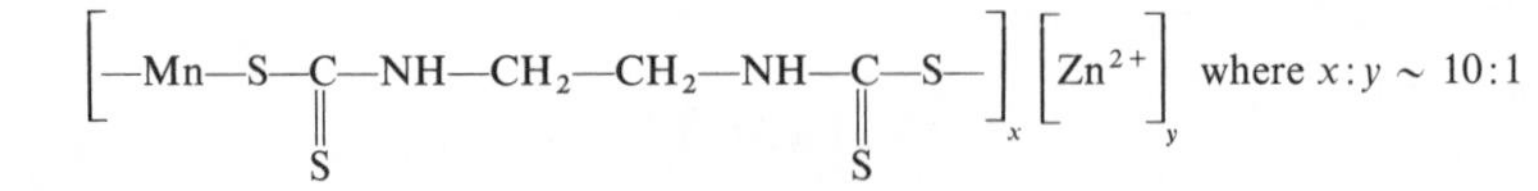

$$\left[\text{—Mn—S—} \underset{\underset{S}{\|}}{C} \text{—NH—CH}_2\text{—CH}_2\text{—NH—} \underset{\underset{S}{\|}}{C} \text{—S—} \right]_x \left[\text{Zn}^{2+} \right]_y \quad \text{where } x:y \sim 10:1$$

Figure 1.

The zinc in this coordination structure is firmly bound and incapable of being washed away preferentially from the polymeric salt. Because of the low solubility and polymeric nature of this chemical the classical methods of purification and structure determination are not applicable. Formulations are not prepared from an essentially pure base diluted with additives as with most pesticide formulations. A high purity product can be obtained by careful attention to purity of reactants and by careful post-washing of the insoluble polymer. The commercial product Dithane M-45 has a label claim of 80 per cent active and represents about the highest concentration economically feasible.

Infra-red, x-ray, ultra-violet absorption, polarographic data. physical separation studies and biological evaluations have demonstrated Dithane M-45 to be a unique member of the dithiocarbamate family of fungicides. All studies reported in this work were with Dithane M-45. No studies have been conducted to determine whether the fate of maneb or zineb or other related products is identical. Presently there is no experimental basis for extrapolating these findings on Dithane M-45 to any other dithiocarbamate fungicides.

To aid in the study of the metabolic fate of Dithane M-45, three radioactively tagged samples were synthesized. These were based on ^{14}C-labelled ethylenediamine, on ^{35}S-labelled carbon disulphide, and a doubly labelled sample based on ^{3}H-labelled ethylenediamine and ^{35}S-labelled carbon disulphide.

METABOLISM AND FATE OF RESIDUE STUDIES

Preliminary chemical studies

Studies *in vitro* with 0.10 to 3.0 per cent slurries of Dithane M-45 in distilled water showed that the material is subject to oxidative degradation, yielding water-soluble and water-insoluble products. The former included zinc and manganous ions, thiosulphate ion and ethylene thiourea (ETU). Insoluble products included elemental sulphur and lesser amounts of the compound heretofore known as ethylenethiuram monosulphide[5, 6]. This compound has been shown by nuclear-magnetic-resonance and isotope-exchange experiments not to conform with the ETM formula shown in *Figure 2*, but is now considered to have structure A or B, and is hereafter referred to as ethylenebisisothiocyanate sulphide (EBIS). Both ethylene-thiuram disulphide (ETD) and ethylenebisisothiocyanate sulphide (EBIS) may occur as intermediates in the oxidative process.

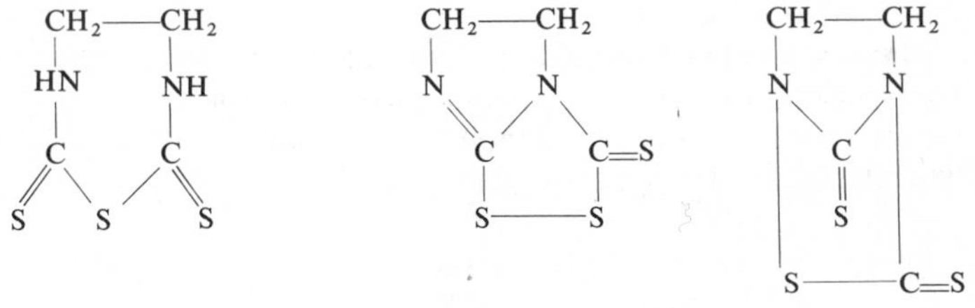

Figure 2.

No more than trace amounts of ethylenethiuram disulphide (ETD[6]) were detected.

Fate of Dithane M-45 in and on plants

Dithane M-45 labelled with radioisotopes (^{3}H, ^{14}C or ^{35}S) was applied to leafy plants (sugar beets, lettuces or turnips) grown outdoors under normal conditions of weather. In a relatively short-term study, radioactivity was

Table 1 Compounds detected in plant residues two weeks after application of labelled Dithane M-45*

Compound	Percentage of ^{3}H activity
Ethylene urea (EU)	17
Ethylenediamine	11
Dithane M-45[7]	9
2-Imidazoline†	
N-Formyl ethylenediamine†	8
Ethylenebisisothiocyanate sulphide	7
Ethylene thiourea	6
Jaffe's base‡	4
Total	62 (of ~ 200 p.p.m. as Dithane M-45)

* Exaggerated application rates were used to assure detectable residues for identification
† These compounds are interconvertible under some experimental conditions.
‡ Jaffe's base: 3-(2-imidazolin-2-yl)-2-imidazolidinethione.

accounted for, by using reverse isotope-dilution techniques, *Table 1*, 13 days after application.

Elemental sulphur, EBIS, ETU and sulphate ion were all detected on leaf surfaces which had been treated with ^{35}S-labelled Dithane M-45. Elemental sulphur and sulphate ion were shown as forming about 30 per cent of the total ^{35}S activity.

It should be recognized that the quantitative figures in *Table 1* are only an example, and not intended to indicate a typical distribution of the percentages of the residues present.

In a full-season experiment with two varieties of potatoes grown outdoors, ^{14}C-labelled Dithane M-45 was applied each week from early in the growing season until near harvest. *Table 2* shows the amount of Dithane M-45 applied and the residues detected.

Table 2. ^{14}C-labelled residues in potatoes treated with ^{14}C-labelled Dithane M-45

	Cobbler	Katahdin	
Foliar sprays, at 1.5 lb/acre	6	5	
Foliar sprays, at 2 lb/acre	5	5	
Total, lb of Dithane M-45/acre	19	17.5	
Weeks from last spray to harvest	3	3	6
Total ^{14}C-labelled residue in tubers, p.p.m.	1.4	1.2	1.4

By reverse isotope-dilution techniques only trace quantities of ethylene thiourea and ethylene urea were detected in Cobbler potatoes, as follows: ETU 0.0022 p.p.m.; EU 0.0056 p.p.m.

A substantial portion (55 per cent) of the ^{14}C activity present was found in starch isolated from Cobbler potatoes. Hydrolysis of the starch to glucose followed by its conversion into glucosazone did not change the specific activity on a molar basis. A small amount (three per cent) of the ^{14}C activity was isolated as glycine by a reverse isotope-dilution method. After overnight refluxing in 9N-sulphuric acid, ^{14}C activity detectable as ethylenediamine was 20 to 25 per cent (three weeks sample) or nine per cent (six weeks sample).

In a separate experiment, in which a single treatment of ^{14}C-labelled Dithane M-45 was applied to radish and tomato plants, which were then kept in a greenhouse, the conversion of total ^{14}C (determined by combustion and radioassay) into ethylenediamine by acid hydrolysis was progressively lower with time, as shown in *Table 3*.

Table 3. ^{14}C-labelled residue in radish foliage

Days after treatment	0 and 7	14	20	28	35
Conversion into EDA, per cent	*ca.* 90	55	47	43	30

From these experiments it is concluded that Dithane M-45 on or in plants is converted through a series of intermediate steps into ethylenediamine, which in turn is oxidized to glycine. This naturally-occurring amino acid, by known metabolic processes, may be converted into a host of different natural substances. The conversion of carbon atoms once present as Dithane M-45 into starch in the potato also strongly supports this conclusion.

Metabolism in animals

Rat feeding study with ^{14}C-labelled Dithane M-45

Six rats were each dosed via a stomach tube with 20 mg of ^{14}C-labelled Dithane M-45 (from [^{14}C]ethylenediamine) each day for seven days. (The specific radioactivity of the ^{14}C-labelled Dithane M-45 was 23.1 μCi/g and was the same material as used in the work on plants.) This dosage corresponds approximately to 100 mg/kg body weight or 1 000 p.p.m. based on total diet. The rats were killed one day after the final dose. Radioassay of excreta and tissues gave the distribution shown in *Table 4* for ^{14}C activity fed.

Table 4 ^{14}C-labelled Dithane M-45 material balance in rats

Material	[14]C, percentage of total dosage
Faeces	70.9
Urine	15.5
Cage washings	3.98
Intestinal washings	0.18
Organ and tissue samples	0.31
Carcasses	0.96
Total recovery	91.8

Analysis of urine and faeces samples, by the reverse isotope-dilution technique, for specific components of residues, which had been identified originally in or on leafy plants, gave the results shown in *Table 5*.

Table 5. Percentage of ^{14}C activity in rat excreta present as known transformation products of Dithane M-45

Material	Percentage of urine [14]C	Percentage of faeces [14]C	Percentage of recovered [14]C*
Dithane M-45[7]	—	47.0	36.8
EBIS	5.6	7.5	7.1
ETU	28.0	6.0	10.8
EU	12.0	2.0	4.1
N-Acetyl EDA	19.0	—	4.1
N-Formyl EDA	1.0	—	0.1
EDA	3.5	—	0.7
	69.1	62.5	63.7

* In urine, faeces and cage washings (^{14}C in cage washings is assumed to be derived from urine).

247

Radioassay of selected tissue samples gave information shown in *Table 6*.

Table 6. Analysis of rat tissues by radioassay

Tissue sample	Percentage of total dose given	Total wt * (g)	Amount as Dithane M-45, p.p.m.
Muscle	0.014	17.3	6.8
Fat	0.010	10.7	7.4
Liver	0.193	65.6	24.8
Kidney	0.076	12.6	51.6
Thyroid	0.003	0.032	865.0
Heart	0.005	5.45	8.2
Brain	0.003	9.67	2.2
Spleen	0.007	5.29	10.7
Total	0.314		

* Total weight of tissue taken from six rats fed 1 000 p.p.m. in diet.

No work was done to determine the chemical form of the ^{14}C activity in any of the tissue samples.

It is concluded from the information obtained from this study that elimination is remarkably prompt and complete, in view of the relatively massive dose administered. Considering that there was no withdrawal period after dosing and that Dithane M-45 is metabolized to naturally occurring substances in cows (see below), the residue levels found in tissues are relatively low, except in the thyroid.

It is well known that this class of compounds commonly produces thyroid hyperplasia in rat-feeding studies and the comparatively high residue level found in the above rat study is not surprising. A number of toxicity tests have been conducted to evaluate the effect of Dithane M-45 on animals. In three months sub-acute studies on rats fed with Dithane M-45, the threshold level for detectable thyroid hyperplasia was determined to be 100 to 150 p.p.m. in the total diet. However, in two years of chronic studies on rats and dogs fed with 0, 25, 100 and 1 000 p.p.m. of Dithane M-45 in the diet, thyroid hyperplasia was limited only to some of the rats (fed with 1 000 p.p.m.). No effect was noted in dogs, either grossly or histologically. Neither rats nor dogs showed any reduction in protein-bound ^{131}I uptake. It can be considered that the 1 000 p.p.m. feeding level of Dithane M-45 in the daily diet did not have an adverse effect on thyroid function. Aside from the thyroid hyperplasia in rats (with no discernible adverse effect on thyroid function), the 1 000 p.p.m. diet level in both rats and dogs was a no-effect dosage in the above studies and in reproduction studies.

The above metabolic studies on Dithane M-45 show that the breakdown in plants and in animals is quite similar. The metabolites excreted in the rat urine provide good evidence that the animal was exposed metabolically to these various decomposition products of Dithane M-45. The above-mentioned sub-acute and chronic toxicity studies therefore not only provide a measure of the toxicity of Dithane M-45 but also a measure of the toxicity of the total terminal residue products that are found in or on plants treated with Dithane M-45.

Cow feeding study with ^{14}C-labelled Dithane M-45

One lactating Guernsey cow was dosed twice daily with ^{14}C-labelled Dithane M-45 (from [^{14}C]ethylenediamine) for three successive 14 day periods at 1 p.p.m., 5 p.p.m. and 25 p.p.m. levels respectively, based on 20 kg daily feed. Milk samples were taken each day. Collections of urine and faeces for 24 h were made once during the second week of each test period. The cow was killed and selected tissues were sampled for analysis at the end of the project.

The recovery of ^{14}C in excreta for the day of collection, compared with the ^{14}C administered per day for each dose level, is given in *Table 7*.

Table 7. ^{14}C-labelled Dithane M-45 material balance in cows

Dose (p.p.m.)	Residue in excreta (p.p.m., as Dithane M-45)			Recovery (per cent)
1	Urine	0.50		13.9
	Faeces	0.47		86.1
			Total	100.0
5	Urine	4.75		31.6
	Faeces	1.49		54.4
			Total	86.0
25	Urine	19.7		32.8
	Faeces	10.4		68.2
			Total	101.0

The average level in milk during the second week of each test period was directly related to the dosing level, as shown in *Table 8* and *Figure 3*.

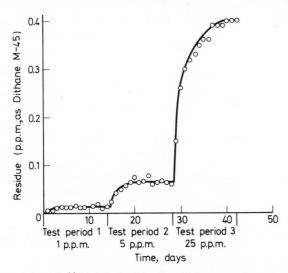

Figure 3. ^{14}C-labelled residues in milk from experimental cow

249

Table 8. ^{14}C in milk versus dose level

Dose (p.p.m.)	Residue in milk (p.p.m.)	Ratio p.p.m. (milk) / p.p.m. (dose)
1.0	0.014	0.014
5.0	0.066	0.013
25.0	0.390	0.016

(All values are calculated as Dithane M-45)

The occurrence of ^{14}C-containing residues in tissues on the day after the last day of dosing at 25 p.p.m. (no withdrawal period) was as shown in Table 9.

Table 9. Analysis of cow tissues by radioassay (Feeding level: 25 p.p.m. of Dithane M-45)

Tissue	p.p.m. (as Dithane M-45)	Tissue	p.p.m. (as Dithane M-45)
Bone (hard tissue)	0.03	Liver	5.6
Bone (marrow)	NDR*	Kidney	1.4
Muscle (thigh)	0.10	Thyroid	14.7
Muscle (flank)	0.15	Heart	0.25
Muscle (triceps)	0.11	Brain	0.19
Fat (mesentery)	NDR	Tripe	0.22
Fat (kidney)	NDR	Tongue	0.19
Fat (heart)	NDR	Lung	0.43
Fat (flank)	0.07	Blood	0.32

* NDR: No detectable residue (< 0.01 p.p.m. for tissues).

Studies were conducted to determine the chemical nature of the ^{14}C-containing residues in milk and urine (from the 25 p.p.m. dosing period) by analysing for specific substances and determining the percentage of the total ^{14}C activity found in the form of naturally occurring materials (Table 10).

Table 10. ^{14}C activity in the milk and urine of cows fed with 25 p.p.m. of Dithane M-45

Substance	Milk		Urine	
	p.p.m.	Percentage of ^{14}C	p.p.m.	Percentage of ^{14}C
Ethylene thiourea	0.03	23	0.06	0.84
Ethylene urea	0.01	10	0.79	12
Urea	—	—	—	3
Oxalic acid	—	—	—	3
Glycine	—	—	—	12
Fat	—	5	—	—
Protein	—	7	—	—
Lactose	—	15	—	—

From these studies it is concluded that a high percentage of Dithane M-45 ingested by a cow is promptly excreted, that extensive metabolism occurs leading, ultimately, to the incorporation of some of the carbon atoms into naturally occurring materials. The level of [14C]-containing materials in milk was about 1.5 per cent of the concentration ingested. Again, the thyroid tissue showed the highest level of [14C]-containing residues, as with rats.

Cow feeding study with [14C]ethylene thiourea

The presence of ethylene thiourea as a possible terminal residue or a transitional residue is of interest. Its fate in the animal body was studied in the cow. Three cows were each dosed for a period of 14 days with [14C]ethylene thiourea at different levels based on 20 kg of total feed. The concentrations of [14C]-labelled residues found in milk, excreta and selected tissues were as shown in Table 11.

Table 11. Analysis of milk, excreta and tissues from cows fed with [14C]ethylene thiourea

Material	Dose of ETU		
	0.01 p.p.m.	0.10 p.p.m.	1.00 p.p.m.
Milk	NDR*	0.003	0.036
Urine	0.030	0.138	1.76
Faeces	NDR	0.010	0.127
Kidney	NDR	0.009	0.127
Liver	0.007	0.043	0.670
Bladder	0.011	0.088	0.381
Thyroid	0.019	0.148	1.55

* NDR: No detectable residue
(< 0.0025 p.p.m., milk : < 0.006 p.p.m., other samples).

Other tissues (same list as the Dithane M-45 cow-feeding study) had no detectable residue at the two lower doses, but detectable residue ranging from 0.01 to 0.04 p.p.m. at the 1.0 p.p.m. dosage.

The distribution of [14C] activity among materials which were isolated and identified from milk and urine from the cow dosed at 1.0 p.p.m. with ETU is shown in Table 12.

Table 12. [14C] activity in the milk and urine of cows fed with 1 p.p.m. of [14C]ethylene thiourea

Material	Conc. (p.p.m.)	Milk % of total [14C]	Conc. (p.p.m.)	Urine % of total [14C]
Ethylene thiourea	0.011	31	0.12	7
Ethylene urea	0.0025	8	0.27	18
Ethylenediamine	—	—	0.14	14
Glycine	—	—	—	6
Oxalic acid	—	—	—	12
Urea	—	—	—	11
Fat	—	3	—	—
Protein	—	18	—	—
Lactose	—	16	—	—
Totals (per cent)		76		68

From this experiment with ethylene thiourea, it is concluded that the level of total ^{14}C residues is related to dose in each substance analysed. It is further concluded that ethylene thiourea is metabolized to progressively simpler substances, such that carbon from this molecule eventually enters the general metabolic pool.

ANALYTICAL METHODS FOR DITHANE M-45 RESIDUES
Carbon disulphide method
An analytical method of long standing for the determination of residues from ethylenebisdithiocarbamate fungicides is the measurement of carbon disulphide generated by treating the sample with hot mineral acid. Various modifications of this method have been widely used for many years. The modification used in Rohm and Haas Co. laboratories has been referred to previously[7].

Ethylenediamine method
It is clear from examination of the chemical structures listed in the section above on the fate of Dithane M-45 in plants that many of the known components of Dithane M-45 residues are incapable of producing carbon disulphide and hence are not determinable by that method. Further consideration of the structures shows that ethylenediamine is the most logical moiety common to these substances on which to base a total residue analytical method.

Extensive work has led to the successful development of such a residue analytical method for which the chemical basis is as follows. The sample is digested in mineral acid to convert all components of residues into ethylenediamine. This then is converted into the bispentafluorobenzamide, which, after separation of interfering substances by liquid column chromatography, is determined by gas chromatography with an electron capture detector.

The sensitivity of detection for this method is 0.01 p.p.m. (as EDA) or 0.05 p.p.m. (as Dithane M-45). The average recovery of fortifications of various components of Dithane M-45 residues in reagents and in two different substrates is as shown in *Table 13*.

Table 13. Recovery of Dithane M-45 and metabolites in EDA method

Fortification	Average percentage recovery		
	Reagents	Potatoes	Milk
Dithane M-45	87	77	67
Ethylenediamine (EDA)	82	82	72
Ethylene urea (EU)	78	78	66
Ethylene thiourea (ETU)	94	15	19
Ethylenebisisothiocyanate sulphide (EBIS)	49	57	40
N-Acetyl ethylenediamine	79	68	72

Ethylene thiourea method
In the data given in *Table 13* for the recovery of fortifications in the EDA

252

method, it is to be noted that ethylene thiourea, while recovered in high percentage from reagents, was not recovered well from substrates. The reason is as yet unknown. Because of this, and the interest in knowing the magnitude of this particular component of residue, a separate method for the determination of ethylene thiourea, specifically, has been developed. In this method the ethylene thiourea is solvent-extracted from the sample, separated from gross interferences by liquid chromatography and converted into a derivative which is ultimately determined by gas chromatography with a flame-photometric detector.

The sensitivity of detection of ETU by the present method is 0.01 p.p.m. for milk and cow tissues and 0.05 p.p.m. for potatoes. (It should be noted that a method[8] different from the one described here was presented at the 84th Annual Meeting of the Association of Official Analytical Chemists (Washington, D.C.; 13 October 1970).

RESIDUE STUDIES

Studies have been conducted utilizing these new procedures in determining residues in potato tubers from potato plants sprayed with Dithane M-45, and in cows fed with aged Dithane M-45 residues on alfalfa. Potatoes were selected because this is one of the major worldwide crop usages for Dithane M-45. Treating alfalfa with Dithane M-45 is not a normal commercial practice but this served as a convenient crop on which to collect and age residues of Dithane M-45 for subsequent feeding to dairy cows.

Potato analyses

Over 300 samples of potatoes from about 40 different growers in eleven states in the USA were collected. Treatments ranged from 1 to 3 lb of Dithane M-45 (80 per cent active)/acre and the number of treatments ranged from 3 to 13, with total quantities of Dithane M-45 applied ranging from 8 to 36 lb/acre during the season. The interval between the final treatment and harvest ranged from 0 to 55 days.

Analyses by the carbon disulphide procedure[7] of a selected number of samples of potato tubers detected no residues in excess of 0.10 p.p.m. (calculated as Dithane M-45).

Analyses of all samples were conducted with the new EDA procedure. There was no obvious correlation between the residues found and the way in which the various fields were treated. The highest residue found was 0.78 p.p.m. in a sample treated eight times (20 lb in total of Dithane M-45 during the season) with no time interval between the last application and harvest. No detectable residues were found in two of the sets (34 and 46 days from last application until harvest). The grand average of all treated samples analysed was 0.17 p.p.m., calculated as Dithane M-45.

Selected samples from among those analysed by the EDA method were also analysed specifically for ethylene thiourea by the new ETU method. Seventy nine treated and thirty five control samples were analysed. No residues could be detected in any of the treated samples by this ETU procedure, as shown in *Table 14*.

253

Table 14. Analyses of potato tubers for ethylene thiourea residues (samples from potato fields commercially treated with Dithane M-45)

Potato tuber samples	No. treated	Average chromatograph peak height (mm)
Non-treated controls	35	3 ± 2
Treated (with Dithane M-45)	79	3 ± 3
Fortified (0.05 p.p.m. ETU)	18	17 ± 8
Fortified (0.10 p.p.m. ETU)	11	32 ± 7

The fact that no detectable residue of ETU ($<$ 0.05 p.p.m.) was found in these potato tubers is in complete agreement with the ^{14}C experiments reported earlier in this paper in which a level of 0.0022 p.p.m. was detected by using the reverse isotope-dilution technique.

Feeding of aged Dithane M-45 residues to cows

This experiment, conducted between November 1969 and January 1970, involved feeding 15 lactating cows with alfalfa treated weekly the previous summer with Dithane M-45 at 3 lb/acre. The hay was stored in bales, then ground and homogenized. This ground hay was analysed for Dithane M-45 residues by the EDA method and used as the source of residue in the cow experiment. Amounts of treated and untreated hay were varied among the cows to provide five groups (three cows per group): food doses 0, 0.78, 9.7, 38.9 and 97.2 p.p.m., calculated as Dithane M-45. Within each group one cow was terminated after two weeks, three weeks, and four weeks, at which time tissue samples were taken for analysis. Representative samples of milk produced each day were collected for analysis. Urine and faecal samples were collected for one 24 h period during the second week on the test feed.

Analysis of milk revealed no detectable residue in cows on the 0.78 p.p.m. feed level. Barely detectable residues were found in about half the milk samples from cows on the 9.7 p.p.m. feed level. Detectable residues averaging 0.11 p.p.m. were found in the milk from cows on the 38.9 p.p.m. feed level, and 0.32 p.p.m. from cows on the 97.2 p.p.m. level.

Milk samples from the three highest feeding levels were analysed specifically for ethylene thiourea by the new method (sensitive to 0.01 p.p.m.). Samples significantly different from the controls were found only at the 97.2 p.p.m. feeding level.

From these milk analyses it can be concluded that ingestion of aged Dithane M-45 residues, such as might occur on leafy crops, will not lead to residues in milk until the level ingested exceeds 10 p.p.m., calculated as Dithane M-45, based on the total quantity of feed consumed. Obviously the feeding of commercially sprayed potatoes to livestock will not result in detectable residues in milk of either Dithane M-45 or its metabolites.

The analysis of excreta from these cows fed with aged residue of Dithane M-45 showed as expected that the residues in urine and faeces were related to the levels fed. However, less than half the residues fed could be accounted for in the excreta. This was not unexpected in view of the findings in the tracer experiments that metabolism in the animal can convert these materials

254

into substances within the metabolic pool which are incapable of conversion into ethylenediamine.

Tissues from each cow from each of the three upper feed levels and control cows were analysed by both the EDA and ETU analytical procedures. The tissues analysed were muscle (three locations), fat (three locations), liver, kidney and thyroid.

These analyses detected no appreciable residues in muscle or fat at any feeding level except the highest (97.2 p.p.m.). Significant residues in the liver and kidney were found at the 38.9 p.p.m. feeding level. These ranged from 0.10 to 0.85 p.p.m. by the EDA method, and 0.02 to 0.10 p.p.m. by the ETU method. Residue values in the thyroid from treated cows were different from the controls only at the highest feeding level (97.2 p.p.m.).

FATE OF DITHANE M-45 IN THE ENVIRONMENT

This exhaustive study on the fate of Dithane M-45 is being continued with residue studies on various other crops and with investigations on the fate of Dithane M-45 in the environment. Several findings from the research reported in this paper bear directly on this subject. It has been shown that oxidative degradation of Dithane M-45 occurs readily in water. It has also been shown that, in both plants and animals, the fungicide is degraded and metabolized until the carbon atoms from the ethylenediamine moiety enter the metabolic pool of the organism and are incorporated into naturally occurring substances such as carbohydrates, fats, proteins, urea and carbon dioxide. It is reasonable to assume that micro-organisms present in soil and natural waters will also hasten the degradation of residues in these media. Preliminary findings from incubation of soil into which ^{14}C-labelled Dithane M-45 has been incorporated have shown a detectable amount of carbon dioxide to be produced within one week. It can be concluded from the available knowledge at this time, that Dithane M-45 will not be persistent in any part of the environment.

ACKNOWLEDGEMENT

It is acknowledged that the work reported briefly in this report is the result of a cooperative effort of many individuals working over an extended period of time. It is expected that the work will be reported in a series of detailed publications, with the particular individuals who conducted the research as authors. The author of this report has only compiled the information available at this time for easy reference and review.

REFERENCES

[1] P. S. Larson, Personal communications (1964–66).
[2] Rohm and Haas Co., Philadelphia, USA. Unpublished reports.
[3] *Code of Federal Regulations.* Title 21, part 120.176. The National Archives of the USA.
[4] *US Pat. No. 3379610.* (Agdoc No. G-2034).
[5] G. D. Thorn and R. A. Ludwig, *Canad. J. Chem.* **32**, 872 (1954).

6 G. D. Thorn and R. A. Ludwig, *The Dithiocarbamates and Related Compounds*. Elsevier: New York (1962).

7 C. F. Gordon, R. J. Schuckert and W. E. Bornak, *J. Assoc. Offic. Anal. Chem.* **50**, 1102–1108 (1967).

8 J. H. Onley and G. Yip, *J. Assoc. Offic. Anal. Chem.* **50**, 165–169 (1971).

CHEMISTRY AND METABOLISM OF THIOPHANATE FUNGICIDES

T. NOGUCHI, K. OHKUMA and S. KOSAKA

Nisso Institute for Life Science, Oiso, Japan

ABSTRACT

Thiophanates, dialkyl 4,4'-*o*-phenylene bis (3-thioallophanate) are recently developed novel types of systemic fungicides. These compounds are weakly acidic, stable in acidic medium but fairly unstable in alkaline medium at room temperature. Thiophanates, synthesized by the reaction of *o*-phenylenediamine and isothiocyanoformic acid esters, were converted into 2-alkoxycarbonyl-aminobenzimidazoles under reflux in acetonitrile with calcium oxide. Dynamic patterns of biotransformation of thiophanates were examined in plants and animals by using ^{14}C- and ^{35}S-labelled thiophanates and a new radiotracer technique of co-TLC–radioautography and whole-body radioautography. The systemic metabolism of the compound was studied in French beans, grapes, cucumbers, apples and mice. Enzymological behaviour of thiophanates was examined in a cell-free system or rat liver microsomes. The differences in the metabolic pattern observed between ^{14}C- and ^{35}S-labelled thiophanates in both studies clearly indicated that cleavage of the bonds between carbon and sulphur atoms readily took place. The main resulting metabolites were identified as 2-alkoxycarbonylaminobenzimidazoles by co-TLC–radioautography in animals and plants. The benzimidazole derivatives were hydroxylated at the 5-position of the benzene ring and eliminated rapidly as conjugates in mouse urine. Thiophanate and thiophanate-methyl had similar biotransformation patterns; however, the urinary elimination rate of thiophanate-methyl was higher than that of thiophanate.

INTRODUCTION

IN a series of investigations[1-6] on the selective toxicity of organosulphur compounds, naphthiomates were found to be specifically active against *Trycophyton* spp. by Noguchi *et al.*[7]. Naphthiomate-T, to which an alternative name (tolnaftate) was given by the American Medical Society, is now in world-wide use as an effective chemotherapeutic agent for athlete's foot.

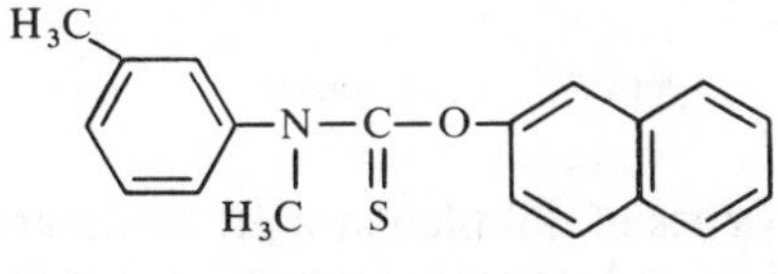

Naphthiomate-T (Tolnaftate).

257

K

Further extension of the work to arylthiocarbamides from arylthiono-carbamates led in 1968 to the invention of the compounds named thio-phanates[8, 9], which were very effective against many important fungal diseases in plants.

Thiophanates have been highly evaluated in the successful field trials in Japan and many other countries in Europe and America[10] (*Table 1*).

Table 1. Effectiveness

NH·C·NH·COO·R (with S double bonds) R; CH₃, C₂H₅ Thiophanates	Apple scab (*Venturia inaequalis*) Pear scab (*Venturia nashicola*) Peach, plum and cherry brown rot (*Sclerotinia cinerea*) Grape grey mould (*Botrytis cinerea*) Citrus scab (*Elsinoe fawcetti*) Strawberry grey mould (*Botrytis cinerea*) and powdery mildew (*Sphaerotheca humuli*) Vegetables grey mould (*Botrytis cinerea*) Sclerotinia rot (*Sclerotinia sclerotiorum*) and powdery mildew (*Sphaerotheca fuliginea*) Sugar beet Cercospora leaf spot (*Cercospora beticola*) Common hop grey mould (*Botrytis cinerea*) and downy mildew (*Pseudoperonospora humuli*) Apple, peach and citrus post-harvest decay (*Penicillium* sp. and *Botrytis* sp.)

CHEMISTRY OF THIOPHANATES

Some confusion over the nomenclature of thiophanates is worthwhile mentioning here. The efficacy of diethyl 4,4'-*o*-phenylene bis(3-thioallo-phanate) was discovered first and this compound was named thiophanate. A little later dimethyl 4,4'-*o*-phenylene bis (3-thioallophanate) was found to be superior and was named thiophanate-methyl. Therefore it is incorrect to say methyl thiophanate for thiophanate-methyl.

Thiophanates are crystalline substances obtainable in quantitative yield by the reaction of *o*-phenylenediamine and alkyl isothiocyanoformate.

$$Na \cdot SCN + Cl \cdot COOR \xrightarrow[\text{in AcOEt}]{\text{Reflux}} SCN—COO \cdot R$$

Synthesis of thiophanates.

Physicochemical properties of thiophanates are summarized in *Table 2*.

They are weakly acidic substances, forming water-soluble salts with sodium and potassium ions and sparingly water-soluble salts with calcium,

Table 2. Physicochemical properties of thiophanates

	Thiophanate	Thiophanate-methyl
m.pt	192 ∽ 193°C (decomp.)	177 ∽ 178°C (decomp.)
λ_{max} (chloroform)	271 mμ	271 mμ
ε_{max}	18 000	19 000
pK'_a	10·5	10·2
Solubility at 25°C (%)		
Water	Sparingly soluble	Sparingly soluble
n-Hexane	Sparingly soluble	Sparingly soluble
Methanol	2·0	3·0
Chloroform	4·6	2·7
Acetone	2·9	5·9
Acetronitrile	20·0	2·5
Cyclohexanone	10·0	4·4

barium and cupric ions. Solubilities of thiophanates in most of the common solvents are relatively low.

As shown in *Figure 1* they are stable in acidic but unstable in alkaline solution at room temperature.

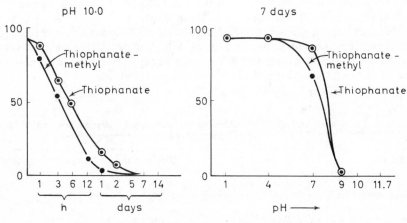

Figure 1. Stability of thiophanates at different pH values.

259

Chemical reactivities of thiophanates are summarized in the scheme:

Chemical reaction of thiophanates.

Most remarkable reaction among those shown is the degradative cyclization to 2-alkoxycarbonylaminobenzimidazoles. This reaction takes place nearly quantitatively when thiophanates are refluxed with calcium oxide in acetonitrile, boiled with cupric acetate in 50 per cent acetic acid[11] or merely heated in dimethylformamide to 80°C. The reaction is important since it is involved in the biotransformation of thiophanates.

The reaction does not proceed at all when thiophanates are kept in methanol or chloroform for 50 days at 24°C but proceeds to some extent when thiophanates are kept at pH 7·0 in water for seven days, as measured by colorimetric assay with bromocresol purple (*Table 3*).

Table 3. Transformation rate of thiophanates to 2-alkoxycarbonylaminobenzimidazoles in non-biological systems

Condition	Thiophanate	Thiophanate–methyl
In phosphate buffer pH 7·4 at 37°C for 2 h	<1%	<1%
In phosphate buffer pH 7·0 at 25°C for 7 days	2%	4%
In methanol at 24°C for 50 days	0·0	0·0
In chloroform at 24°C for 50 days	0·0	0·0

The reaction may be accelerated slightly on contact of thiophanates with adsorbents such as silica gel or alumina. However, it was confirmed that diatomaceous earth, having been used for formulation, did not accelerate this reaction at all at temperatures ranging from 20° to 50°C.

METABOLISM OF THIOPHANATES

Taking the above-described chemical properties of thiophanates into account, chemodynamic transformation patterns of thiophanates both in plant and animal were investigated with ^{14}C- and ^{35}S-labelled compounds.

Synthesis of radioisotopically labelled thiophanate

Three kinds of labelled thiophanates were synthesized as shown in the scheme.

Scheme for synthesis of labelled thiophanates.

The positions of labelling are: (1) ^{14}C at one of the thioureido groups; (2) ^{14}C at one of the alkyl groups of esters; (3) ^{35}S at one of the thioureido groups. Urethane labelled at the ester carbon atom was also prepared. The specific radioactivities of the compounds are shown in *Table 4*.

Table 4. Specific radioactivities of labelled thiophanates and urethanes

R	thiourea-^{14}C	thiourea-^{35}S	alkyl-^{14}C	urethane-^{14}C
C_2H_5	1.42 µCi/mg	4.75 µCi/mg	1.62 µCi/mg	0.883 µCi/mg
CH_3	1.35 µCi/mg	2.67 µCi/mg	0.883 µCi/mg	0.361 µCi/mg

Chemodynamic transformation pattern of thiophanates in plants

Labelled thiophanates were applied either to one of the primary leaves of French bean seedlings (*Phaseolus vulgaris*), by dotting, or to the hypocotyl,

261

by injection, and each radioautogram was developed 21 days after application. An example of such a radioautogram is shown in *Figure 2*.

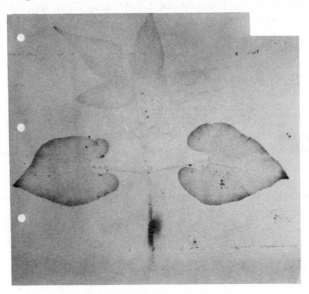

Figure 2. Radioautogram of bean treated with [^{14}C]-thiophanate-methyl. Stem injection: 21 days.

Radioactivities distributed in each part of the plant and that escaping as gas were determined by a liquid scintillation spectrophotometer. The results with thiophanate-methyl are shown in *Table 5*.

Table 5. R.I. recovery in parts of bean plant and expired gas 14 days after foliar dotting in metabolic cage

	Thiophanate-methyl			
	Thiourea-^{14}C		Thiourea-^{35}S	
	d.p.m.	%	d.p.m.	%
Applied radioactivity	6.62×10^5	(100)	4.84×10^5	(100)
Treated leaf	47.9×10^4	72.4	31.2×10^4	64.4
Trapped gas	6.33×10^4	9.6	8.09×10^4	16.7
Stem. Untreated leaf	5.72×10^4	8.6	4.43×10^4	9.1
Root	1.34×10^4	2.1	2.21×10^4	4.6
Total activity	6.13×10^5	92.7	4.59×10^5	94.8

Most of the radioactivity (72.4 per cent) remained in the primary leaf treated, eight to nine per cent was translocated to the rest of the plant and ten to seventeen per cent escaped as gas. This last portion was significantly greater than that found with the ^{14}C-labelled compound; suggesting that degradation took place at the C=S bond.

Similar patterns of distribution of radioactivity were obtained with grapes and apples.

CHEMISTRY AND METABOLISM OF THIOPHANATE FUNGICIDES

To elucidate the metabolic fate of thiophanates, *Phaseolus* seedlings treated with ^{14}C- and ^{35}S-labelled compounds were extracted with chloroform. The extracts were subjected to TLC–radioautography, and the results are shown in *Figure 3* and *Figure 4*.

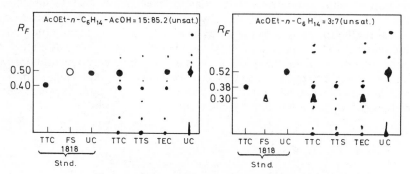

From medium of water culture (bean plant, 7 days).
Nearly the same patterns were obtained from: bean plant: foliar dotting, stem injection, homogenate. Cucumber plant: foliar dotting, stem injection, water culture. Grape and apple: foliar dotting, stem injection.

Figure 3. Thin-layer chromatography–radioautograms of chloroform-extractable metabolites of thiophanate in plants.

TTC, ^{14}C-thiophanate labelled at one of the thioureido carbon atoms;
FS1818, 2-ethoxycarbonylaminobenzimidazole;
UC, ^{14}C-labelled urethane;
TTS, ^{35}S-thiophanate labelled at one of the thioureido sulphur atoms;
TEC, ^{14}C-thiophanate labelled at ester carbon atoms.

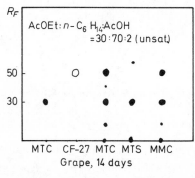
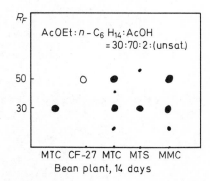

From treated leaf of foliar dotting.
Nearly the same patterns were obtained from: grape: stem injection. Apples: stem injection, foliar dotting. Bean plant: stem injection, water culture.

Figure 4. Thin-layer chromatography–radioautograms of chloroform-extractable metabolites of thiophanate–methyl in plants.

MTC, ^{14}C-thiophanate–methyl labelled at one of the thioureido carbon atoms;
CF27, 2-methoxycarbonylaminobenzimidazole;
MTS, ^{35}S-thiophanate–methyl labelled at one of the thioureido sulphur atoms;
MMC, ^{14}C-thiophanate–methyl labelled at one of the ester carbon atoms.

263

The results indicated that the main metabolite (metabolite A) did not contain a sulphur atom but did contain carbon from thiocarbamide and ester. It was also expected from the behaviour of the metabolite on TLC, namely a lower R_f value than that of thiophanate (with tailing), when developed with a relatively less-polar solvent (ethyl acetate–n-hexane; 3:7, v/v), that major metabolites were more polar than thiophanates, probably due to the loss of one ester group. These main metabolites from thiophanate and thiophanate-methyl are identified respectively as 2-ethoxy-carbonylaminobenzimidazole (ECAB) and 2-methoxycarbonylaminobenz-imidazole (MCAB) by means of thin-layer co-chromatography and identities of i.r. spectra of isolated crystals with those of authentic samples which were synthesized via an independent route (*Figure 5* and *Figure 6*).

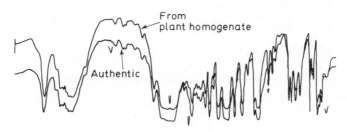

R : CH_3 or C_2H_5

Synthesis of 2-alkoxycarbonylaminobenzimidazoles.

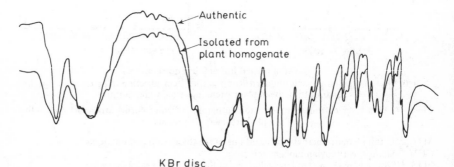

KBr disc

Figure 5. Infra-red spectra of metabolite A and synthetic standard ECAB.

KBr disc

Figure 6. Infra-red spectra of metabolite A and synthetic standard MCAB.

264

The amount of the metabolites formed varied from 30 per cent to 90 per cent of the total radioactive materials recovered by chloroform extraction, depending on how the plant was treated (*Table 6*).

Table 6. Conversion rate of thiophanates into 2-alkoxycarbonylaminobenzimidazole in plants (foliar treatment)

	French bean	Grape	Apple
Thiophanate	30.0% (67.5%*)	41.6%	36.7%
Thiophanate-methyl	34.3% (87.5%*)	48.8%	62.7%

* Absorption from root in water culture

Feeding thiophanates through the roots to the plant was more efficient than foliar application in converting thiophanates into metabolite A.

Chemodynamic transformation pattern of thiophanates in animals

Mice (dd-Y strain), which were kept in a metabolic cage, were given orally

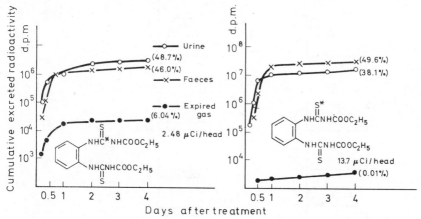

Figure 7. Balance study of thiophanate in mice.

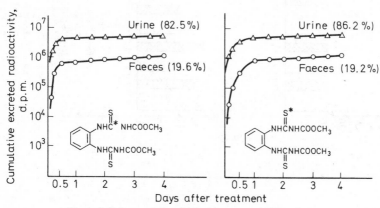

Figure 8. Balance study of thiophanate–methyl in mice.

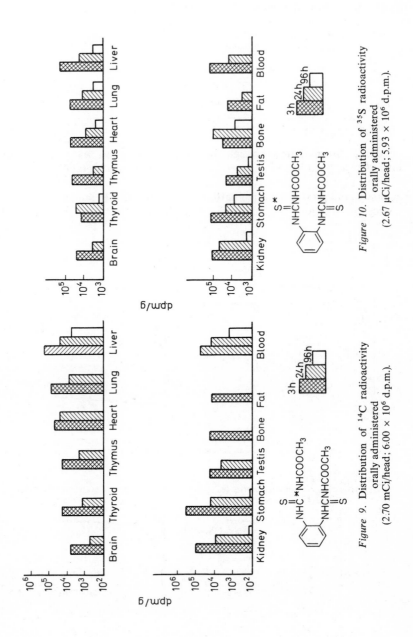

Figure 9. Distribution of ^{14}C radioactivity
orally administered
(2.70 mCi/head; 6.00 × 10^6 d.p.m.).

Figure 10. Distribution of ^{35}S radioactivity
orally administered
(2.67 μCi/head; 5.93 × 10^6 d.p.m.).

administered ^{14}C- or ^{35}S-labelled thiophanates. Radioactivities in faeces, urine and expired gas were measured at certain intervals (*Figure* 7 and *Figure 8*).

Thiophanate was eliminated in the faeces in greater amount than thiophanate-methyl, indicating that thiophanate was less adsorbed through the gastrointestinal tract into the cardiovascular system, whereas thiophanate-methyl was absorbed more efficiently and eliminated rapidly in the urine.

Time-course distributions of radioactivity in each organ and tissue of mice treated with thiophanate were studied with whole-body radioautography. With the ^{14}C-labelled compound all the radioactivity was excreted in 42 h and no accumulation was observed. With the ^{35}S-labelled compound a small

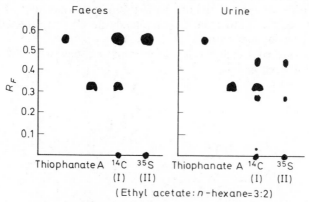

Figure 11. Thin-layer chromatography–radioautogram of chloroform-soluble metabolites of thiophanate in mice.

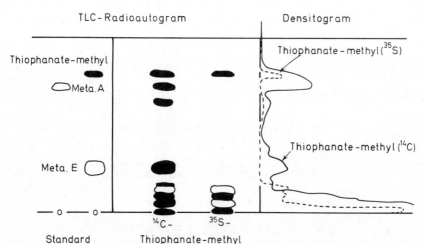

Figure 12. Thin-layer chromatography–radioautogram and densitogram of metabolites in urine of mice treated with ^{14}C- or ^{35}S-labelled thiophanate–methyl.

267

amount of ^{35}S remained in some cartilages, indicating that organic sulphur was metabolized to inorganic sulphate and incorporated into cartilage as chondroitin sulphate.

A liquid scintillation spectrophotometer was used for the determination of the time-course distributions of radioactivity in each organ and tissue with respect to thiophanate-methyl (*Figure 9* and *Figure 10*). In line with the above results from the radioautographic study of thiophanate, almost all the radioactivity disappeared within 96 h from any organ and tissue with the ^{14}C-labelled compound.

Metabolites of thiophanates in faeces and urine were studied with TLC–radioautography. With thiophanate, 2-ethoxycarbonylaminobenzimidazole was detected as a major metabolite in the faeces (*Figure 11*).

In the urine of mouse treated with thiophanate-methyl, 5-hydroxy-2-methoxycarbonylaminobenzimidazole (metabolite E) was detected together with unhydroxylated compound (*Figure 12*).

It was identified by thin-layer co-chromatography with the authentic sample synthesized as follows[12].

Synthesis of 5-hydroxy-2-alkoxycarbonylaminobenzimidazole.

The hydroxylated benzimidazole derivative appeared to be largely present as conjugate, since treatment of urine with enzyme (glucuronidase and sulphatase) greatly increased its amount (*Figure 13*).

Enzymological behaviour of thiophanates in rat liver microsomes was also studied. Thiophanate gave a fair amount of ECAB in this system and 5-hydroxy-2-methoxycarbonylaminobenzimidazole along with MCAB was detected with thiophanate-methyl.

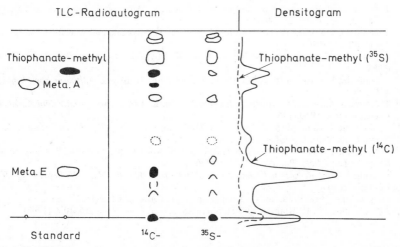

Figure 13. Thin-layer chromatography–radioautogram and densitogram of metabolites in enzyme-treated urine of mice given orally ^{14}C- or ^{35}S-labelled thiophanate–methyl. (Enzyme: β-glucuronidase and sulphatase).

Evidence for enzyme induction could not be obtained with liver microsomes prepared from rats which had been fed daily with 640 p.p.m. of thiophanate-methyl for 3 months (*Figure 14*).

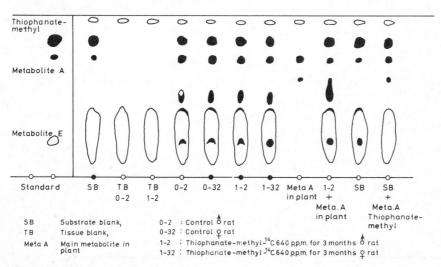

Figure 14. Thin-layer chromatography–radioautogram of metabolites in liver microsomes of rats fed on a control diet or given 640 p.p.m. of thiophanate–methyl in food.

REFERENCES

[1] T. Noguchi, Y. Hashimoto, K. Miyazaki and A. Kaji. *J. Pharm. Soc., Japan.* **88**, 227 (1968).
[2] T. Noguchi, Y. Hashimoto, K. Miyazaki and A. Kaji. *J. Pharm. Soc., Japan.* **88**, 335 (1968).

³ T. Noguchi, Y. Hashimoto, S. Kosaka, M. Kikuchi, K. Miyazaki, R. Sakimoto and K. Kaji. *J. Pharm. Soc., Japan,* **88**, 344 (1968).
⁴ T. Noguchi, S. Kosaka, Y. Hashimoto, M. Kikuchi, K. Miyazaki and A. Kaji. *J. Pharm. Soc., Japan,* **88**, 353 (1968).
⁵ T. Noguchi, Y. Hashimoto, K. Kikkawa and K. Miyazaki. *J. Pharm. Soc., Japan,* **88**, 465 (1968).
⁶ T. Noguchi, Y. Hashimoto, T. Makita, K. Miyazaki and K. Miyagi. *J. Pharm. Soc., Japan,* **88**, 473 (1968).
⁷ T. Noguchi, A. Kaji, Y. Igarashi, A. Shigematsu and K. Taniguchi. *Antimicrobial Agents and Chemotherapy,* p 259 (1962).
⁸ T. Noguchi, K. Khomoto, Y. Yasuda, S. Hashimoto, K. Kato, K. Miyazaki and S. Kano. (Nippon Soda Co. Ltd.), *Belg. Pat. No. 722080* (1969).
⁹ T. Noguchi, Y. Yasuda, M. Asada, S. Hashimoto, K. Kato, K. Miyazaki and S. Kano.(Nippon Soda Co. Ltd.), *Belg. Pat. No. 734742* (1969).
¹⁰ K. Ishii. *VIIth International Congress of Plant Protection, Paris* (21–25 September 1970). Résumés, p 200.
¹¹ H. A. Selling, J. W. Vonk and A. Kaars Sijpesteijn. *Chem. and Ind.* 1625 (1970).
¹² J. A. Gardiner, R. K. Brantley and H. Sherman. *J. Agr. Food Chem.* **16**, 1050 (1968).

THE FATE OF CARBOXIN IN SOIL, PLANTS AND ANIMALS

W. T. Chin, G. M. Stone and A. E. Smith

Uniroyal Chemical, Elm Street, Naugatuck, Conn. 06770, USA

ABSTRACT

The systemic fungicidal activity of carboxin, 5,6-dihydro-2-methyl-1,4-oxathiin-3-carboxanilide (Vitavax), was reported by von Schmeling and Kulka in 1966. It has proved most useful as a seed treatment for small grains, cotton and peanuts, to control smuts, bunts and seedling blights. Carboxin is absorbed by germinating seeds and moves upwards in the seedling. It travels with the transpiration stream and moves into lower stem and first leaves of the plant. It does not redistribute into new growth as the plant develops. The molecule is surprisingly resistant to hydrolysis, but is readily oxidized to the sulphoxide in water, soil, plants and animals. Young plants contain carboxin, its sulphoxide and traces of the sulphone, as well as bound anilide complexes. Residues in mature plants, including seed, are less than 0·2 p.p.m., the sensitivity of analytical methods. Animals excrete carboxin and its degradation products rapidly; no accumulation in tissues is indicated, even after two-year feeding tests. Analytical techniques used in this work, and preliminary fate studies on oxycarboxin are also discussed.

INTRODUCTION

The systemic fungicidal activity of carboxin (Vitavax®) has been reported by von Schmeling and Kulka[1]. Carboxin has proved most useful as a seed treatment for small grains, cotton and peanuts to control smuts, bunts and seedling blights. It is particularly effective against basidiomycete-type fungi.

Since it is systemic, and is used on food crops, it was important to study residues in plants and animals, as well as its fate in the environment. Both ^{14}C-radioactivity and non-radioactive techniques were used in this work.

EXPERIMENTAL

Two samples of ^{14}C-labelled carboxin (I) were used in these studies, one labelled uniformly in the aniline ring, the other labelled in the 2 position of the oxathiin ring.

Specific activity was about 1 mCi/m-mol. Plants grown from treated seed gave satisfactory radioautograms after a few days exposure. Quantitative data on amounts of radio residues in various tissues were obtained by wet

® Uniroyal Inc. Registered Trademark.

(I) Carboxin

(5,6-Dihydro-2-methyl-1,4-oxathiin-3-carboxanilide)

oxidation and scintillation counting. It was possible to detect 0.05 p.p.m., calculated as carboxin.

Thin-layer-chromatographic (TLC) techniques were developed for carboxin and six of its possible hydrolysis and oxidation products, since hydrolysis of the anilide linkage and/or oxidation at the bivalent sulphur seemed likely[2]. The products considered were carboxin (I), its sulphoxide (II) and sulphone (III), the three corresponding heterocyclic carboxylic acids and aniline. With silica-gel plates and chloroform development good separation was given for most of the samples encountered. Alternative systems were also developed. Visualization was satisfactory under u.v. illumination after a fluorescein spray.

Specific determination of carboxin by gas–liquid chromatography (GLC) is possible since carboxin can be separated from its degradation products and determined quantitatively in plant extracts with a short, inert GLC column and a specific sulphur detector[2]. Residue methods are based on the fact that carboxin and its derived residues in soil, plants and animals can be hydrolysed to liberate aniline, which is steam-distilled. The steam-distillate is subjected to conventional cleaning techniques and determined by a colorimetric method[3] or by GLC, using a specific nitrogen detector[4].

(a) The colour method is useful for direct caustic hydrolysis of green plant samples. The aniline is distilled and coloured with a p-dimethylaminobenz-aldehyde. This method is sensitive to 0.05–0.20 p.p.m.; the interference level (apparent residue in an untreated sample) varies with the tissue. Recoveries are usually between 80 and 100 per cent. Recent adaptations make it possible to analyse meat, milk and eggs.

(b) Unfortunately the colorimetric method is not useful for low residue levels in most kinds of seeds, because the untreated sample blanks show about 1 p.p.m. for apparent carboxin. To analyse such samples, the GLC method has been developed. This procedure involves grinding the sample, Soxhlet extraction with methanol, and conventional cross-extraction cleaning techniques. The sample is then subjected to caustic hydrolysis, the aniline is steam-distilled, extracted, concentrated and analysed by GLC, using a microcoulometric nitrogen detector. Reagent blanks vary from 0.04–0.1 p.p.m., and crop samples from untreated plots range from 0.0–0.2 p.p.m. The method has been used for small grains, peanuts, sorghum, corn and cotton, and adapted for vegetable oils, seed meals and dry mature plants.

FATE IN WATER AND SOIL

By using unlabelled carboxin and the TLC techniques reported, it was found that carboxin is readily oxidized to the sulphoxide in water; at pH 2 half was oxidized in a few weeks and further oxidation to the sulphone could be detected after about two months. Oxidation was much slower at pH values in the range 4 to 8, but after six months the sulphoxide and traces of sulphone were detected. At pH 10 no change was noted even after four years. Surprisingly, hydrolysis was not observed under any of these conditions.

In soil even more rapid oxidation to the sulphoxide has been noted[2]. In one typical soil (pH 6) the half-life of carboxin was only about one week. Although microbial activity may be a factor, it has been shown that carboxin is readily oxidized (presumably by dissolved oxygen) in sterilized water, soil and in a variety of organic solvents.

The presence of thiram or captan in fungicidal formulations has had little or no effect on the rate of oxidation of carboxin in soils tested.

Further oxidation to the sulphone is difficult and slow in soil, but traces of sulphone have been detected in some cases by TLC techniques.

FATE IN PLANTS

The fate of carboxin in plants was investigated from three main viewpoints: (a) uptake and distribution of [^{14}C]carboxin (effects of plant species, age and position of ^{14}C-label); (b) chemical nature of residues; (c) magnitude of residues (effect of crop, plant part and test conditions).

Uptake and distribution

Seeds of several plant species were treated with normal and exaggerated doses of [^{14}C]carboxin, both the aniline ring- and heterocyclic-labelled materials being used. When the seeds are planted and germinate, ^{14}C-labelled chemicals are absorbed and move upward in the seedling.

1. Wheat, cotton and peanuts show similar distribution patterns. Cotton and wheat (two-week seedlings) are shown in *Figure 1*. The heaviest concentration is in the basal portion of the cotton hypocotyl and the first leaves. Movement up into the next leaves can be seen; the activity moves in the vascular tissues and tends to concentrate at leaf margins and tips, indicating typical apoplastic movement. Wheat shows an analogous pattern. Similar conclusions have been reached by Snel and Edgington[6].

2. Radioautograms of seedling plants at various growth stages show the ^{14}C is not re-translocated from the lower leaves; trace residues found in the third set of leaves are probably from continued uptake and movement with the transpiration stream. Essentially no ^{14}C could be detected in new growth made after a few weeks.

3. Radioautograms of 2- to 8-week seedlings of several crops were made, comparing the distribution of ^{14}C from the heterocyclic- and aniline-labelled carboxin treatments. The patterns show no significant differences. This indicates that the two ring systems remain attached to each other during absorption and movement.

Chemical nature of the residues

The rapid oxidation of carboxin in water and soil would suggest the sulphoxide (II) as a likely plant residue, and the immobility of ^{14}C-labelled

273

Photograph   Radioautograph

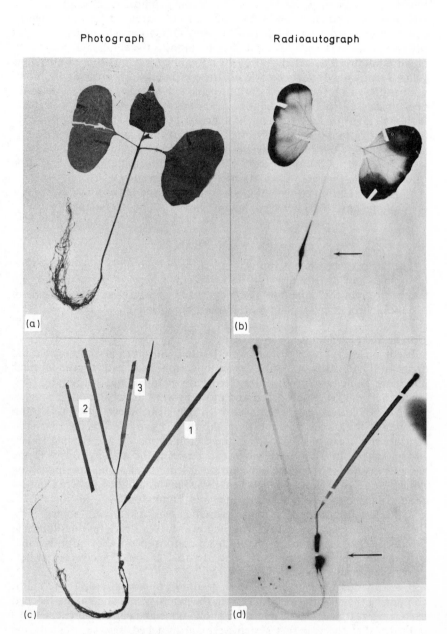

Figure 1. Distribution of ^{14}C in cotton and wheat.
(a) Two-week cotton: (b) Arrow denotes the hypocotyl; (c) Two-week wheat: 1 first leaf; 2 second leaf; 3 third leaf; (d) Arrow denotes the crown.

274

residues in the hypocotyl and lower leaves suggests the possibility of complex-formation.

An extraction procedure was used to separate and identify residues in plants grown from carboxin-treated seed[5]. Similar work has been done with [14C]carboxin, but suitable non-radioactive techniques made it possible to do much of the work on field grown crops without using 14C.

Extracts of plants grown from [14C]carboxin treated seed showed carboxin and the sulphoxide by TLC, as expected. This work also showed that both extractable and non-extractable residues could be hydrolysed to give aniline, so the colorimetric test was used to measure total residues in the young plant, and the unextracted residue. The extractable residues were separated by TLC; the separated products were scraped from the plate and analysed by the colour test. Alternatively the carboxin could be determined directly, in the extract, without separation. This was done by gas–liquid chromatography under conditions that allowed carboxin to come off the column well ahead of the sulphoxide.

The nature of the extractable residues in young plants is illustrated in *Table 1*. These data show exaggerated residues from high rate greenhouse

Table 1. Change in composition with time of extractable residues from barley in greenhouse

Analysis for	Analytical method		Residues (p.p.m.)				
		Time (weeks) 1	2	4	6	15
Total anilides	Colour	28	17	6	1	0
Carboxin	Direct MCGC	3	1	0.3	0	0
Sulphoxide	TLC + colour	19	15	6	0.5	0

treatments, but are useful to show that even at one week after crop emergence the main residue is the sulphoxide.

The trends noted from the above data and from experiments involving 14C-radioactivity and non-radioactive studies in the greenhouse and the

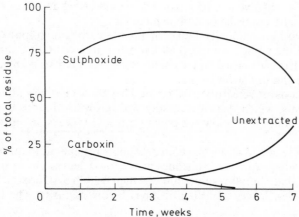

Figure 2. Typical composition of residues in barley and wheat.

field are illustrated graphically in *Figure 2*. Results are plotted to show the change, with time, of the relative amounts of carboxin, sulphoxide and bound complex. It does not show the total p.p.m. of residue; that will be discussed below.

The unextracted residue has been analysed by direct caustic hydrolysis to liberate aniline, but has not been separated from plant tissue in a form to allow full characterization. It is associated with the lignin fraction and appears to represent a detoxication mechanism of the plant, since at exaggerated doses large amounts are bound. The structure is not known, but the complex can be hydrolysed by acids[6] and bases[5] to liberate aniline, and it is not effective as a fungicide. Since the unextracted residue contains ^{14}C whether the aniline- or heterocyclic-labelled form is used, we believe that both moieties are involved in the anilide complex.

Since the predominant extractable residue in plants is the sulphoxide it is of interest to know whether it is absorbed from the soil, or whether carboxin is oxidized in the plant to give the sulphoxide. We have shown that both routes occur: (a) plants take up [^{14}C]sulphoxide (II) from soil; (b) plants whose roots are immersed in a suspension of carboxin show predominantly (II) in their foliage even though the suspension shows only carboxin.

Small amounts of oxycarboxin (III, the sulphone) have been detected in cotton and small grains. It may come from the soil or be formed in the plant. It is difficult to detect except in the ^{14}C studies, since there is much less of it than of the sulphoxide, and plant interference is a problem in the TLC work.

These results are on wheat and barley, but similar results have been obtained on cotton and other crops. Cleavage to liberate aniline and the heterocyclic acid has not been detected in our work.

Amount of residues

The possibility of residues in food under conditions of practical use has been investigated with both ^{14}C-labelling and other residue methods.

The ^{14}C studies, with both labelling positions used, have been run in the greenhouse and the field. The crops were grown to maturity. Harvested cotton, wheat, sorghum and barley showed no detectable residue in the seed. This method is sensitive to 0·05 p.p.m. and would detect any form of residue containing the heterocyclic or aniline moieties.

Since the residues actually found in plants (carboxin, sulphoxide, oxycarboxin and the anilide complex) all hydrolyse to give aniline, most of the residue work has been based on the colour test (green plants) and the MCGC* method (seed and dry straw).

These methods are sensitive to 0·2 p.p.m. They show relatively high residues in young plants, which decrease rapidly with growth dilution. Under field conditions residues fall below 0·2 p.p.m. in 6 to 10 weeks, as illustrated in *Figure 3*.

Analyses of seed and straw show no detectable residues at maturity for the field crops studied. Any trace residues in the lower leaves are so diluted by plant growth that overall residues are less than 0·2 p.p.m. Under field conditions these oldest leaves are often dropped before maturity. The harvested

---

* MCGC: microcoulometric gas chromatography.

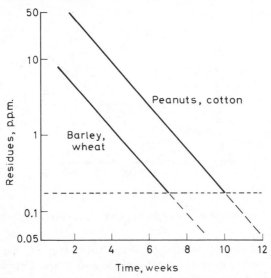

Figure 3. Residues in plant foliage.

seeds show no detectable residues (less than 0·2 p.p.m.) in field studies, and the ^{14}C work indicates that residues are not more than 0·05 p.p.m.

FATE IN ANIMALS*

Rats given a single oral dose of [*phenyl*-^{14}C]carboxin (about 10 to 20 mg/kg) were found to excrete over 90% of the ^{14}C within two days, mainly as sulphoxide in the urine. No ^{14}C was detected in expired air, and only traces of radioactivity were left in tissues. After the animals were killed (four days), the livers contained about 0·15 per cent of the ingested activity (even at the high dose administered this is equivalent to only a fraction of a p.p.m. calculated as carboxin) and even smaller amounts were present in muscle, fat and other organs tested, as shown in *Table 2*.

Table 2. Material balance in rats given [^{14}C]carboxin

Sample	% of administered dose recovered	
	48 h	96 h
Expired air	0.0	0.0
Urine†	60	60 +
Faeces	35	35 +
Liver		0.14
Kidney		0.02
Blood		0.10
Rest of carcass (including hair etc.)		0.20
Total		96

† Mainly as sulphoxide based on TLC.

* Animal studies run by Industrial Biotest Laboratories Inc., Northbrook, Ill.

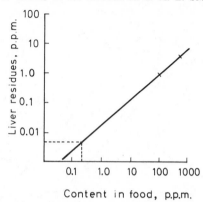

Figure 4. Relationship between feeding level and residues in liver for dogs.

One group of dogs from the two-year toxicology studies was fed with 600 p.p.m. of carboxin in the total diet for two years. This was a no-effect level, and feeding was continued to killing. Organs and excreta from these dogs were analysed to study excretion routes and possible storage in dogs; data are summarized in *Table 3*.

Table 3. Analysis of tissues from dogs fed with carboxin for two years
(600 p.p.m. in total diet)

Tissue	Total residue	Comments
Fat	None detectable	⎰ Method sensitive
Muscle	None detectable	⎱ to 0.5 p.p.m.
Kidney	Trace	About 0.5 p.p.m.
Liver	5 p.p.m.†	⎰ 1 p.p.m. from dogs ⎱ fed 100 p.p.m.

† About 2 p.p.m. carboxin, 1 p.p.m. sulphoxide and 2 p.p.m. polar anilides.

There is no accumulation or storage in the tissues. The small amounts in the liver are believed to be in transit, since animals were fed until they were killed. In any case these low residues at high feeding levels indicate virtually no residues in liver if feeding levels are reduced to 0.2 p.p.m. This is illustrated in *Figure 4*; indicated residues in liver are less than 0.01 p.p.m.

Analysis of the excreta showed elimination in both faeces and urine. The faeces contained more carboxin than sulphoxide; the urine contained polar complexes, sulphoxide and some carboxin.

OXYCARBOXIN

The fate of oxycarboxin (Plantvax®), the sulphone, in plants has been studied briefly since it is of interest as a possible commercial seed treatment on safflower and other crops, and because traces are found in soil and plants from use of carboxin.

278

Work so far indicates that its translocation pattern is similar to that of carboxin. When taken up from the soil it moves into the developing leaves, and tends to accumulate at leaf edges and leaf tips; it does not retranslocate into new growth.

Oxycarboxin is also of interest as a mid-season foliar spray (on wheat, for example, to control rust). In this case residues may be found in foliage. However, in seed treatment and foliar spray work, with ^{14}C and non-radio-active techniques, no evidence of residues has been found in harvested seed. Crops investigated include green beans, safflower and wheat.

SUMMARY

Carboxin (Vitavax) is a systemic fungicide, useful as a seed treatment. The principal reaction of carboxin in water and in soil is oxidation to the sulphoxide. Further oxidation to the sulphone (oxycarboxin) has been detected but is quite limited and slow. Hydrolysis does not appear to be a significant factor.

Plant seedlings take up both carboxin and its sulphoxide from soil. The carboxin is oxidized in the plant also, giving more sulphoxide and traces of sulphone. The chemicals move in the transpiration stream to the margins of the lower leaves. No redistribution is indicated. Part of the residues is bound as a complex, probably with lignin. No residues are detected in the seeds or upper leaves of crops grown from treated seed. The methods used are sensitive from 0·05 to 0·2 p.p.m.

Rats treated with a single oral dose of [^{14}C]carboxin excrete over 90 per cent of the radioactivity within two days, mainly in the urine, as sulphoxide. No respiratory ^{14}C was detected. No accumulation in any tissue was indicated. Tissues from dogs fed with 600 p.p.m. of carboxin in their total diet for two years (a no-effect level) were analysed by TLC and colour techniques. No accumulation in any tissue was indicated; excretion was as carboxin, the sulphoxide and as more-polar derivatives.

Preliminary work on oxycarboxin (Plantvax) shows that it is more stable than carboxin in soil and plants, but that its distribution is similar. No residues have been found in beans or grain harvested from crops treated with oxy-carboxin as a seed, soil or mid-season foliar treatment.

REFERENCES

[1] B. von Schmeling and M. Kulka, *Science*, **142**, 659 (1966).
[2] W. T. Chin, G. M. Stone and A. E. Smith, *J. Agr. Food Chem.* **18**, 731 (1970).
[3] J. R. Lane, *J. Agr. Food Chem.* **18**, 409 (1970).
[4] H. R. Sisken and J. E. Newell, *J. Agr. Food Chem.* In press.
[5] W. T. Chin, G. M. Stone and A. E. Smith, *J. Agr. Food Chem.* **18**, 709 (1970).
[6] M. Snel and L. V. Edgington, *Phytopathology*, **60**, 1708 (1970).

THE TOXICITY OF ORGANOTIN FUNGICIDES

M. S. Rose

M.R.C. Toxicology Unit, Woodmansterne Road,
Carshalton, Surrey, UK

ABSTRACT

Triethyltin does not interact with high affinity with a general class of biological molecules. It does interact with high affinity with a few distinct proteins—two of these being rat haemoglobin and an unidentified protein from guinea-pig liver supernatant. In both of these the binding sites appear to consist of two histidine residues and in the complex so formed the tin atom is penta-coordinate. The tendency to penta-coordination in the group IV metals decreases in the order Pb > Sn > > > Ge and this is in agreement with (a) the decrease in the toxicity of the trialkyl derivatives of these elements, (b) the decrease in their fungicidal activity, (c) the decrease in their ability to interact with rat haemoglobin, and (d) the decrease in their ability to inhibit mitochondrial oxidative phosphorylation. We think therefore that just as we may be able to explain the effects of the dialkyltin derivatives by their reactivity towards dithiols, the toxicological and fungicidal activity of the trialkyltins may reside in their very specific affinity for binding sites containing two histidine residues.

INTRODUCTION

Organotins are widely used for their biocidal activities. Triphenyltin is used as an agricultural fungicide, as an industrial fungicide in paints and has been demonstrated to have a chemosterilant activity against flies. Tributyltin is mainly used as an industrial fungicide, owing to its higher mammalian toxicity.

There are four classes of organotins which have the general structures $RSnX_3$, R_2SnX_2, R_3SnX and R_4Sn, where R can be an alkyl or aryl group and X is an anion, usually sulphate, acetate, chloride or hydroxide. Each class has its own properties, chemical and toxicological, which are dependent on the number of R groups attached to tin, and are largely independent of the nature of X[1].

TOXICOLOGY AND METABOLISM

Monoalkyltins

Little is known generally about the monoalkyltins, but monoethyltin trichloride has a low toxicity in rats when administered either intraperi-toneally or intravenously. A dose of 150 mg/kg body wt given intravenously is not fatal[1]. On oral administration of monoethyltin trichloride to rats at a dose of 25 mg/kg body wt over 90 per cent of the tin was excreted in the

281

faeces[2]. After intraperitoneal injection at a dose of 12.5 mg/kg body wt it was largely excreted in the urine unchanged[2].

Dialkyltins

The dialkyltins are more toxic than the monoalkyltins. The toxicity decreases with increasing size of the R group and doses of 400 mg/kg body wt of dioctyltin can be given to rats orally for three to four successive days without any apparent harmful effects[3]. The dibutyltin salts, and to a lesser extent the other homologues, produce a lesion of the bile duct in rats, which may cause death, and severe lesions of the skin can be produced in rats or guinea-pigs on topical application of these compounds to exposed skin. The effects of dialkyltins are antagonized by 2,3-dimercaptopropanol (British Anti-Lewisite or BAL)[1,4]. The effect of 2,3-dimercaptopropanol in lowering the toxicity of diethyltin suggested that the dialkyltins may act in a similar way to the tervalent arsenicals. This was confirmed by Aldridge and Cremer in 1955, who demonstrated with a rat brain preparation and rat liver mitochondria that diethyltin behaved in an analogous fashion to phenylarsenious acid in inhibiting the oxidation of α-keto acids[4]. These effects *in vitro* were also prevented by suitable concentrations of 2,3-dimercaptopropanol[4].

The inhibition of α-keto acid oxidation by arsenicals and dialkyltins occurs through their ability to react with the dithiol groups of lipoic acid and possibly also dithiol groups present in lipoic acid dehydrogenase. That diethyltin can interact with dithiols directly was demonstrated by following the oxidation of 2,3-dimercaptopropanol by the dye 2,6-dichlorophenol-indophenol[4]. The decolorization of the dye is completely prevented by a 40-fold excess of diethyltin over 2,3-dimercaptopropanol and considerably slowed by a two fold excess.

The antibacterial effect of diethyltin dichloride and the dialkyltins in general has been interpreted as arising through such inhibition of α-keto acid oxidation, and it is speculated that the antifungal action of diphenyltin dichloride may also be a consequence of this type of inhibition[5].

Rats given 10 mg/kg body wt of diethyltin dichloride intraperitoneally excreted one-third of the tin in the urine, mostly as monoethyltin and a little as unchanged diethyltin[2]. Similar results were obtained after oral administration[2]. Thus extensive dealkylation of diethyltin can take place, probably with the evolution of ethane since no $^{14}CO_2$ could be detected when ^{14}C-labelled material was administered.

Trialkyl and tetra-alkyltins

The trialkyltins are the most toxic of all the organotin compounds[1]. Unlike the dialkyltins there is no evidence for any dealkylation of triethyltin in tissues of rats, and the toxic effects of triethyltin are not antagonized by 2,3-dimercaptopropanol. The symptoms exhibited by rats after administration of tetraethyltin are delayed in onset, but are identical with those obtained after administration of triethyltin[1]. The only pathological lesion seen in rats poisoned with triethyltin is an oedema of the brain and the spinal cord, and this can also be produced with tetraethyltin[6]. Owing to these similarities it seemed likely that tetraethyltin might be converted into triethyltin *in vivo*.

This was confirmed and it has been possible to detect large amounts of triethyltin in the tissues of rats one hour after administration of tetraethyltin[6]. This metabolism of tetraethyltin has been shown to take place in the microsomal fraction of liver and to a lesser extent in kidney. There is no evidence of any further metabolism down to di- or mono-alkyltin.

The symptoms produced in rats after injection of triethyltin either intraperitoneally or intravenously are a marked weakness of the hind limbs and a drop in the body temperature[1]. The latter can be prevented by keeping the animals at an environmental temperature of $32°C$[7]. This drop in body temperature was responsible for some of the early findings that rat brain phospholipid metabolism was impaired after triethyltin and this was thought to have implications with respect to the production of the cerebral oedema. However, when the animals were kept at an environmental temperature of $32°C$, no inhibition of phospholipid metabolism could be seen, whereas the LD_{50} and the production of oedema were unchanged[7] (*Table 1*).

Table 1. Environmental temperature and the effects of triethyltin

Effect	Control 20°C	Control 32°C	Triethyltin 20°C	Triethyltin 32°C
LD_{50} (mg of triethyltin sulphate/kg body wt)	—	—	5.1	4.7
Water content of brain (g of water/g dry wt)	3.69	3.65	3.98	4.00
$^{32}P_i$ incorporation into brain phospholipids (% control at 20°C)	100	98	76	102

The toxicity of triphenyltin has been extensively studied owing to its use as an agricultural fungicide. It has a very high intrinsic toxicity, i.e. when injected intraperitoneally or intravenously it appears to be as toxic as the lower members of the trialkyl series[8]. However, it is very much less toxic when administered orally to rats, but the guinea-pig still remains quite sensitive. There is some evidence that triphenyltin accumulates in the guinea-pig, since when fed on diets containing different quantities of the compound, the animals tend to die when they have consumed much the same total amount[8]. This possible accumulation, plus the known sensitivity of man to triethyltin, makes any assessment of the safety of triphenyltin as a residue difficult.

BIOCHEMISTRY OF TRIALKYLTINS

Most of the biochemistry of the trialkytins has been carried out with triethyltin since this is the most active of the series and is readily obtained labelled with ^{113}Sn. Early biochemical studies were carried out on brain preparations since the only observable lesion was present in the white matter of the brain and spinal cord. An inhibition of glucose oxidation by brain slices was an early finding[9]. It was later demonstrated that triethyltin was an inhibitor of energy conservation in mitrochondria, i.e. those reactions which link ATP synthesis to the oxidation of substrates[10]. Inhibition of oxidative phosphorylation is common to all the lower homologues, methyl through

283

hexyl, but tri-*n*-octyltin is inactive. Triphenyltin is also an effective inhibitor, which is in agreement with its high intrinsic toxicity.

BINDING AND SPECIFICITY OF TRIETHYLTIN

Triethyltin is a simple organometal, which inhibits oxidative phosphorylation at very low concentrations but has no obvious chemical properties to explain this. It does not react with monothiols, dithiols or metal-chelating agents such as EDTA[4,11]. A survey of the interaction with a variety of molecules, by using its formation of a coloured complex with diphenylthiocarbazone, revealed that it had some affinity for certain phospholipids such as lecithin but no affinity for a wide range of biologically important molecules[12].

An examination of the distribution of [113]Sn-labelled triethyltin in the tissues of three species (rat, guinea-pig and hamster) indicated a highly significant difference between rat and the other two species[13] (*Table 2*).

Table 2. Distribution of triethyltin 4 h after administration of 42 μmoles/kg body wt

	Triethyltin (nmoles/g wet wt)		
	Rat	Hamster	Guinea-pig
Liver	103	124	275
Kidney	52.7	31.4	78.5
Muscle	16.2	26.0	17.8
Brain	21.6	24.6	24.8
Spinal cord	20.7	23.1	24.4
Fat	30.3	48.7	11.2
Blood	224	7.7	8.3

Rat blood contained the highest concentration of triethyltin of all rat tissues even 24 hours after dosing and irrespective of whether the dose was given intravenously or intraperitoneally. Both hamster and guinea-pig blood had only a very low concentration of triethyltin. Investigation of the binding of triethyltin to rat blood led to the finding that triethyltin was tightly bound to rat haemoglobin[13,14] Each molecule of rat haemoglobin binds two molecules of triethyltin with an affinity constant of approximately 3×10^5 M^{-1}. This binding to rat haemoglobin is highly specific and no other species of haemoglobin tested has any affinity for triethyltin, with the possible exception of mouse haemoglobin which has a small affinity (probably in the region of ten per cent of that of rat).

Since only rat haemoglobin binds triethyltin with such high affinity, certain conclusions may be drawn about the nature of the binding site. There are four haem groups per molecule of haemoglobin, but only two triethyltin binding sites, making it unlikely that the haem group alone is responsible. Similarly the species specificity indicates that the binding sites must be located on the protein.

Since the liver contains the highest concentration of triethyltin in the hamster and the guinea-pig and also contains the next highest concentration of triethyltin in the rat, the distribution of triethyltin in subcellular fractions of liver was examined. Both in rat liver and in guinea-pig liver, the most substantial amount of triethyltin present in liver after injection was found to be located in the supernatant fraction obtained after centrifuging down the particulate components of the cell[13] (*Table 3*). This would, of course, be

Table 3. Distribution of triethyltin in fractions of rat liver. Dose: 42 μmoles triethyltin/kg body wt. Animals were killed 2 h after dose

Fraction	Triethyltin		
	(nmole/fraction)		(nmole/mg of protein)
Nuclei debris	353		0.64
		(%)	
Mitochondria	80	10	0.40
Liver mitochondria	47	6	0.66
Microsome	107	13	0.69
Supernatant	565	71	1.09
	799	100	

the expected result if triethyltin were freely distributed in the liver and free in solution in the cell water. However, equilibrium dialysis of the supernatant fraction indicated that the triethyltin was bound to a non-dialysable component. Purification of the supernatant fraction obtained from guinea-pig liver showed that 70 per cent of the triethyltin present in guinea-pig liver after intravenous injection is present bound to a protein fraction, which is at the most a few per cent of the total liver protein. This protein fraction binds triethyltin with an affinity even greater than that of rat haemoglobin (affinity constant 2×10^6 M^{-1})[15].

Binding studies with rat liver mitochondria revealed the existence of triethyltin-binding sites with an affinity of 5×10^5 M^{-1}, i.e. the same order of magnitude as those characterizing the binding to rat haemoglobin and guinea-pig liver supernatant protein[16]. Available evidence to date suggests that these sites are involved in the inhibition of oxidative phosphorylation produced by triethyltin.

Studies with a wide variety of proteins (plus the evidence from sub-fractionation of liver) indicate that triethyltin only binds to a few well-defined

Table 4. Macromolecules with no affinity for triethyltin

DNA	Fumarase
Phosvitin	Papain
Clupein	Insulin
Salmine	Sperm whale myoglobin
Cytochrome *c*	Horse myoglobin
Bovine plasma albumin	Guinea-pig haemoglobin
Chymotrypsin (with and without tryptophan)	Horse haemoglobin
Bovine pancreatic ribonuclease	Rabbit haemoglobin
Creatine phosphokinase	Human haemoglobin

proteins (*Table 4*). It is not a general protein-binding reagent in the same way that, for example, the organomercurials are.

PROPERTIES OF TRIETHYLTIN BINDING

Treatment of rat haemoglobin or guinea-pig liver protein with high concentrations of urea results in loss of triethyltin binding[14, 15]. This contrasts with the binding of organomercury compounds to rat haemoglobin, which increases on treatment of the protein with urea as more thiol groups become available. It therefore appears unlikely that the triethyltin-binding sites would be single amino acid residues.

Decrease in pH inhibits the binding of triethyltin to rat haemoglobin[14]. This inhibition of binding appears to have a pK in the region of 7.1 (*Figure 1*),

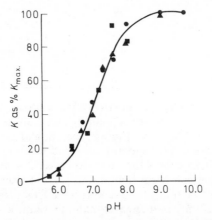

Figure 1. Effect of pH on the association constants of rat haemoglobin for triethyltin (■, ●) and trimethyltin (▲)

which cannot be due to the dissociation of triethyltin itself (which has a pK in the region of 6.6). The binding inhibition data for trimethyltin fall on the same theoretical curve and yet trimethyltin has an even lower pK of 6.2. Thus the pK of 7.1 probably refers to the titration of the binding site on the protein.

In order to identify the chemical nature of the triethyltin binding sites, a procedure which selectively and progressively modifies amino acid residues in proteins was used. The protein under investigation (rat haemoglobin or guinea-pig liver supernatant protein) was photo-oxidized in the presence of a suitable photo-sensitizing dye (either methylene blue or rose bengal). The ability of the protein to bind triethyltin after this procedure was then measured, and the amino acid composition was also measured after hydrolysis to ascertain which amino acids had been lost[14, 15].

After photo-oxidation of haemoglobin there is a net loss of binding sites available to triethyltin, but the affinity of the remaining sites is unaffected[14]. This suggests that general denaturation of the protein is not occurring but specific loss of amino acid concerned in binding is. The rate of loss of binding sites is first order.

The only amino acids that are affected by photo-oxidation are histidine, cysteine, methionine, tryptophan and tyrosine[17]. Only the first three were lost when haemoglobin was photo-oxidized and all three were lost in first-order reactions. Thus the loss of binding sites must be explained in terms of the loss of these three classes of amino acid.

It can be shown that if the activity of an enzyme catalytic site or a binding site is dependent on the presence at that site of two residues X and Y, destruction of either one leading to complete loss of activity, then if these residues are lost in first-order reactions, activity loss will also be first order and $k_a = k_X + k_Y$, where k_a is the first-order rate constant for loss of activity and k_X and k_Y are the first-order rate constants for loss of the classes of residues X and Y respectively[18]. Now the rate constant for loss of triethyltin binding sites in haemoglobin is 0.03 min^{-1}; the rate constant for the loss of histidine residues is 0.015 min^{-1}; the rate constant for the loss of cysteine residues is 0.022 min^{-1}, and the rate constant for the loss of methionine residues varies between 0.005 and 0.01 min^{-1}. Therefore there is no one amino acid which is lost fast enough to account for the loss of binding, and it must be a combination of amino acids that is responsible for binding triethyltin. The rate constant for loss of binding 0.03 min^{-1} could be arrived at by assuming that each site consists of two histidine residues or that each site consists of one cysteine residue plus one methionine residue. The latter combination can be ruled out since (a) complete alkylation of thiol groups with n-ethylmaleimide does not abolish triethyltin binding, and (b) the thiol groups of photo-oxidized haemoglobin can be regenerated with a thiol reagent (dithiothreitol) without any regeneration of triethyltin-binding sites.

Thus the data obtained for triethyltin binding to haemoglobin can be interpreted to indicate that each triethyltin-binding site consists of two histidine residues, and the rate of loss of binding will be twice as fast as the rate of loss of the histidine residues.

The effects of photo-oxidation on guinea-pig liver supernatant protein are more complex in that loss of binding is not first order, but can be analysed into two first-order components. Similarly the loss of histidine can be analysed into two first-order components and the relationship that emerges is the same as that in rat haemoglobin, i.e. binding is lost twice as fast as histidine

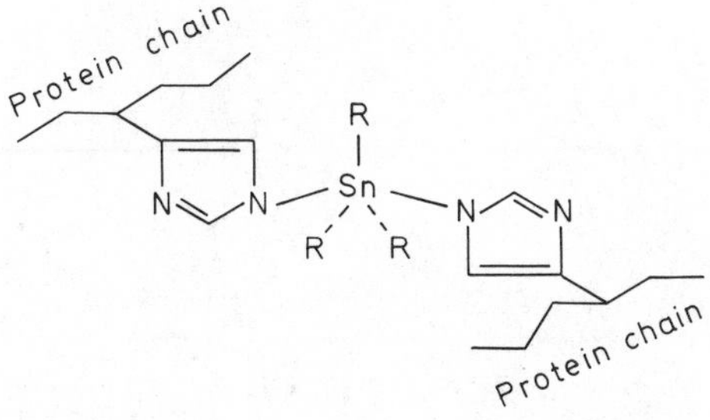

Figure 2. Proposed structure for protein–triethyltin-binding sites

residues, which can be interpreted to indicate that each binding site again consists of two histidine residues[15].

The evidence from both proteins that have been studied that bind triethyltin, fits in well with the work of Professor Van der Kerk and his group in Utrecht, who demonstrated in 1964 that trialkyltins will form stable penta-coordinate complexes with imidazole in non-aqueous solvents[19]. From the structures they propose we think that triethyltin-binding sites in proteins may possess the structure shown in *Figure 2*.

REFERENCES

[1] H. B. Stoner, J. M. Barnes and J. I. Duff, *Brit. J. Pharmacol.* **10**, 16 (1955).
[2] J. W. Bridges, D. S. Davies and R. T. Williams, *Biochem. J.* **98**, 14P (1966).
[3] J. M. Barnes and H. B. Stoner, *Brit. J. Indust. Med.* **15**, 15 (1958).
[4] W. N. Aldridge, and J. E. Cremer, *Biochem. J.* **61**, 406 (1955).
[5] A. Kaars Sijpesteijn, *World Rev. of Pest Control*, **9**, 85 (1970).
[6] J. E. Cremer, *Biochem. J.* **68**, 685 (1958).
[7] M. S. Rose and W. N. Aldridge, *J. Neurochem.* **13**, 103 (1966).
[8] H. B. Stoner, *Brit. J. Indust. Med.* **23**, 222 (1966).
[9] J. E. Cremer, *Biochem. J.* **67**, 87 (1957).
[10] W. N. Aldridge, *Biochem. J.* **69**, 367 (1958).
[11] W. N. Aldridge and J. E. Cremer, *Analyst*, **82**, 37 (1957).
[12] W. N. Aldridge and B. W. Street, *Biochem. J.* **91**, 287 (1964).
[13] M. S. Rose and W. N. Aldridge, *Biochem. J.* **106**, 821 (1968).
[14] M. S. Rose, *Biochem. J.* **111**, 129 (1969).
[15] M. S. Rose and E. A. Lock, *Biochem. J.* **120**, 151 (1970).
[16] W. N. Aldridge and B. W. Street, *Biochem. J.* **118**, 171 (1970).
[17] L. Weil, W. G. Gordon and A. R. Buchert, *Archs. Biochem.* **33**, 90 (1951).
[18] W. J. Ray and D. E. Koshland, *J. Biol. Chem.* **236**, 1973 (1961).
[19] M. J. Janssen, J. G. A. Luijten and G. J. M. Van der Kerk, *J. Organomet. Chem.* **1**, 286 (1964).

THE CHEMISTRY AND METABOLISM OF HERBICIDES AND PLANT-GROWTH REGULATORS

METABOLISM OF PHENOXY HERBICIDES BY PLANTS AND SOIL MICRO-ORGANISMS

M. A. Loos

Department of Microbiology and Plant Pathology,
University of Natal, Pietermaritzburg, South Africa

ABSTRACT

Metabolism of 2,4-D (2.4-dichlorophenoxyacetic acid) and other substituted phenoxyacetic acid herbicides by plants occurs by degradation or lengthening of the acetic acid side chain, hydroxylation and in some cases degradation of the aromatic ring and conjugation with plant constituents. Homologues with longer side chains may be metabolized by β- or ω-oxidation or lengthening of the side chain, as well as by ring hydroxylation. Esters and amides are hydrolysed and nitriles are hydrolysed or α-oxidized, yielding free phenoxy acids. The extent and rate of metabolism is often an important factor in determining the response of specific plants to phenoxy herbicides. Soil micro-organisms metabolize phenoxy herbicides by degrading the side chain and hydroxylating the aromatic ring, which may subsequently be cleaved and further degraded. Degradation pathways in bacteria have recently been elucidated. The chlorines of the ring are liberated as chloride. The side chain of the higher phenoxy-alkanoic acids is β-oxidized, or removed intact from the molecule by cleavage of the ether linkage. The non-herbicidal compound, sodium 2,4-dichloro-phenoxyethyl sulphate (Sesone), is activated in soil by microbial conversion into 2,4-dichlorophenoxyethanol and 2,4-D. Susceptibility to metabolism by soil micro-organisms is of great importance in determining the persistence of phenoxy herbicides in soil.

INTRODUCTION

The substituted phenoxyacetic acid herbicides, 2,4-D (2,4-dichlorophen-oxyacetic acid), MCPA (4-chloro-2-methylphenoxyacetic acid) and 2,4,5-T (2,4,5-trichlorophenoxyacetic acid) were introduced as weedkillers at the end of World War 2, and have since been extensively used in agriculture. Recently, 2,4-D and 2,4,5-T have been employed on a large scale as defoliants in the Vietnam War[1, 2]. The ability of the soil microflora to degrade the phenoxyacetic acid herbicides was recognized soon after their introduction[3]; hence they were not considered to present any environmental hazard if properly used. Recently this complacency has been jolted by reports of teratogenic (foetus-deforming) effects of 2,4,5-T and the iso-octyl ester of 2,4-D[4, 5], although with 2,4,5-T at least, the observed effects may result from contamination of the herbicide with 2,3,7,8-tetrachloro-dibenzo-*p*-dioxin[5, 6]. The possible hazards of using these chemicals are thus being reconsidered, and obviously such factors as the amount and manner in which the herbicides

291

are applied and their degradation in the environment are of great importance.

The present survey of the metabolism of phenoxy herbicides by plants and soil micro-organisms is of necessity brief, and will concentrate on chemical aspects. More detail is available in two recent reviews[7, 8].

METABOLISM BY PLANTS

Phenoxyacetic acids
Side chain degradation

Degradation of the acetic acid side chain of substituted phenoxyacetic acid herbicides is a well-documented mechanism in plants. ^{14}C-labelled carbon dioxide has been liberated by many different plants when whole plants, individual organs or tissues have been treated with *carboxyl-*[14]*C* or *methylene-*[14]*C* labelled 2,4-D, or other phenoxyacetic acid herbicides[9–23]. Tick beans metabolizing 2,4-D[20] and *Galium aparine* (bedstraw or cleavers) metabolizing MCPA[15] released both side chain carbon atoms as carbon dioxide at the same rate, suggesting removal of the side chain as a C_2 unit through cleavage of the molecule at the ether linkage, or release of the methylene carbon atom immediately after the carboxyl carbon. By contrast, bean[11], redcurrant[12], strawberry[13], cotton and sorghum[17] released the carboxyl carbon about twice as fast as the methylene carbon. Such observations may indicate a stepwise degradation of the side chain and it was suggested that in strawberry 2,4-dichloroanisole might be produced as a 'bound' intermediate[13]; on the other hand, the results are not necessarily inconsistent with removal of the side chain as a C_2 unit. The two carbon atoms of acetate, for example, may be released as carbon dioxide by plants at different rates, the carboxyl carbon being released faster than the methyl carbon[24]. In a recently elucidated bacterial pathway, the side chain of 2,4-D was released as glyoxylate, which was subsequently partially decarboxylated and condensed with ammonia to form alanine[25] (*Figure 1*); however, it is not known whether glyoxylate is also the primary product of phenoxyacetic acid side chain metabolism in plants.

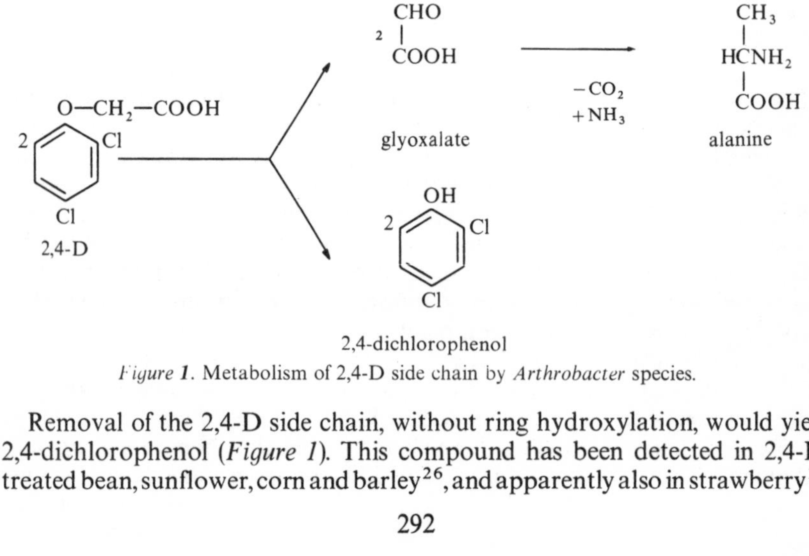

2,4-dichlorophenol

Figure 1. Metabolism of 2,4-D side chain by *Arthrobacter* species.

Removal of the 2,4-D side chain, without ring hydroxylation, would yield 2,4-dichlorophenol (*Figure 1*). This compound has been detected in 2,4-D-treated bean, sunflower, corn and barley[26], and apparently also in strawberry[13].

Side chain lengthening

Lengthening of the 2,4-D side chain, suggested in 1961 by Bach[27], has recently been demonstrated by Linscott and co-workers[28, 29]. Alfalfa added two carbon atoms to the side chain of 2,4-D to yield 4-(2,4-dichlorophenoxy) butyric acid (2,4-DB), which could then add additional C_2 units[28]. Resistant grasses added a single carbon atom to 2,4-D to yield 3-(2,4-dichlorophenoxy) propionic acid[29].

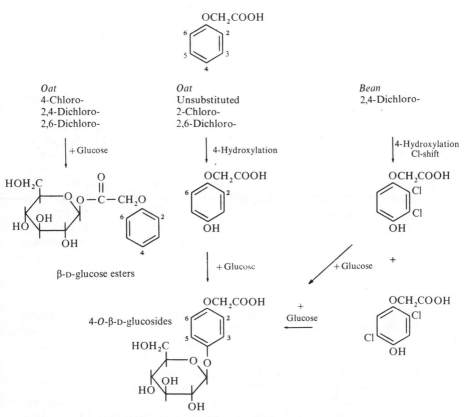

Figure 2. Metabolism of phenoxyacetic acids in oats and beans, involving hydroxylation and conjugation with glucose.

Ring hydroxylation

Hydroxylation of the aromatic ring (*Figure 2*) is an important reaction of phenoxy compounds in plants. Thomas *et al.*[30, 31] at Oxford showed that oats hydroxylated the phenoxy ring in the 4-position if this position was unsubstituted, as in phenoxyacetic acid[30], 2-chlorophenoxyacetic acid (2-CPA) and 2,6-dichlorophenoxyacetic acid (2,6-D)[31]. 2,4,6-Trichlorophenoxyacetic acid, with a substituted 4-position, was hydroxylated in the 3-position, and 2,4-D and 4-chlorophenoxyacetic acid (4-CPA) were not hydroxylated by oats[31]. However, beans hydroxylated 2,4-D in the 4-position with a shift of the

4-chlorine to the 3- or 5-position, to yield 2,3-dichloro- or 2,5-dichloro-4-hydroxyphenoxyacetic acid[32]. These conversions of 2,4-D were also observed in the fungus *Aspergillus niger*[33]. The shift of a hydrogen atom or a substituent from the 4-position to the 3- or 5-position during 4-hydroxylation of an aromatic ring has recently been established as a general reaction of aromatic metabolism (hydroxylation-induced intramolecular migration or the 'NIH shift')[34].

Ring cleavage

Cleavage of the 2,4-D ring, followed by further degradation, is indicated by the production in cucumber of a metabolite with the chromatographic behaviour of chloroacetic acid[35].

Conjugation with plant constituents

Hydroxylated or non-hydroxylated phenoxyacetic acids may conjugate with plant constituents such as glucose, aspartic acid, pectic acid and possibly protein. For example, in oats the hydroxyphenoxyacetic acids, 2-chloro-4-hydroxyphenoxyacetic acid, 2,6-dichloro-4-hydroxyphenoxyacetic acid and 3-hydroxy-2,4,6-trichlorophenoxyacetic acid, formed β-D-glucosides whereas the non-hydroxylated 2,4-D, 2,6-D and 4-CPA formed β-D-glucose esters[31] (*Figure 2*). The dichlorohydroxyphenoxyacetic acids produced from 2,4-D in beans also formed β-D-glucosides[32]. Wheat[36], peas[37], red- and blackcurrants[12], and possibly also wild and cultivated cucumbers[22], produced 2,4-dichlorophenoxyacetylaspartic acid from 2,4-D, and in citrus peel 2,4-D was bound as a conjugate in the pectic acid fraction[38]. The formation of 2,4-D–protein complexes[39] is somewhat controversial[27].

Higher ω-phenoxyalkanoic acids

β-Oxidation

The most important mechanism for the metabolism of higher ω-phenoxyalkanoic acids in plants is β-oxidation[40–53] (*Figure 3*). If β-oxidation is complete, the corresponding phenoxyacetic acids are produced from phenoxyalkanoic acids with an even number of carbon atoms in the side chain, whereas the corresponding phenols are produced from phenoxyalkanoic acids with an odd number of carbon atoms in the side chain[40–44]. However, substituent groups on the phenoxy ring, in particular *o*-chloro- and *o*-methyl substituents, may hinder β-oxidation of the side chain in certain plants so that it stops at the phenoxybutyric (or β-hydroxyphenoxybutyric) or phenoxypropionic acid stage[42].

ω-Oxidation

Large amounts of phenol were produced during the metabolism of 10-phenoxy-*n*-decanoic acid by flax[43]. Oxidation of the ω-carbon of the side chain and hydrolysis of the resulting ester were proposed to explain the formation of this unexpected product.

Side chain lengthening

Linscott and colleagues[28, 54] showed that alfalfa both β-oxidized 2,4-DB to 2,4-D and lengthened the 2,4-DB side chain by C_2 units to form 6-(2,4-

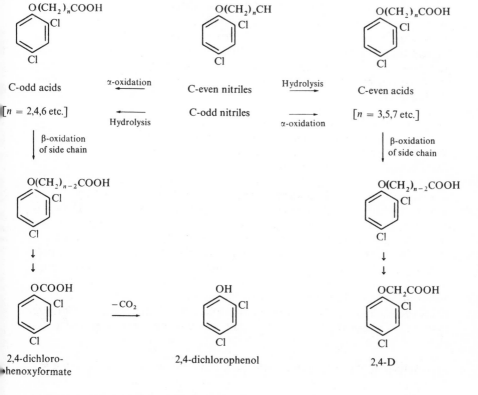

Figure 3. Metabolism of ω-(2,4-dichlorophenoxy)alkanoic acids and ω-(2,4-dichlorophenoxy)-alkane nitriles in plants.

dichlorophenoxy)caproic acid, 10-(2,4-dichlorophenoxy)decanoic acid and apparently other 2,4-dichlorophenoxyalkanoic acid homologues. In addition, esters of 4-(2,4-dichlorophenoxy)crotonic acid and 4-(2,4-dichlorophenoxy)-3-hydroxybutyric acid, which are intermediates in the breakdown of 2,4-DB to 2,4-D, were converted into 2,4-DB and also appeared to undergo side chain lengthening. The two processes of β-oxidation and side chain lengthening are thus in competition in alfalfa metabolizing 2,4-DB. The enzymes responsible for side chain lengthening may normally be concerned with the synthesis of surface waxes.

Ring hydroxylation
   Hydroxylation of the ring, which either preceded or followed β-oxidation of the side chain, was observed during the metabolism of unsubstituted phenoxyalkanoic acids by pea, wheat, oats, barley and corn[42, 55].

Higher α-phenoxyalkanoic acids
   Little is known of the metabolism of α-phenoxyalkanoic acids with three or more side chain carbon atoms, although 2-(4-chloro-2-methylphenoxy)

295

propionic acid (Mecoprop), 2-(2,4-dichlorophenoxy)propionic acid (Dichlor-prop) and 2-(2,4,5-trichlorophenoxy)propionic acid (Silvex) are used as herbicides. Slow decarboxylation of Dichlorprop and Silvex occurred in big leaf maple[19], and in prickly pear Silvex was slowly decarboxylated and metabolized to unidentified metabolites[23]. *Galium aparine*, which readily degraded the side chain of MCPA, was unable to metabolize the side chain of Mecoprop[15].

Ester, amide and nitrile derivatives of phenoxyalkanoic acids

Esters and amides of phenoxyalkanoic acids are hydrolysed by various plants to the corresponding free acids, which may then be β-oxidized if the side chain contains sufficient carbon atoms[41, 56–60].

Fawcett and co-workers[41, 61] proposed two different mechanisms for the metabolism of ω-(2,4-dichlorophenoxy)alkane nitriles by wheat tissue, namely, hydrolysis of the nitrile to the corresponding acid followed by β-oxidation of the acid side chain and, secondly, α-oxidation of the nitrile side chain to yield an acid with one carbon atom less, followed by β-oxidation of this acid (*Figure 3*). Thus all ω-(2,4-dichlorophenoxy)alkane nitriles supplied to wheat tissue, with the exception of the propionitrile, were metabolized to both 2,4-D and 2,4-dichlorophenol. Pea tissue converted the acetonitrile into 2,4-D and possibly the propionitrile into 2,4 dichlorophenol, but was unable to convert ω-(2,4-dichlorophenoxy)alkane nitriles with more than three carbon atoms in the side chain into either a 2,4-dichlorophenoxy-alkanoic acid or into the amide.

Metabolism of phenoxy herbicides in plants in relation to herbicidal activity

The phenoxy herbicides have been developed for selective use against dicotyledonous plants. However, even within this group different species and varieties of plant may differ considerably in their susceptibility to the action of these herbicides. Major factors determining susceptibility and resistance are absorption, translocation and metabolism. Only metabolism will be discussed here.

Plants resistant to a specific phenoxyacetic acid herbicide have often been found to decarboxylate the herbicide, i.e. to degrade the side chain, at a rapid rate[12–15, 20], or to convert the herbicide rapidly into a metabolite or metabolites[12, 17, 22, 39]. However, herbicide decarboxylation and formation of metabolites may also occur in susceptible plants, but in many cases more slowly[11, 13, 16, 17, 27, 39, 62, 63]. Hence, rate of metabolism of the herbicide to inactive products appears to be the determinant of susceptibility or resistance in many plants. This observation has found practical application in the usage of herbicides and growth regulators. For example, *Galium aparine* was resistant to and rapidly degraded MCPA, but was susceptible to and failed to degrade the corresponding 2-phenoxypropionic acid herbicide, Mecoprop[15]. Similarly, 2,4-D was inactive as a growth regulator for McIntosh apples because of rapid decarboxylation, but 2-chloro-4-fluorophenoxy-acetic acid, which was decarboxylated only slowly, was active[14].

Although the rapid metabolism of phenoxyacetic acids usually results in herbicide detoxication, in some cases metabolites with toxic or growth-regulating properties may be produced. Thus 2,4,5-trichlorophenol might be responsible for the toxicity to red-currant of 2,4,5-T, which is rapidly decarboxylated in this plant[12, 13]. A non-acidic metabolite produced from 2,4-D by red- and black-currants, apples and strawberries exhibited auxin activity[12, 13]. Chloroacetic acid, which appeared to be produced during 2,4-D metabolism by cucumber, has growth-stimulating and herbicidal activity[35]. In fact, Tutass[35] has postulated that chloroacetic acid may be the agent responsible for the growth-regulating activity of chlorine-substituted phenoxyacetic acids, which would first have to be degraded to this metabolite.

For many phenoxyalkanoic acids metabolism is an essential activation mechanism. The ω-phenoxyalkanoic acids with more than two, or in some cases three, carbon atoms in the side chain are inactive *per se* as plant growth regulators and they must be metabolized by β-oxidation to the phenoxyacetic or phenoxypropionic acids to show activity; however, the phenoxypropionic acids are often further β-oxidized to inactive phenols[40-49]. The end-product of β-oxidation, and whether it is active or not, depends on the plant and on the substituents on the phenoxyalkanoic acid ring[41-44]. The differences among plants and herbicides may be exploited to achieve greater selectivity in weed control; for example, the phenoxybutyric acid herbicides 2,4-DB and 4-(4-chloro-2-methylphenoxy)butyric acid (MCPB) were introduced for this purpose[45-49, 66].

The lengthening of the side chain of 2,4-D and 2,4-DB in alfalfa[28, 54] provides an explanation for the relative resistance of legumes to 2,4-DB. This resistance was puzzling, as β-oxidation of 2,4-DB to 2,4-D was detected in various legumes against which 2,4-D is active[41, 42, 44, 67]. However, if the concentration of 2,4-D produced from 2,4-DB remained sufficiently low because of the lengthening of the side chain of both the 2,4-D and 2,4-DB in opposition to β-oxidation, the plants would not be affected by the 2,4-D production[28, 54]. On the other hand, direct application of 2,4-D to the legume presumably results in herbicidal 2,4-D concentrations in the plant.

Most ester, amide and nitrile derivatives of phenoxyalkanoic acids are probably not active *per se* as plant growth regulators but require metabolic conversion into an active acid[47, 48]. However, certain amino acid derivatives of Dichlorprop and Silvex might not require hydrolysis to the free phenoxypropionic acid as a prerequisite for activity[68, 69].

METABOLISM BY SOIL MICRO-ORGANISMS
Phenoxyacetic acids

A wide range of substituted phenoxyacetic acids is metabolized by soil micro-organisms, especially species of bacteria[3, 7, 70]. As with plants, breakdown of the side chain and hydroxylation of the ring are important degradation reactions but, in addition, ring cleavage and dehalogenation are well-documented mechanisms of bacteria. Degradation pathways have been most extensively studied in an *Arthrobacter* species and pseudomonads (*Figure 4*).

The *Arthrobacter* sp., which was investigated at Cornell University by Alexander and co-workers[71-79], first removes the side chain of phenoxyacetic acids to yield the corresponding phenol[72-74]. Phenol derived from phenoxyacetic acid with the ether oxygen labelled with ^{18}O, retained all the ^{18}O label in the phenolic hydroxyl group[75]. The C_2 side chain, which was

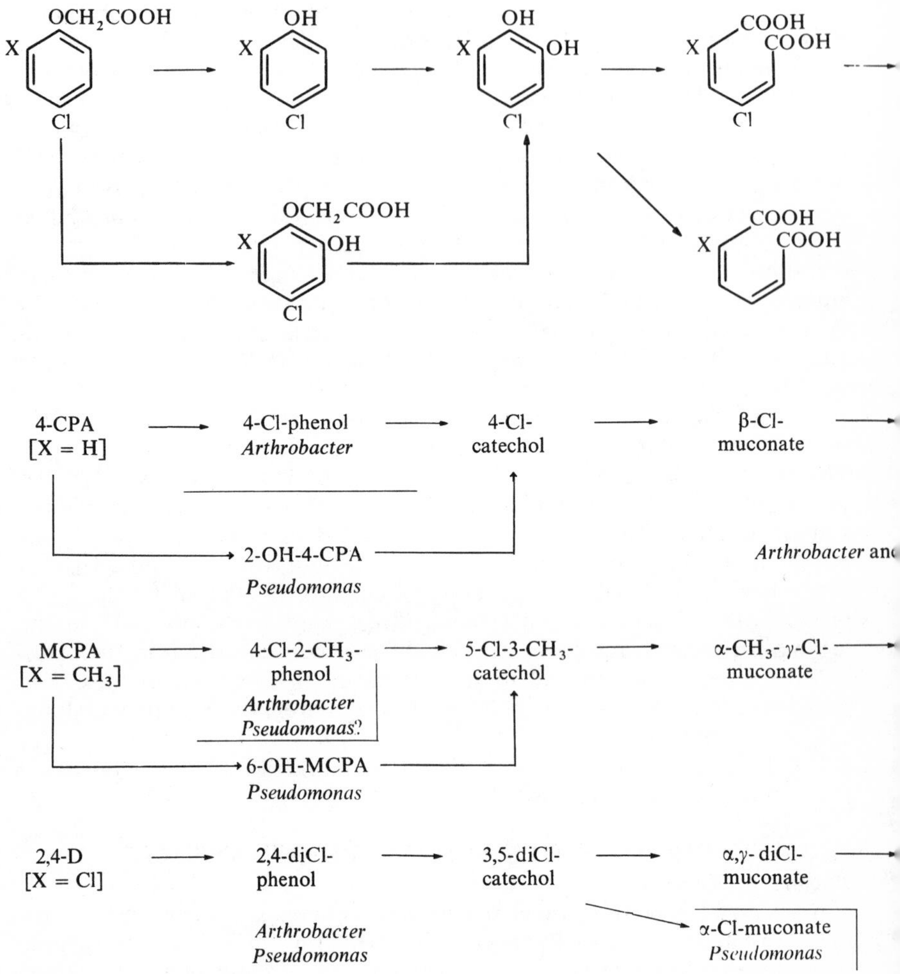

Figure 4. Metabolism of 4-CPA, MCPA and 2,4-D by *Arthrobacter* and *Pseudomonas* species.

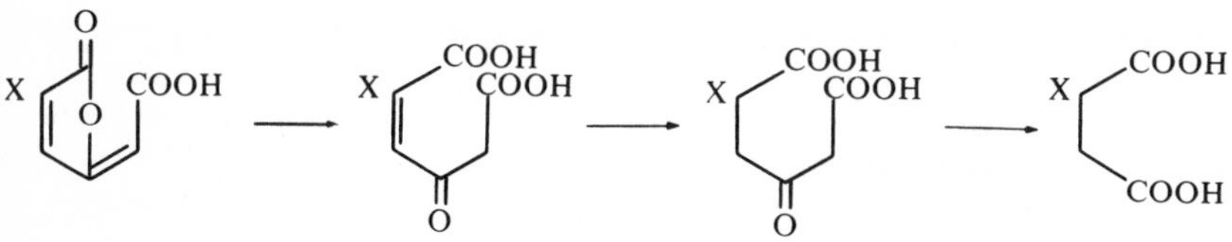

γ-carboxy-   ⟶   maleyl-   ⟶   β-keto-   ⟶   succinate
methylene-   acetate   adipate
Δᵅ-butenolide

Pseudomonas   *Arthrobacter*

α-CH₃-γ-carboxy-   ⟶   α-CH₃-
methylene-   maleyl-
Δᵅ-butenolide   acetate

Pseudomonas

α-Cl-γ-carboxy-   ⟶   Cl-maleyl-   ⟶   α-Cl-γ-keto-   ⟶   Cl-succinate
methylene-   acetate   adipate   and
Δᵅ-butenolide   succinate

Arthrobacter

removed apparently as glyoxylic acid, was condensed with partial decarboxylation and incorporation of ammonia, to yield alanine (*Figure 1*)[25].

The phenols produced from 4-CPA, 2,4-D and MCPA were further metabolized[74, 76]. Pathways were established for the metabolism of 4-chloro- and 2,4-dichloro-phenol[76-79]. The 4-chlorophenol was *ortho*-hydroxylated to 4-chlorocatechol, which was then metabolized via β-chloromuconic acid and γ-carboxymethylene-Δ$^{\alpha}$-butenolide to maleylacetic acid. The maleylacetic acid was converted, apparently via β-keto-adipic acid, into succinic acid. The 2,4-dichlorophenol was metabolized via identical steps, but retaining the 2-chlorine in the intermediates, to chloromaleylacetic acid, then to succinic acid, probably via α-chloro-γ-keto-adipic acid and chlorosuccinic acid.

In the pseudomonads studied by Evans and his colleagues[80-85], the initial step in the degradation of 4-CPA and MCPA was *ortho*-hydroxylation of the ring to yield a hydroxyphenoxyacetic acid[80, 81]. This was followed by removal of the side chain to yield a catechol, which was then cleaved and further degraded. Thus 4-CPA appeared to be degraded via 2-hydroxy-4-chlorophenoxyacetic acid to 4-chlorocatechol[80, 82], then to maleylacetic acid via the same sequence as in the *Arthrobacter*[82, 83]. Similarly, MCPA was apparently metabolized via 6-hydroxy-4-chloro-2-methylphenoxyacetic acid (6-hydroxy-MCPA), 5-chloro-3-methylcatechol, α-methyl-γ-chloromuconic acid, α-methyl-γ-carboxymethylene-Δ$^{\alpha}$-butenolide and presumably α-methylmaleylacetic acid[81]. However, as 4-chloro-2-methylphenol was detected during MCPA metabolism[81], the MCPA might also have been metabolized to 5-chloro-3-methylcatechol via the corresponding phenol, as an alternative to the 6-hydroxy-MCPA pathway. There is no satisfactory evidence that 6-hydroxy-2,4-dichlorophenoxyacetic acid (6-hydroxy-2,4-D) was produced during the metabolism of 2,4-D[80, 84], breakdown appearing to occur via 2,4-dichlorophenol[83, 85], 3,5-dichlorocatechol[83] and α-chloromuconic acid[85].

These results with *Arthrobacter* and *Pseudomonas* species clearly indicate two alternative basic reaction sequences between the phenoxyacetic acid and the catechol, and thereafter a single basic reaction sequence, with the exception of α-chloromuconic acid production during the metabolism of 2,4-D by a pseudomonad (*Figure 4*).

In contrast to the bacteria, *Aspergillus niger* hydroxylated the ring of 2-CPA, 4-CPA, MCPA and 2,4-D in various positions without subsequent ring cleavage, but in some cases involving dechlorination or a chlorine shift[33, 86-90].

Little is known of the breakdown of 2,4,5-T in soil. However, it is degraded with cleavage of the aromatic ring and liberation of the chlorines as chloride[8, 91]. The kinetics of degradation indicate that micro-organisms are responsible[8, 92] but metabolic studies with isolated organisms have not yet been reported.

Higher phenoxyalkanoic acids

As in plants, β-oxidation is an important mechanism for the metabolism of ω-phenoxyalkanoic acids by soil micro-organisms[93-97]. An *o*-chloro or *o*-methyl substituent on the ring tends to hinder β-oxidation; other ring substituents may affect it favourably or unfavourably[94, 96]. β-Oxidation may also be retarded by introducing a methyl substituent on the ω-carbon of the side chain[95], but it is promoted by lengthening the methylated or non-methylated side chain[95, 96]. Phenoxyalkanoic acids with 10 or 11 carbon atoms in the side chain may undergo α- as well as β-oxidation[96].

Aspergillus niger metabolized 4-phenoxybutyric acid and 5-phenoxyvaleric acid by β-oxidation accompanied by *ortho* or *para* ring hydroxylation[86].

A *Flavobacterium* species, isolated from soil, cleaved 2,4-dichlorophenoxy-alkanoic acids at the ether linkage to yield the corresponding fatty acid and 2,4-dichlorophenol[98, 99].

Sodium 2,4-dichlorophenoxyethyl sulphate

Sodium 2,4-dichlorophenoxyethyl sulphate (Sesone) is nonherbicidal *per se* and has no effect if applied to the foliage of 2,4-D-susceptible plants. However, it is herbicidal for such plants if applied to the soil in the root zone[100], on account of its conversion by soil micro-organisms into 2,4-dichloro-phenoxyethanol and 2,4-D[101-103]. In soils of pH 4.0 or lower, Sesone is converted non-biologically into 2,4-dichlorophenoxyethanol[104].

Persistence of phenoxy herbicides in soils

Substituents on the ring greatly affect the ability of soil micro-organisms to degrade phenoxy herbicides[3, 70, 105, 106]. Chlorine substitution in the *para* position promotes degradation of phenoxyacetic acids, but in the *ortho* and *meta* positions hinders it. The o-methyl group of MCPA is more 'de-activating' than the o-chlorine of 2,4-D. Among the higher phenoxyalkanoic acids, the ω-phenoxy acids are more readily degraded than the α-phenoxy acids, but lengthening of the side chain tends to reduce the persistence of the latter[105, 106]. The breakdown of the higher phenoxyalkanoic acids is also hindered by *meta*-substitution[105, 106]

Organisms degrading phenoxy herbicides are not particularly abundant in soils. Thus, seven Natal soils contained, by most probable number count, from 1 to 184 2,4-D-decomposing organisms and from 0.17 to 1 402 MCPA-degrading organisms per gramme of soil[8, 91]. However, soil perfusion studies[92, 107, 108] and the use of the enrichment culture technique to isolate such organisms[71, 80, 109-114] indicate that they readily proliferate when soils are treated with the appropriate herbicides. Investigations of 2,4,5-T-degrading microbial populations in the Natal soils are still in progress, but 50 g samples from two soils, and 500 g samples from two others, degraded 2,4,5-T within 200 days[91]. Disappearance of the 2,4,5-T ultra-violet-absorption spectrum occurred within 50–100 days in the most active samples. This result agrees with those of Brownbridge (see ref. 70) and Burger *et al.*[106], but is in contrast to the observations of Alexander and Aleem[105], which suggested that 2,4,5-T was particularly recalcitrant in respect of microbial breakdown[115, 116]. However, it appears that the organisms which 'rapidly' degrade 2,4,5-T are scarce in soils[91], and hence were not present in the 4 g soil samples used by Alexander and Aleem[105].

CONCLUSION

To sum up, the commonly used phenoxy herbicides, with the possible

301

exception of the inadequately studied α-phenoxypropionic acids, are readily degraded in the environment. There seems to be no danger that these chemicals or their degradation products will cause lasting environmental pollution. However, dioxin contamination and teratogenicity problems, such as occur with 2,4,5-T, have to be resolved.

REFERENCES

1 E. W. Pfeiffer, *Science J.* **5**, 34 (1969).
2 F. H. Tschirley, *Science* **163**, 779 (1969).
3 L. J. Audus. In *Herbicides and the Soil*. pp 1–19. Ed. by E. K. Woodford and G. R. Sagar. Blackwell: Oxford (1960).
4 B. Nelson, *Science* **166**, 977 (1969).
5 K. D. Courtney, D. W. Gaylor, M. D. Hogan, H. L. Falk, R. R. Bates and I. Mitchell, *Science* **168**, 864 (1970).
6 P. H. Abelson, *Science* **170**, 495 (1970).
7 M. A. Loos. In *Degradation of Herbicides*, pp 1–49. Ed. by P. C. Kearney and D. D. Kaufman. Marcel Dekker: New York (1969).
8 M. A. Loos, *J. S. Afr. Chem. Inst.* **22** (Spec. Issue), S71 (1969).
9 R. W. Holley, F. P. Boyle and D. B. Hand, *Arch. Biochem. Biophys.* **27**, 143 (1950).
10 R. L. Weintraub, J. W. Brown, M. Fields and J. Rohan, *Am. J. Bot.* **37**, 682 (1950).
11 R. L. Weintraub, J. W. Brown, M. Fields and J. Rohan, *Plant Physiol.* **27**, 293 (1952).
12 L. C. Luckwill and C. P. Lloyd-Jones, *Ann. Appl. Biol.* **48**, 613 (1960).
13 L. C. Luckwill and C. P. Lloyd-Jones, *Ann. Appl. Biol.* **48**, 626 (1960).
14 L. J. Edgerton and M. B. Hoffman, *Science* **134**, 341 (1961).
15 E. L. Leafe, *Nature, Lond.* **193**, 485 (1962).
16 R. L. Weintraub, J. H. Reinhart and R. A. Scherff. In *A Conference on Radioactive Isotopes in Agriculture*, pp 203–208. A.E.C. Rept. TID—7512 (1956).
17 P. W. Morgan and W. C. Hall, *Weeds* **11**, 130 (1963).
18 E. Basler, *Weeds* **12**, 14 (1964).
19 L. A. Norris and V. H. Freed, *Weed Res.* **6**, 212 (1966).
20 M. J. Canny and K. Markus, *Austr. J. Biol. Sci* **13**, 486 (1960).
21 M. C. Williams, F. W. Slife and J. B. Hanson, *Weeds* **8**, 244 (1960).
22 F. W. Slife, J. L. Key, S. Yamaguchi and A. S. Crafts, *Weeds* **10**, 29 (1962).
23 P. N. Chow, O. C. Burnside, T. L. Lavy and H. W. Knoche, *Weeds* **14**, 38 (1966).
24 H. Beevers, *Respiratory Metabolism in Plants*, pp 54–57. Row, Peterson: Evanston, Illinois (1961).
25 J. M. Tiedjie and M. Alexander, *J. Agr. Food Chem.* **17**, 1080 (1969).
26 D. I. Chkanikov, N. N. Pavlova and D. F. Gertsuskii, *Khim. v Sel'skom Khoz.* **3**, 56 (1965); *Chem. Abstr.* **63**, 8250c (1965).
27 M. K. Bach, *Plant Physiol.* **36**, 558 (1961).
28 D. L. Linscott and R. D. Hagin, *Weed Sci.* **18**, 197 (1970).
29 R. D. Hagin, D. L. Linscott and J. E. Dawson, *J. Agr. Food Chem.* **18**, 848 (1970).
30 E. W. Thomas, B. C. Loughman and R. G. Powell, *Nature, Lond.* **199**, 73 (1963).
31 E. W. Thomas, B. C. Loughman and R. G. Powell, *Nature, Lond.* **204**, 286 (1964).
32 E. W. Thomas, B. C. Loughman and R. G. Powell, *Nature, Lond.* **204**, 884 (1964).
33 J. K. Faulkner and D. Woodcock, *Nature, Lond.* **203**, 865 (1964).
34 G. Guroff, J. W. Daly, D. M. Jerina, J. Renson, B. Witkop and S. Udenfriend, *Science* **157**, 1524 (1967).
35 H. O. Tutass, *PhD. Thesis*, University of California, Davis (1967).
36 H. D. Klämbt, *Planta* **57**, 339 (1961).
37 W. A. Andreae and N. E. Good, *Plant Physiol.* **32**, 566 (1957).
38 W. R. Meagher, *J. Agr. Food Chem.* **14**, 599 (1966).
39 J. S. Butts and S. C. Fang. In *A Conference on Radioactive Isotopes in Agriculture*, pp 209–214. A.E.C. Rept. TID-7512 (1956).
40 M. E. Synerholm and P. W. Zimmerman. *Contrib. Boyce Thompson Inst.* **14**, 369 (1947).
41 C. H. Fawcett, H. F. Taylor, R. L. Wain and F. Wightman, *Proc. Roy. Soc. B*, **148**, 543 (1958).

42 C. H. Fawcett, R. M. Pascal, M. B. Pybus, H. F. Taylor, R. L. Wain and F. Wightman, *Proc. Roy. Soc.* B, **150**, 95 (1959).
43 C. H. Fawcett, J. M. A. Ingram and R. L. Wain, *Proc. Roy. Soc.* B, **142**, 60 (1954).
44 R. L. Wain and F. Wightman, *Proc. Roy. Soc* B, **142**, 525 (1954).
45 R. L. Wain, *Ann. Appl. Biol.* **42**, 151 (1955).
46 R. L. Wain, *J. Agr. Food Chem.* 3, 128 (1955).
47 R. L. Wain, *Advan. Pest Control Res.* 2, 263 (1958).
48 R. L. Wain. In *The Physiology and Biochemistry of Herbicides*, pp 465–481. Ed. by L. J. Audus. Academic Press: New York (1964).
49 D. L. Linscott, *J. Agr. Food Chem.* **12**, 7 (1964).
50 P. G. Balayannis, M. S. Smith and R. L. Wain, *Ann. Appl. Biol.* **55**, 261 (1965).
51 C. A. Bache, D. J. Lisk and M. A. Loos, *J. Ass. Offic. Agr. Chemists* **47**, 348 (1964).
52 L. A. Norris and V. H. Freed, *Weed Res.* **6**, 283 (1966).
53 S. N. Fertig, M. A. Loos, W. H. Gutenmann and D. J. Lisk, *Weeds* **12**, 147 (1964).
54 D. L. Linscott, R. D. Hagin and J. E. Dawson, *J. Agr. Food Chem.* **16**, 844 (1968).
55 M. Wilcox, D. E. Moreland and G. C. Klingman, *Physiol. Plantarum* **16**, 565 (1963).
56 C. E. Hagen, C. O. Clagett and E. A. Helgesen, *Science* **110**, 116 (1949).
57 A. S. Crafts, *Weeds* **8**, 19 (1960).
58 D. J. Morré and B. J. Rogers, *Weeds* **8**, 436 (1960).
59 S. S. Szabo, *Weeds* **11**, 292 (1963).
60 E. A. Erickson, B. L. Brannaman and C. W. Coggins, *J. Agr. Food Chem.* **11**, 437 (1963).
61 C. H. Fawcett, R. C. Seeley, H. F. Taylor, R. L. Wain and F. Wightman. *Nature, Lond.*, **176**, 1026 (1955).
62 E. G. Jaworski and J. S. Butts, *Arch. Biochem. Biophys.* **38**, 207 (1952).
63 S. C. Fang, *Weeds* **6**, 179 (1958).
64 M. K. Bach and J. Fellig. In *Plant Growth Regulation, 4th Intern. Conf. Plant Growth Regulation*, pp 273–287. Iowa State University Press: Ames (1961).
65 M. K. Bach and J. Fellig, *Plant Physiol.* **36**, 89 (1961).
66 W. C. Shaw and W. A. Gentner, *Weeds*, **5**, 75 (1957).
67 S. N. Fertig, M. A. Loos, W. H. Gutenmann and D. J. Lisk, *Weeds* **12**, 147 (1964).
68 C. F. Krewson, T. F. Drake, J. W. Mitchell and W. H. Preston, *J. Agr. Food Chem.* **4**, 690 (1956).
69 C. F. Krewson, J. F. Carmichael, T. F. Drake, J. W. Mitchell and B. C. Smale, *J. Agr. Food Chem.* **8**, 104 (1960).
70 L. J. Audus. In *The Physiology and Biochemistry of Herbicides*, pp 163–206. Ed. by L. J. Audus. Academic Press: New York (1964).
71 M. A. Loos, R. N. Roberts and M. Alexander, *Canad. J. Microbiol.* **13**, 679 (1967).
72 M. A. Loos, R. N. Roberts and M. Alexander, *Canad. J. Microbiol.* **13**, 691 (1967).
73 M. A. Loos, J.-M. Bollag and M. Alexander, *J. Agr. Food Chem.* **15**, 858 (1967).
74 J.-M. Bollag, C. S. Helling and M. Alexander, *Appl. Microbiol.* **15**, 1393 (1967).
75 C. S. Helling, J.-M. Bollag and J. E. Dawson, *J. Agr. Food Chem.* **16**, 538 (1968).
76 J.-M. Bollag, C. S. Helling and M. Alexander, *J. Agr. Food Chem.* **16**, 826 (1968).
77 J.-M. Bollag, G. G. Briggs, J. E. Dawson and M. Alexander, *J. Agr. Food Chem.* **16**, 829 (1968).
78 J. M. Tiedjie, J. M. Duxbury, M. Alexander and J. E. Dawson, *J. Agr. Food Chem.* **17**, 1021 (1969).
79 J. M. Duxbury, J. M. Tiedjie, M. Alexander and J. E. Dawson, *J. Agr. Food Chem.* **18**, 199 (1970).
80 W. C. Evans and B. S. W. Smith, *Biochem. J.* **57**, xxx (1954).
81 J. K. Gaunt and W. C. Evans, *Biochem. J.* **79**, 25P (1961).
82 W. C. Evans and P. Moss, *Biochem. J.* **65**, 8P (1957).
83 W. C. Evans. In *Encyclopedia of Plant Physiology*, Vol. 10, pp 474–476. Ed. by W. Ruhland. Springer: Berlin (1958).
84 J. P. Brown and E. B. McCall, *J. Chem. Soc.* 3681 (1955).
85 H. N. Fernley and W. C. Evans, *Biochem. J.* **73**, 22P (1959).
86 R. J. W. Byrde and D. Woodcock, *Biochem. J.* **65**, 682 (1957).
87 J. K. Faulkner and D. Woodcock, *J. Chem. Soc.* 5397 (1961).
88 J. K. Faulkner and D. Woodcock, *J. Chem. Soc.* 1187 (1965).
89 D. R. Clifford and D. Woodcock, *Nature, Lond.* **203**, 763 (1964).
90 S. M. Bocks, J. R. Lindsay-Smith and R. O. C. Norman, *Nature, Lond.* **201**, 398 (1964).

91 M. A. Loos. Unpublished data.
92 L. J. Audus, *Plant Soil* **3**, 170 (1951).
93 D. M. Webley, R. B. Duff and V. C. Farmer, *Nature, Lond.* **179**, 1130 (1957).
94 D. M. Webley, R. B. Duff and V. C. Farmer, *J. Gen. Microbiol.* **18**, 733 (1958).
95 D. M. Webley, R. B. Duff and V. C. Farmer, *Nature, Lond.* **183**, 748 (1959).
96 H. F. Taylor and R. L. Wain, *Proc. Roy. Soc.* B, **156**, 172 (1962).
97 W. H. Gutenmann, M. A. Loos, M. Alexander and D. J. Lisk, *Proc. Soil Sci. Soc. Amer.* **28**, 205 (1964).
98 I. C. MacRae, M. Alexander and A. D. Rovira, *J. Gen. Microbiol.* **32**, 69 (1963).
99 I. C. MacRae and M. Alexander. *J. Bacteriol.* **86**, 1231 (1963).
100 L. J. King, J. A. Lambrech and T. P. Finn, *Contrib. Boyce Thompson Inst.* **16**, 191 (1951).
101 A. J. Vlitos, *Contrib. Boyce Thompson Inst.* **16**, 435 (1952).
102 A. J. Vlitos, *Contrib. Boyce Thompson Inst.* **17**, 127 (1953).
103 L. J. Audus, *Nature, Lond.* **170**, 886 (1952).
104 R. B. Carroll. *Contrib. Boyce Thompson Inst.* **16**, 409 (1952).
105 M. Alexander and M. I. H. Aleem, *J. Agr. Food Chem.* **9**, 44 (1961).
106 K. Burger, I. C. MacRae and M. Alexander, *Proc. Soil Sci. Soc. Amer.* **26**, 243 (1962).
107 L. J. Audus, *Plant Soil* **2**, 31 (1949).
108 L. J. Audus, *J. Sci. Food Agr.* **3**, 268 (1952).
109 L. J. Audus, *Nature, Lond.* **166**, 356 (1950).
110 H. L. Jensen and H. I. Petersen, *Nature, Lond.* **170**, 39 (1952).
111 R. L. Walker and A. S. Newman, *Appl. Microbiol.* **4**, 201 (1956).
112 T. I. Steenson and N. Walker, *Plant Soil* **8**, 17 (1956).
113 M. H. Rogoff and J. J. Reid, *J. Bacteriol.* **71**, 303 (1956).
114 G. R. Bell, *Canad. J. Microbiol.* **3**, 821 (1957).
115 M. Alexander. In *Principles and Applications in Aquatic Microbiology*, pp 15–38. Ed. by H. Heukelekian and N. C. Dondero. Wiley: New York (1964).
116 M. Alexander, *Proc. Soil Sci. Soc. Amer.* **29**, 1 (1965).

METABOLISM OF SUBSTITUTED UREA HERBICIDES

Hans Geissbühler and Günther Voss

CIBA—GEIGY Agrochemical Division, Basle, Switzerland

ABSTRACT

The metabolism of substituted urea herbicides is critically reviewed with regard to the formation of terminal residues. It is pointed out that degradation processes by which these herbicides are affected, are regulated by physical/chemical and physiological features, such as water solubility, photochemical decomposition, leaching and adsorption in soils, and translocation in plants. The metabolic transformations of urea herbicides are discussed in terms of phase I reactions (introduction of relatively polar, biochemically reactive groups into the molecule) and phase II reactions (conjugation or complexing with endogenous animal, soil or plant constituents). Phase I reactions comprise the following mechanisms: (1) N-demethylation has been demonstrated to occur in animals, plants and soils. The resulting monomethyl or demethyl derivatives may be more abundant in plants and soil environments than the corresponding parent compounds. (2) N-demethoxylation represents a metabolic pathway for methylmethoxy ureas. (3) Ring-hydroxylation of the unchanged ureas as well as their N-dealkylated metabolites has been detected in animals. The position of the OH-moiety on the phenyl nucleus apparently depends on steric effects of the original substituents. (4) Aniline formation, one of the key steps in urea herbicide metabolism with regard to terminal residues, has so far not been demonstrated to be a major metabolic pathway. (5) The formation of aniline conversion products, such as substituted nitrobenzenes, acetanilides, or ring-hydroxylated anilines should be confirmed by additional experiments. (6) Azobenzenes do not represent significant terminal residues of urea herbicides. (7) Conjugate and complex formation, phase II transformation processes, give rise to water soluble metabolites, such as glucuronides or ester sulphates, which are readily excreted from the animal body in the urine. In plants, similar conjugating or complexing systems apparently do exist, but they have not yet been clearly defined. One type of plant conjugate is most probably the β-D-glucoside of the N-methylol derivative of substituted ureas.

INTRODUCTION

Since their discovery in the early 'fifties[1] the substituted ureas have grown into one of the most prominent and diversified groups of herbicides. Even now the addition of new types of molecules to this group continues at the rate of two to three compounds each year, which reach the late development or marketing stage. A recent list of accepted common names of pesticides issued by the International Standards Organisation mentions more than 20 urea derivatives[2] (*Table 1*).

Whereas the first important phenylureas were chlorine-substituted dimethyl

305

Table 1. Common and chemical names of substituted urea herbicides

Common name	Chemical name
Benzthiazuron	3-(2-benzothiazolyl)-1-methylurea
Buturon	3-(4-chlorophenyl)-1-isobutinyl-1-methylurea
Chlorbromuron	3-(4-bromo-3-chlorophenyl)-1-methoxy-1-methylurea
Chloroxuron	3-4-(4-chlorophenoxy)phenyl-1,1-dimethylurea
Chlortoluron	3-(3-chloro-4-methylphenyl)-1,1-dimethylurea
Cycluron	3-cyclo-octyl-1,1-dimethylurea
Difenoxuron	3-4-(4-methoxyphenoxy)phenyl-1,1-dimethylurea
Diuron	3-(3,4-dichlorophenyl)-1,1-dimethylurea
Fenobenzuron	3-benzoyl-3(3,4-dichlorophenyl)-1,1-dimethylurea
Fenuron	3,3-dimethyl-1-phenylurea
Fenuron TCA	3,3-dimethyl-1-phenyluronium trichloroacetate
Fluometuron	3-(3-trifluoromethylphenyl)-1,1-dimethylurea
Linuron	3-(3,4-dichlorophenyl)-1-methoxy-1-methylurea
Methabenzthiazuron	3-benzothiazol-2-yl-1,3-dimethylurea
Metobromuron	3-(4-bromophenyl)-1-methoxy-1-methylurea
Metoxuron	3-(3-chloro-4-methoxyphenyl)-1,1-dimethylurea
Monolinuron	3-(4-chlorophenyl)-1-methoxy-1-methylurea
Monuron	3-(4-chlorophenyl)-1,1-dimethylurea
Monuron TCA	3-(4-chlorophenyl)-1,1-dimethyluronium trichloroacetate
Neburon	3-(3,4-dichlorophenyl)-1-butyl-1-methylurea
Noruron	3-(hexahydro-4,7-methanoindan-5-yl)-1,1-dimethylurea
Siduron	3-(2-methylcyclohexyl)-1-phenylurea
Trimeturon	3-(4-chlorophenyl)-2,1,1-trimethylisourea

derivatives with a high order of inherent phytotoxicity, in more recent compounds, ring substituents, ring structures and alkyl moieties have become increasingly complex (*Figure 1*). These structural modifications have led to more subtle differences among the molecules with regard to their behaviour in soil and plant environments.

Since our review of the metabolism of substituted ureas[3] a number of additional and significant contributions have been made which extend our knowledge on the transformation pathways of this class of compounds in plants, animals and soils. Since the present Symposium specifically deals with terminal residues of pesticides, emphasis will be placed on those metabolic pathways that seem to be involved in the formation of relatively persistent metabolites and which have to be taken into account when evaluating the residue situation of urea compounds. To generate a meaningful discussion we shall not refrain from making a few critical remarks with regard to some data and interpretations published on this topic.

FACTORS AFFECTING DEGRADATION OF UREAS

Before turning to a detailed description of the metabolic pathways of ureas, we shall briefly mention some physical/chemical and physiological features which affect the behaviour of these compounds in various environments and hence determine the conditions under which they are most likely affected by degradation processes.

Most of the ureas, exceptions being fenuron and cycluron, are only sparingly

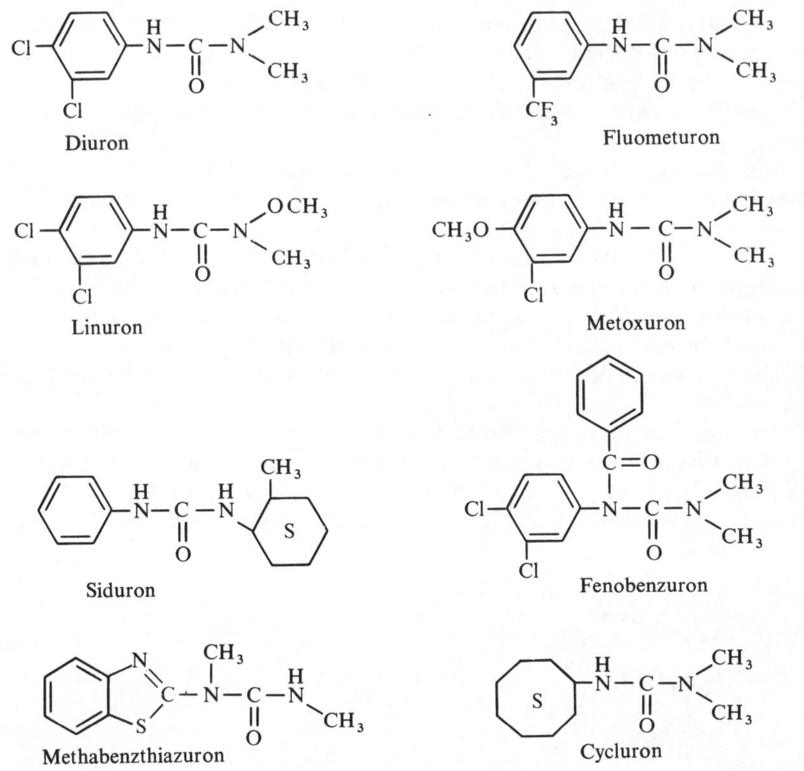

Figure 1. Chemical structures and common names of typical representatives of urea herbicides

soluble in water, solubilities ranging from a few to no more than 400 p.p.m.[3]. This low water solubility and the resulting unfavourable partitioning coefficients between water and organic phases are factors which limit the movement of most ureas in plant and soil systems. Losses by rapid leaching through soil profiles or by evaporation with water from plant surfaces and hence significant contamination of sites removed from those of application have so far not been demonstrated for the class of compounds discussed.

The movement of ureas or their availability in aqueous solutions is further controlled by adsorption of these compounds to various soil and plant constituents. The degree of adsorption not only varies from substrate to substrate, but also from compound to compound. In a particular soil the less strongly adsorbed herbicides are more readily available in soil solution and normally more rapidly decomposed by micro-organisms. In plants, the less strongly adsorbed compounds are more easily translocated from roots to shoots and leaves. These phenomena do not only affect the site of terminal residues, but also the physical and biochemical environment to which the herbicides are exposed.

Although no extended data on the chemical stability of urea herbicides under field conditions are available, it appears that purely chemical mechanisms such

307

as oxidations, reductions or hydrolyses are not important in controlling the rate of degradation of these compounds. Hance[4] has determined the velocity constants of the decomposition reactions undergone by diuron and linuron at high temperatures when present in aqueous slurries of soil and clay. The values extrapolated to 20°C showed that for both compounds examined decomposition by purely chemical means was unlikely to be an important pathway of degradation, as their half-lives at 20°C were found to be of the order of 10–70 years.

In contrast to their chemical stability, urea herbicides are more readily decomposed by photochemical means. Such processes seem to be of practical importance to herbicide degradation under field conditions, especially in arid regions exposed to intense sunlight[5, 6]. In an investigation by Crosby and Tang[7] the decomposition of monuron in dilute aqueous solution amounted to roughly six per cent when exposed for 14 days to summer sunlight conditions in California. The most interesting feature of this study as regards potential residues was the observation that the products of monuron decomposition are essentially analogous to those obtained by metabolic, i.e. by biochemical, transformations (*Figure 2*). It will be demonstrated below that this pheno-

VII   III   I   II   IV   red pigments polymers   VI   V

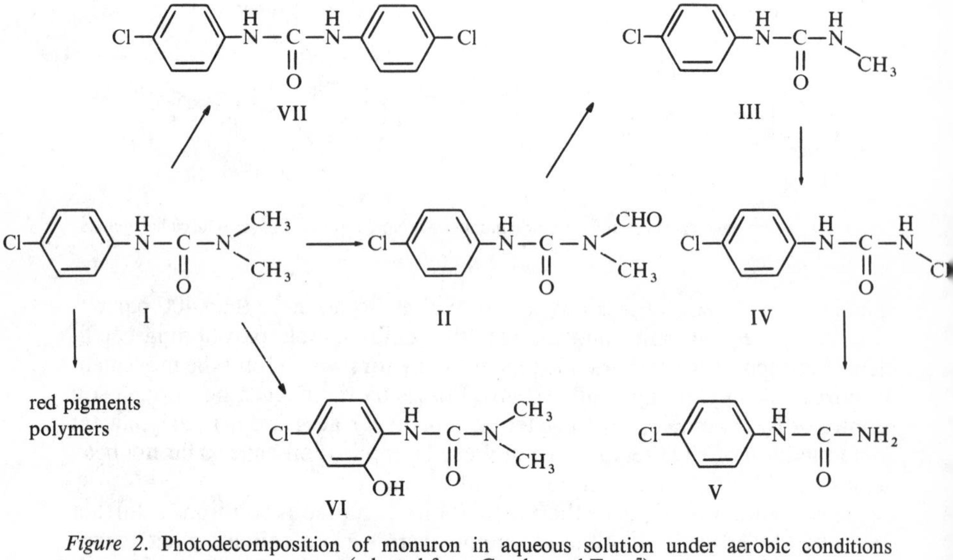

Figure 2. Photodecomposition of monuron in aqueous solution under aerobic conditions (adapted from Crosby and Tang[7])

menon certainly applies to the demethylated and hydroxylated transformation products, but not to the formyl derivatives observed. In spite of these small discrepancies we strongly recommend the initiation of metabolism experiments on urea herbicides by appropriate photodecomposition studies, which may give significant leads as to the most labile sites of a particular herbicide molecule.

METABOLIC TRANSFORMATIONS

A survey of the present literature on the metabolism of urea herbicides

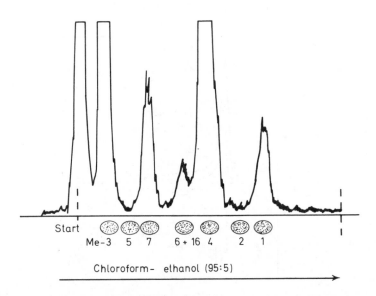

^{14}C-labelled metobromuron
Tobacco, leaves
Ether phase
Silica gel

Start

Me-3 5 7   6 + 16 4   2   1

Chloroform- ethanol (95:5)

Figure 3. Separation by thin-layer chromatography of metobromuron metabolites derived from tobacco plants after application of the ^{14}C-ring-labelled herbicide[35]

demonstrates that pathways of transformations in plants, animals and soils have sufficient common features to obviate separate discussion of degradation in the three substrates. On the other hand, in presenting the principal degradation mechanisms, we shall follow Parke's suggestion to distinguish between phase I and phase II reactions[8, 9]. By phase I reactions we mean oxidative, reductive or hydrolytic transformations of a foreign compound, which introduce or lead to relatively polar and biochemically reactive groups (such as —NH$_2$, —OH and —COOH) in the molecule. In phase II reactions these reactive groups are then bound or conjugated to endogenous animal, soil or plant metabolites.

The phase I transformations elucidated so far for substituted ureas comprise the following mechanisms: *N*-demethylation, *N*-demethoxylation, ring-hydroxylation and, to a smaller extent, aniline formation. Before describing these main pathways in some detail we should like to make some remarks on the methodology of metabolite identification. In most recent publications on urea herbicide degradation, thin-layer chromatography has been the most prominent and often only means for separation and so-called 'identification' of metabolites. Although adequate separation of some metabolites may actually be achieved by this procedure (*Figure 3*), the determination of only one or two R$_F$ values is far from being sufficient to identify degradation products positively. Further separation techniques such as liquid or gas chromatography (*Figure 4*)

309

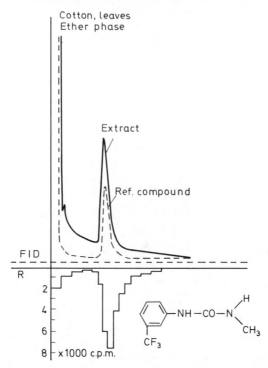

Figure 4. Separation and purification of ^{14}C-labelled metabolite of fluometuron by flame ionization gas chromatography. Radioactivity was determined by fraction collection and subsequent scintillation counting

are required to get the metabolites clean enough for infra-red, nuclear-magnetic-resonance or mass-spectral analyses. The latter spectral procedures are essential for positive identification of transformation products and the spectra of crucial metabolites should not only be mentioned but actually be published and interpreted in the literature.

N-Demethylation

Since our first experiments with chloroxuron[10] the mechanism of stepwise *N*-demethylation of dimethyl derivatives and one-step *N*-demethylation of methyl-methoxy compounds has now been demonstrated to occur in animals, soils and plants with a considerable number of phenylureas, including monuron, diuron, monolinuron, linuron, fluometuron, metobromuron and chlorbromuron[11-21] (*Figure 5*). Recently we have tentatively identified the methylol or hydroxy-methyl derivative of fluometuron as a short-lived intermediate in cotton plants, and Dr D. S. Frear apparently also has observed the same intermediate metabolite. Frear *et al.*[22,23] have further shown that the plant enzyme system involved in *N*-demethylation is a mixed-function oxidase, which is located in the microsomal fraction of plant extracts and which requires molecular oxygen and either NADPH or NADH as cofactors.

From the terminal residue point of view it is important to realize that

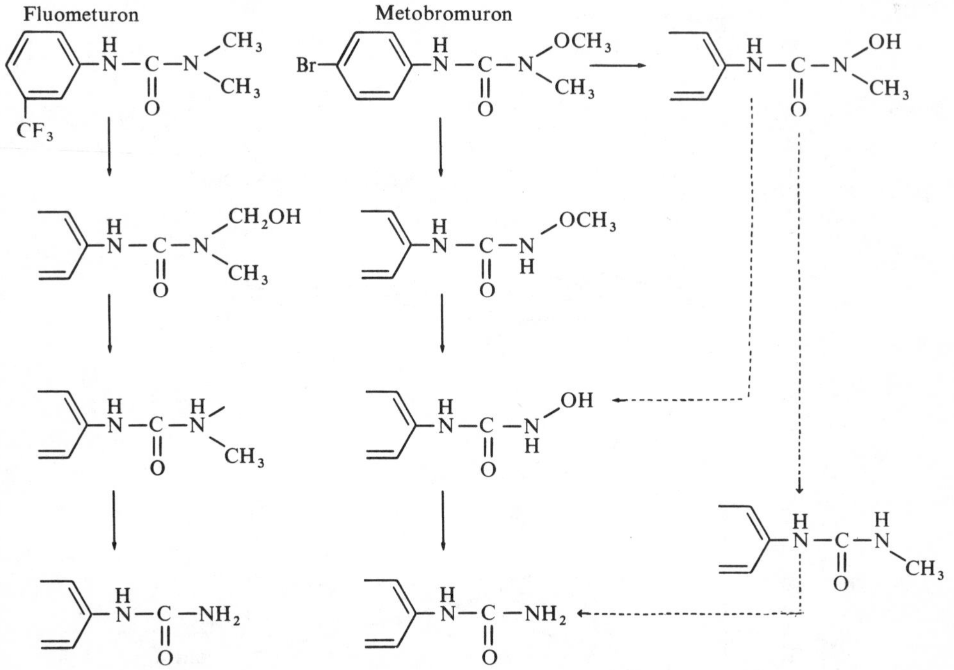

Figure 5. N-Demethylation and N-demethoxylation mechanisms of biodegradation of dimethyl- and methyl-methoxy-substituted phenylureas

depending on the plant species involved and the time elapsing between application and harvest, the monomethyl or demethyl derivatives may be more abundant in plant and soil environments than the parent compound (*Figure 6*). Consequently any residue method designed for phenylureas has to account for the N-demethylated metabolites, as shall be discussed in a separate paper during the present congress.

N-Demethoxylation

Methylmethoxy ureas such as linuron, monolinuron, metobromuron and chlorbromuron have been less extensively investigated than dimethyl compounds. However, there are a number of definite results which demonstrate that these herbicides are subjected to N-demethoxylation or O-demethylation in plants, animals and soils[3, 17, 18, 20, 24-26] (*Figure 5*). The exact pathway of N-demethoxylation is still unknown, although in our own experiments with metobromuron we had some indication that the corresponding hydroxylamides are present as transient intermediates. It might be difficult to detect such intermediates as the related arylhydroxylamines have been demonstrated to be rapidly reduced to the corresponding amines in animal tissues[27]. The methyl-methoxy compounds mentioned apparently are more accessible to N-demethylation than N-demethoxylation, since the N-methoxy metabolites

311

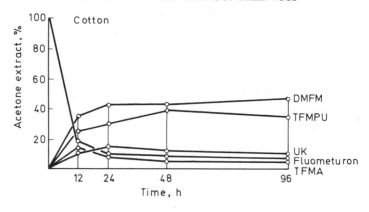

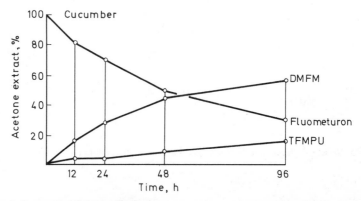

Figure 6. Amounts of ^{14}C-labelled fluometuron and its radioactive metabolites as a function of time in cotton and cucumber leaves[16]. DMFM, 3-(3-trifluoromethylphenyl)-1-methylurea; TFMPU, 3-trifluoromethylphenylurea; TFMA, 3-trifluoromethylaniline; UK, unknown metabolite

have consistently been found to be more abundant in plant tissue than either the *N*-methyl derivative or the unsubstituted urea.

Ring hydroxylation

Although not working with herbicides, Bray *et al.*[28], when investigating the animal degradation of aryl ureas, had already demonstrated in 1949 that the ureido grouping was biologically rather stable and that ring-hydroxylation in the *ortho* position was a prominent pathway with these compounds. In 1965 Ernst and Böhme[24, 25] reported on their extensive degradation experiments in animals with monuron, diuron, monolinuron and linuron and showed that all of these herbicides, in addition to being *N*-dealkylated, were ring-hydroxylated by the rat (*Figures 7* and *8*). The orientation of the hydroxyl moieties on the phenyl nucleus apparently followed steric effects: position 2 was strongly preferred by the monochloro compounds monuron and monolinuron, whereas the dichloro compounds diuron and linuron were mainly converted into the 6-hydroxy derivatives.

312

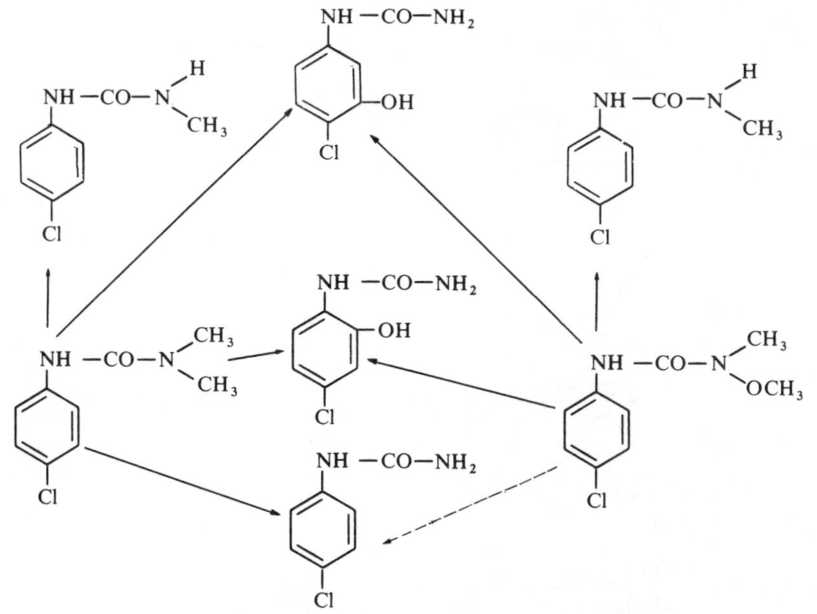

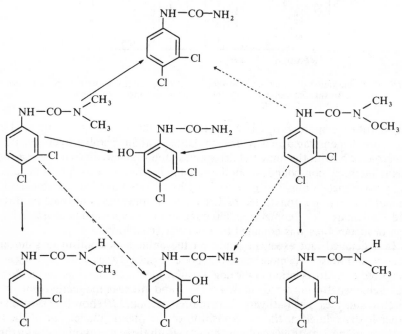

Figure 7. Pathways of mammalian degradation of monuron (left) and monolinuron (right) (adapted from Ernst and Böhme[24])

Figure 8. Pathways of mammalian degradation of diuron (left) and linuron (right) (adapted from Böhme and Ernst[25])

313

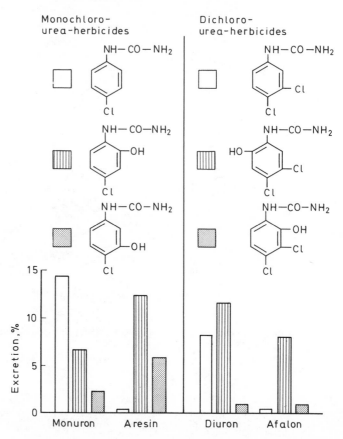

Figure 9. Quantitative distribution of metabolites derived from urea herbicides in rat urine. Aresin = monolinuron, Afalon = linuron (adapted from Ernst[29])

Quantitative analyses by Ernst and Böhme of the metabolites eliminated in rat urine demonstrated that N-demethylation without parallel hydroxylation occurred only with the dimethyl derivatives monuron and diuron, whereas the methylmethoxy compounds monolinuron and linuron were mainly eliminated as hydroxy metabolites[29] (*Figure 9*). Ring-hydroxylation of urea herbicides in animal tissues as demonstrated by Ernst and Böhme was confirmed by Boyd and Fogleman[30] for fluometuron, although in these experiments characterization of metabolites was confined to thin-layer separation.

In a detailed and excellent study on the animal metabolism of siduron, Belasco and Reiser[31] demonstrated that both the phenyl and cyclohexyl ring are subjected to hydroxylation in the dog. Positive identification of the metabolites was achieved by infra-red, mass-spectral and nuclear-magnetic-resonance spectral analyses. The pathways as proposed in *Figure 10* show that siduron is either hydroxylated at the *para*-position of the phenyl nucleus or at the 4-position of the 2-methylcyclohexyl moiety. Both these metabolites are further hydroxylated to form 1-(4-hydroxy-2-methylcyclohexyl)-3-(*p*-hydroxy-

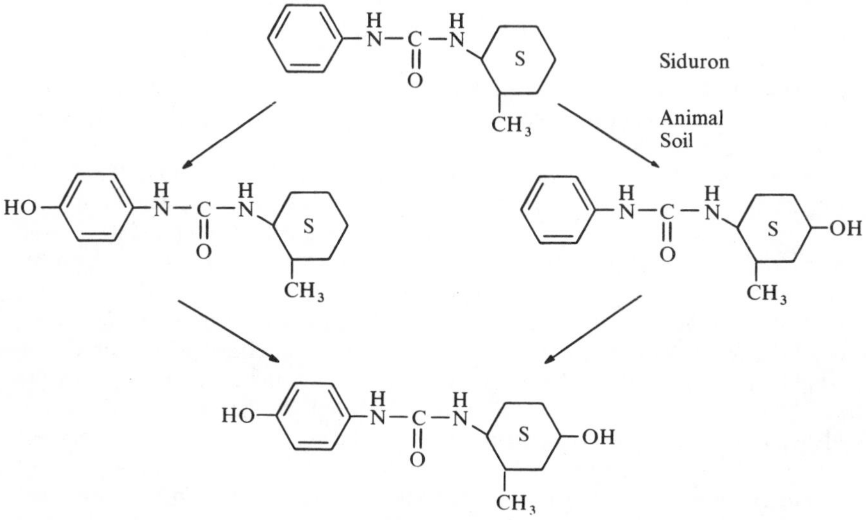

Figure 10. Pathways of mammalian transformation of siduron (adapted from Belasco and Reiser[31])

phenyl) urea. All three metabolites identified apparently were eliminated in the urine as highly water-soluble conjugates. Analyses of urine samples for aminophenol and aniline respectively after suitable hydrolyses further showed that hydroxylation of the phenyl moiety was more prominent in the rat than in the dog.

In a second study in which the *carbonyl-*[14]C-labelled compound was applied, Belasco and Langsdorf[32] showed that microbial degradation was the major route of siduron disappearance in the soil. The metabolites separated on thin-layer plates had the same characteristics as those identified in animal urine and the authors therefore concluded that ring-hydroxylation was also operative in soil environments. Since siduron is hydroxylated in both animals and soil, claims by Splittstoesser and Hopen[33] that this herbicide is not metabolized in plants appear to be somewhat doubtful.

In view of the general mechanisms of microbial degradation of aromatic compounds it is surprising that ring-hydroxylation of phenylureas has not been observed more frequently in soil environments. Since hydroxylation mechanisms are the generally accepted preliminary steps in enzymatic fission of aromatic nuclei[34] a more thorough study of ureas with regard to such mechanisms appears to be highly desirable. In plants, ring hydroxylation has so far not been demonstrated to be a pathway of urea herbicide transformation. We have recently isolated a metabolite of metobromuron from tobacco tissue which fulfils a number of criteria for a ring-hydroxylated compound; however, positive identification has not yet been terminated.

Aniline formation

One of the key problems of urea herbicide metabolism with regard to terminal residues is the occurrence and extent of aniline formation. Although in

315

many publications stepwise demethylation has been claimed to be followed by further degradation to the aniline, the evidence for such a degradation step has been rather circumstantial[10-12, 14, 18, 20]. In animal[24, 25, 36] and plant[14, 15, 17, 20] experiments the quantities of free aniline detected were consistently small and characterization of these trace quantities was in most studies limited to some sort of chromatographic separation on thin-layer plates. In our own extensive plant experiments with several compounds labelled with ^{14}C in either the phenyl ring itself or in one of its substituents, the free anilines were not observed at all or were present in such small traces that positive identification was impossible[15, 35]. In these experiments special precautions were taken to prevent any loss of these very volatile compounds by evaporation. In addition, as we shall discuss below, we have no definite indication for rapid conversion or conjugation of free anilines into other major metabolites, which processes would mask the intermediate formation of the aromatic amines. From the evidence present at this time, we therefore conclude that, in animals and in plants, degradation of urea herbicides to the corresponding anilines does not represent a major pathway of transformation.

The situation in regard to aniline formation apparently is somewhat different in soils, although the various data presented are not much more extensive or convincing than those derived from animals and plants. In several studies indirect evidence for aniline formation in soil by microbial suspensions was obtained by the formation of radioactive carbon dioxide from carbonyl-labelled urea compounds[10, 17, 37]. The measured rates of evolution of carbon dioxide varied within considerable limits and in those experiments in which formation of the gas was apparently rapid the amounts of free aniline detected were far below the ones to be expected. Such results, of course, can be explained by rapid further conversions of the aromatic amines or by the evaporation of these compounds from the systems to which they were exposed. In view of the apparent lack of definite information on the rate of aniline formation in soil environments, an establishment of a detailed balance of radioactivity derived from ring-labelled ureas is urgently required.

In a series of papers Wallnöfer[37-39] showed that the methylmethoxy ureas monolinuron, linuron and metobromuron, but not the dimethyl derivatives examined, were rapidly decomposed by a strain of *Bacillus sphaericus* or by a cell-free extract derived from induced cells of this organism. The author did not

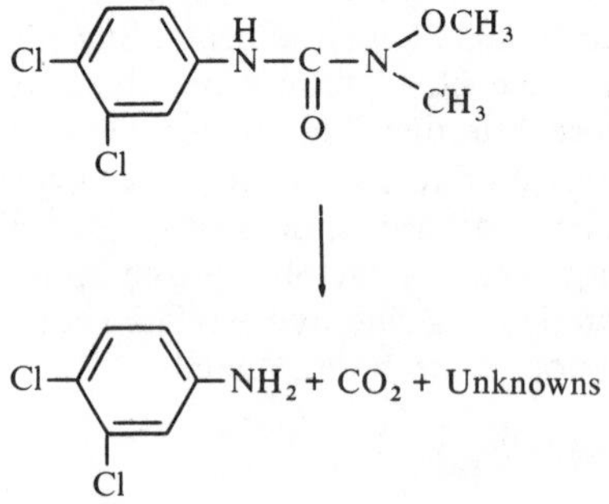

Figure 11. Degradation of linuron by *Bacillus sphaericus* as proposed by Wallnöfer[38]

only claim that considerable amounts of aromatic amines accumulated in the culture media, but that degradation of the ureas to the anilines proceeded directly without intermediate formation of demethylated derivatives (*Figure 11*). The mechanism of degradation was not exactly defined but it was suggested that the cell-free system prepared had an 'amidase' activity, which would yield phenylcarbamic acid and an unidentified metabolite as first intermediates. Unfortunately the analytical details given in these papers are far from being sufficient to preclude definitely the presence of metabolites other than the anilines.

Aniline conversions

Provided that anilines are formed to some extent from substituted ureas, they should either accumulate or be converted into other metabolites. Evidence for the presence of such conversion products is not very extensive at this time (*Figure 12*).

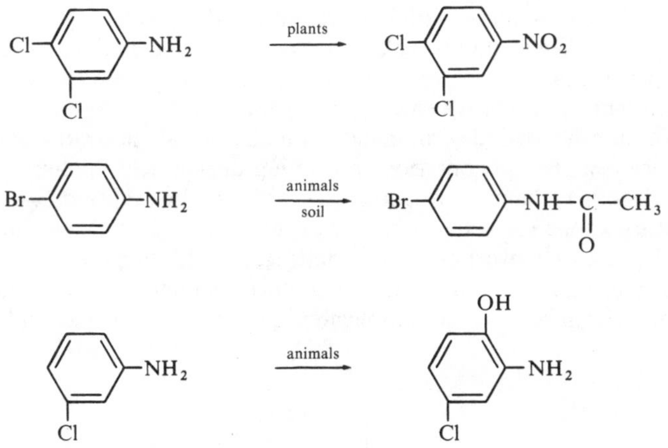

Figure 12. Biotransformation reactions of halogenated anilines

In corn seedlings Onley *et al.*[14], who applied ^{14}C-labelled diuron by nutrient solution, identified 3,4-dichlorobenzene in addition to small quantities of 3,4-dichloroaniline and thus proposed N-oxidation of the latter compound. Unfortunately the authors were not in a position to decide if nitrobenzene formation represented a chemical or enzymatic process in plants, the buildup of an artefact or a combination of these processes. In our own plant experiments with labelled fluometuron and metobromuron we have so far not been able to confirm nitrobenzene formation, although we have carefully checked for the presence of these compounds[35].

A second aniline transformation reaction, which has been known for some time to occur in animals is acetylation[27, 40] (*Figure 12*). This mechanism, which represents a phase II reaction, has been postulated for the urea herbicide metobromuron after exposure of this compound to suspensions of the fungus

317

Talaromyces wortmanii[21, 41]. In these experiments Tweedy *et al.* isolated from the culture media *p*-bromoacetanilide and thus proposed conversion of *p*-bromoaniline into the former metabolite. Since purification procedures applied in these experiments were not very extensive, occurrence of acetylation as a pathway of urea herbicide transformation should be confirmed by additional experiments.

A third aniline transformation reaction is ring-hydroxylation[27, 40, 42]. This oxidative conversion has been demonstrated for *m*-chloroaniline and, to a smaller extent, for *p*-chloroaniline when these compounds were administered to rats, rabbits and mice. However, at this time there is no experimental evidence for the formation of ring-hydroxylated anilines derived from ureas, although such mechanisms have been observed to be valid for phenylcarbamate herbicides[43].

Azobenzene formation

In the last few years a number of investigators, who have joined the azobenzene bandwaggon, have felt obliged to implicate urea herbicides in the formation of such compounds without presenting corresponding experimental evidence[38, 44, 45]. We certainly acknowledge the significance and meaning of model experiments in which relatively high concentrations of compounds are exposed to various oxidative enzyme and photosensitizing systems; however, we do not approve of indiscriminate extrapolation of the results obtained in such experiments to the conditions prevailing during field application and to compounds other than those actually examined. In addition, we feel that investigators who are so active in setting up model experiments, which, from the analytical point of view, pose few problems, should afterwards share in the much more demanding task of detecting, purifying and identifying azo compounds at the p.p.b. level in complicated biological substrates and environments.

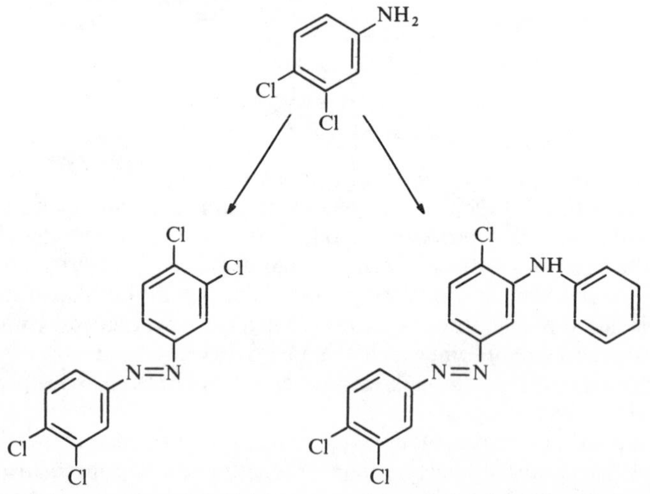

Figure 13. Formation of symmetrical and asymmetrical azobenzene derivatives from anilines after peroxidatic catalysis *in vitro* (adapted from Linke[49])

Although the formation of symmetrical and asymmetrical halogenated azo-benzenes from relatively high concentrations of anilines and from certain anilide herbicides appears to be well established[46-49] (*Figure 13*), we are not aware of any experimental data which show that urea herbicides are converted into azobenzenes under model or field conditions. On the contrary, extensive analyses by Belasco and Pease[50], Maier-Bode[51] and ourselves[52] did not reveal detectable residues of azobenzenes in a large number of soil samples that had

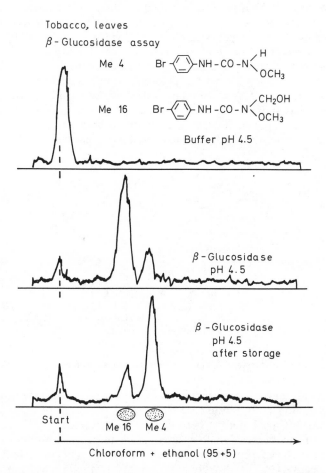

Figure 14. Thin-layer separation on silica gel of water-soluble metabolite of ^{14}C-ring-labelled metobromuron before and after incubation with β-glucosidase (adapted from Geissbühler *et al.*[35])

been treated with different urea herbicides under field conditions. In laboratory experiments we administered high concentrations of ^{14}C-labelled fluometuron and metobromuron to strongly irradiated cotton and tobacco plants, but were not able to detect labelled azobenzene derivatives. From the data at present available we therefore conclude that azobenzenes do not represent significant terminal residues of urea herbicides in either soils or plants.

Conjugate- and complex-formation

By enzymatic or mineral acid cleavage it was shown that the above-described hydroxylated animal metabolites of dimethyl- and methyl-methoxy ureas and of siduron are mainly eliminated by the urine as glucuronides or ester sulphates[24, 25, 31]. Formation of these conjugates represents phase II reactions that lead to very water-soluble metabolites, which are readily eliminated from the animal body by the urinary tract. So far the chemical structure of these conjugates has not been verified by actual synthesis of references.

In plants, similar conjugating or complex-forming systems apparently do exist but these have not yet been clearly defined. In the first study on urea herbicide metabolism, Fang et al.[53] observed the formation of a monuron complex in bean plants. Upon acid hydrolysis, this complex, which was later speculated to be of peptide nature[54], yielded the unchanged herbicide. That a fraction of urea herbicides taken up by plants may be bound to certain protein constituents has more recently been indicated by the work of Nashed and Ilnicki[19, 20], who applied linuron and chlorbromuron to corn plants. After exhaustive extraction of the herbicide-treated plant material, additional quan-

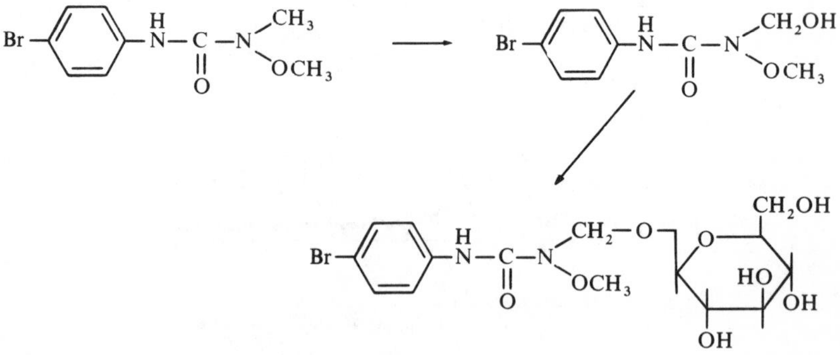

Figure 15. Tentative scheme of conjugate formation of metobromuron in tobacco tissue[35]

tities of aniline-containing compounds were released from the residue either by alkaline digestion or by proteinase treatment. Unfortunately these so-called 'bound materials' have not yet been further characterized.

We have recently made some progress in identifying conjugates of fluometuron and metobromuron, which are major metabolites in cotton and tobacco plants respectively[35]. These highly water-soluble metabolites, which by alkaline hydrolysis were shown to contain the unchanged aniline structure, were purified by thin-layer and column chromatography on Sephadex. When the conjugate derived from metobromuron was incubated with a sample of purified β-glucosidase, a hydrolysis product appeared which co-chromatographed with the methylol derivative of the herbicide (*Figure 14*). Upon storage, the labile hydrolysis product was slowly converted into the corresponding demethyl compound. The fluometuron conjugate in cotton exhibited the same properties. Although identification by comparison with synthetic references and spectral analysis is not yet completed, we feel rather confident that the mentioned conjugates are the β-D-glucosides of the methylol compounds (*Figure 15*). Similar plant conjugates have earlier been shown to occur with the phosphoric acid crotonamide insecticides monocrotophos and dicrotophos[55, 56].

In concluding our review on urea herbicide metabolism, we should like to emphasize that, in spite of the considerable progress made during the last few years, we still ignore some important aspects of the biodegradation of this class of herbicides. The occurrence and extent of aniline formation should be more clearly defined, and in case this pathway really turns out to be a significant one the further degradation of aromatic amines under field conditions should be more extensively investigated. Furthermore, the various 'complexes' and conjugates that have consistently cropped up in the literature should be subjected to more detailed characterization. Finally, some of the more recent urea compounds, which contain different or additional ring structures or nonhalogenated ring substituents, must certainly be included in metabolism studies.

REFERENCES

[1] H. C. Bucha and C. W. Todd, *Science*, **114**, 453 (1951).
[2] *Common names of pesticides*, PANS, **15**, 293 (1969).
[3] H. Geissbühler, in *Degradation of Herbicides*. Ed. by P. C. Kearney and D. D. Kaufman. Marcel Dekker Inc., New York (1969).
[4] R. J. Hance, *J. Sci. Food Agric.* **18**, 544 (1967).
[5] R. D. Comes and F. L. Timmons, *Weeds*, **13**, 81 (1965).
[6] L. S. Jordan, J. D. Mann and B. E. Day, *Weeds*, **13**, 43 (1965).
[7] D. G. Crosby and C. S. Tang, *J. Agr. Food Chem.* **17**, 1041 (1969).
[8] D. V. Parke, *The Biochemistry of Foreign Compounds. Int. Ser. of Monographs in Pure and Applied Biology. Division Biochem.*, vol. 5, Pergamon Press, Oxford (1968).
[9] D. V. Parke and R. T. Williams, *Brit. Med. Bull.* **25**, 256 (1969).
[10] H. Geissbühler, C. Haselbach, H. Aebi and L. Ebner, *Weed Res.* **3**, 277 (1963).
[11] R. L. Dalton, A. W. Evans and R. C. Rhodes, *Weeds*, **14**, 31 (1966).
[12] J. W. Smith and T. J. Sheets, *J. Agr. Food Chem.* **15**, 577 (1967).
[13] C. R. Swanson and H. R. Swanson, *Weed Sci.* **16**, 137 (1968).
[14] J. H. Onley, G. Yip and M. H. Aldridge, *J. Agr. Food Chem.* **16**, 426 (1968).
[15] G. Voss and H. Geissbühler, *Proc. 8th Brit. Weed Control Conf.*, vol. 1, 266 (1966).
[16] R. L. Rogers and H. H. Funderburk, *J. Agr. Food Chem.* **16**, 434 (1968).
[17] H. Börner, *Z. Pfl. Krankh. Pfl. schutz*, **74**, 135 (1967).
[18] H. Börner, H. Burgemeister and M. Schroeder, *Z. Pfl. Krankh. Pfl. schutz*, **76**, 385 (1969).
[19] R. B. Nashed and R. D. Ilnicki, *Weed Sci.* **18**, 25 (1970).
[20] R. B. Nashed, S. E. Katz and R. D. Ilnicki, *Weed Sci.* **18**, 122 (1970).
[21] B. G. Tweedy, C. Loeppky and J. A. Ross, *J. Agr. Food Chem.* **18**, 851 (1970).
[22] D. S. Frear, *Science*, **162**, 674 (1968).
[23] D. S. Frear, H. R. Swanson and F. S. Tanaka, *Phytochemistry*, **8**, 2157 (1969).
[24] W. Ernst and C. Böhme, *Food Cosmet. Toxicol.* **3**, 789 (1965).
[25] C. Böhme and W. Ernst, *Food Cosmet. Toxicol.* **3**, 797 (1965).
[26] H. Kuratle, E. M. Rahn and C. W. Woodmanssee, *Weed Sci.* **17**, 216 (1969).
[27] C. T. Williams, *Detoxification Mechanisms*, Chapman and Hall, London (1949).
[28] H. G. Bray, H. J. Lake and W. V. Thorpe, *Biochem. J.* **44**, 136 (1949).
[29] W. Ernst, *J. South African Chem. Inst.* **22**, 879 (1969).
[30] V. F. Boyd and R. W. Fogleman, *Amer. Chem. Soc.*, 15 3td Meeting Miami (April 1967).
[31] I. J. Belasco and R. W. Reiser, *J. Agr. Food Chem.* **17**, 1000 (1969).
[32] I. J. Belasco, and W. P. Langsdorf, *J. Agr. Food Chem.* **17**, 1004 (1969).
[33] W. E. Splittstoesser and H. J. Hopen, *Weed Sci.* **16**, 305 (1968).
[34] D. T. Gibson, *Science*, **161**, 1093 (1968).
[35] H. Geissbühler, D. Gross and G. Voss, Unpublished data, (1971).
[36] H. C. Hodge, W. L. Downs, B. S. Panner, D. W. Smith and E. A. Maynard, *Food Cosmet. Toxicol.* **5**, 513 (1967).

M

37 P. Wallnöfer, *Mitt. Biol Bundesanst. Land- u. Forstwirtsch.* **132**, 69 (1969).
38 P. Wallnöfer, *Weed Res.* **9**, 333 (1969).
39 P. Wallnöfer, *Appl. Microbiol.* **19**, 714 (1970).
40 C. Böhme and W. Grunow, *Food Cosmet. Toxicol.* **7**, 125 (1969).
41 B. G. Tweedy, C. Loeppky and J. A. Ross, *Science,* **168**, 482 (1970).
42 L. A. Elson, F. Goulden and F. L. Warren. *Brit. J. Cancer,* **12**, 108 (1958).
43 W. Grunow, C. Böhme and B. Budczies, *Food Cosmet. Toxicol.* **8**, 277 (1970).
44 R. Bartha, H. A. B. Linke and D. Pramer, *Science,* **161**, 582 (1968).
45 J. D. Rosen, M. Siewiersky and G. Winnett, *J. Agr. Food Chem.* **18**, 494 (1970).
46 R. Bartha and D. Pramer, *Science,* **156**, 1617 (1967).
47 R. Bartha, *J. Agr. Food Chem.* **16**, 602 (1968).
48 P. C. Kearney, J. R. Plimmer and F. B. Guardia, *J. Agr. Food Chem.* **17**, 1418 (1969).
49 H. A. B. Linke, *Naturwissenschaften,* **57**, 307 (1970).
50 I. J. Belasco and H. L. Pease, *J. Agr. Food Chem.* **17**, 1414 (1969).
51 H. Maier-Bode, Personal communication (1971).
52 V. F. Boyd and J. A. Guth. Unpublished data (1971).
53 S. C. Fang, V. H. Freed, R. H. Johnson and D. R. Coffee, *J. Agr. Food Chem.* **3**, 400 (1955).
54 V. H. Freed, M. Montgomery and M. Kief, *Proc. Northeast Weed Control Conf.* **15**, 6 (1961).
55 D. L. Bull and D. A. Lindquist, *J. Agr. Food Chem.* **12**, 310 (1964).
56 D. A. Lindquist and D. L. Bull, *J. Agr. Food Chem.* **15**, 267 (1967).

METABOLISM OF s-TRIAZINES AND ITS SIGNIFICANCE IN BIOLOGICAL SYSTEMS

R. H. Shimabukuro, G. L. Lamoureux, D. S. Frear and J. E. Bakke

*Metabolism and Radiation Research Laboratory,
US Department of Agriculture, ARS, Fargo, North Dakota 58102, USA*

ABSTRACT

Most of our information on metabolism of s-triazines in biological systems is based on studies with substituted 2-chloro-s-triazines with alkylamino groups in the 4- and 6-positions. Glutathione conjugation and subsequent metabolism seem to be the most significant metabolic pathway for 2-chloro-s-triazine degradation in plants. This reaction also occurs in animals. Glutathione conjugation of atrazine is the primary factor responsible for the resistance of higher plants to atrazine injury. N-Dealkylation of side chains seems to occur in plants, animals and soil micro-organisms. This reaction occurs in s-triazines with chlorine, methoxy, hydroxyl and methylmercapto substituents in the 2-position. However, complete dealkylation at a significant rate seems to require substituents other than the hydroxyl group in the 2-position. Hydrolysis of 2-chloro-s-triazines to their 2-hydroxy derivatives seems to be significant in a few selected plant species and as a mechanism for detoxication in soil. In plants the incorporation of s-triazine derivatives into methanol-insoluble residue is more significant than ring cleavage and oxidation of ring carbon atoms to carbon dioxide. The nature of the terminal residues of s-triazines in plants is still unknown.

INTRODUCTION

The first report of herbicidal activity in s-triazines appeared in 1955[1]. Since that time, rapid development of s-triazines as selective herbicides has given us some of the most effective and widely used herbicides. Simazine, atrazine, propazine and prometryne are some of the better-known s-triazines in use today. Owing to its effectiveness and outstanding selectivity, atrazine is one of the most widely used herbicides and today has the highest sales among all pesticides in the United States[2].

The structures, chemical names, original code numbers, common names and some chemical and physical data on the more important s-triazine herbicides have been published[3]. The chemistry of s-triazine herbicides and and their structure-activity relationships have been thoroughly reviewed[4,5]. This paper will primarily review the metabolism of s-triazine herbicides in plants, animals and micro-organisms. The elucidation of new metabolic pathways for s-triazine degradation within the last 4 years, their physiological significance and their contribution to terminal residues in the environment will be discussed. Earlier research on the metabolism of s-triazines has been presented in previous reviews and will not be discussed in detail[4-9].

Some of the more common s-triazines discussed in this report are given in *Table 1*. Several s-triazines are still in the experimental stages of development, but they are included in this report to illustrate new degradation reactions occurring in biological systems. Very little information is available on the metabolism and degradation of 2-methoxy- and 2-methylmercapto-s-triazines. Therefore this review on s-triazine metabolism deals primarily with substituted 2-chloro-s-triazines with alkylamino groups in the 4- and 6-positions.

Table 1. Chemical structures of several s-triazines

X	R_1	R_2	Common name*
Cl	—CH$_2$CH$_3$	—CH$_2$CH$_3$	Simazine
Cl	—CH$_2$CH$_3$	—CH(CH$_3$)$_2$	Atrazine
Cl	—CH(CH$_3$)$_2$	—CH(CH$_3$)$_2$	Propazine
Cl	—CH$_2$CH$_3$	—CH—CH$_2$ (cyclopropyl, CH$_3$)	S-9115†
Cl	—CH$_2$CH$_3$	—C—C≡N (CH$_3$, CH$_3$)	SD-15418†
Cl	—CH$_2$CH$_3$	—C—CH$_3$ (CH$_3$)	GS-13529†
OCH$_3$	—CH(CH$_3$)$_2$	—CH(CH$_3$)$_2$	Prometone
OCH$_3$	—CH$_2$CH$_3$	—CHCH$_2$CH$_3$ (CH$_3$)	GS-14254†
SCH$_3$	—CH$_2$CH$_3$	—CH(CH$_3$)$_2$	Ametryne
SCH$_3$	—CH(CH$_3$)$_2$	—CH(CH$_3$)$_2$	Prometryne

* Common names assigned by Weed Science Society of America.
† Experimental compounds.

METABOLISM AND DEGRADATION IN BIOLOGICAL SYSTEMS

Hydrolysis. Dechlorination of atrazine (I) and simazine in corn to their 2-hydroxy derivatives (hydroxyatrazine and hydroxysimazine) was the first degradation reaction of 2-chloro-s-triazine herbicides identified in plants[4,10–12] (*Figure 1*). The active constituent in corn that catalyses the conversion of simazine into hydroxysimazine was isolated and identified as 2,4-dihydroxy-7-methoxy-1,4-benzoxazine-3-one (Benzoxazinone) (II) or its glucoside[13–15] (*Figure 1*). Incubation of atrazine and simazine in either a protein-free extract or homogenate of corn, or in a solution of pure benzoxazinone, resulted in the formation of hydroxyatrazine (III) and hydroxy-simazine[4,10–12].

The conversion of 2-chloro-s-triazines into 2-hydroxy-s-triazines has been accepted as a primary factor in determining the resistance of plants to herbicidal injury. However, the hydroxylation of 2-chloro-s-triazines seems

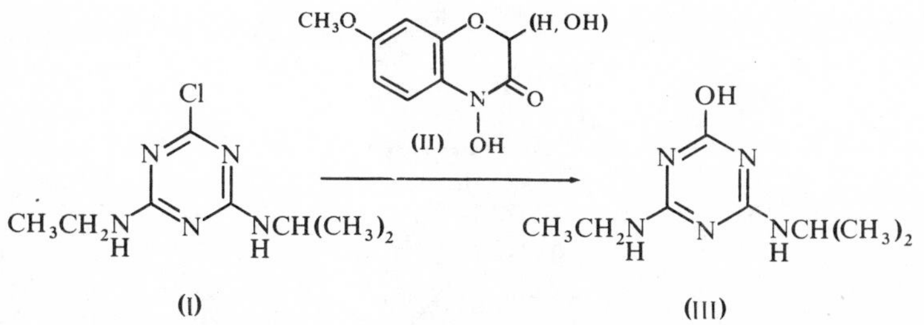

Figure 1. Hydrolysis of 2-chloro-s-triazine catalysed by benzoxazinone

to be limited to benzoxazinone-containing species such as resistant corn and *Coix lacryma-jobi*, and susceptible wheat and rye[16,17]. Resistant species such as sorghum, intermediately susceptible pea and cotton, and susceptible oat, barley and soybean, did not form the 2-hydroxy derivatives[16,17,20]. None of these plants contain benzoxazinone. Current results[18,19] indicate that alternative metabolic pathways effectively detoxify 2-chloro-s-triazines. Therefore hydroxylation contributes to total detoxication, but it is not essential for resistance even in crop plants such as corn[19].

Hydroxyatrazine is formed in soil principally as a result of chemical hydrolysis[3]. One example of a micro-organism that hydrolyses atrazine to hydroxyatrazine has been reported[21]. In these studies the soil fungus, *Fusarium roseum* (L.K), Snyder and Hansen, and atrazine were incubated for 60 days. Paper chromatography indicated that hydroxyatrazine was the predominant metabolite. The same organism was found to evolve $^{14}CO_2$ from chain-labelled simazine under similar incubation conditions.

Hydroxylation of 2-chloro-s-triazines in animals does not seem to occur very readily. However, small amounts of hydroxyatrazine were detected in the faeces and urine of rats dosed with ring-^{14}C-labelled atrazine[22]. Hydroxylated derivatives of atrazine, propazine and simazine were also reported to be formed in rats[3].

N-Dealkylation. The first evidence for oxidative removal of the alkyl side chain was reported for chain-^{14}C-labelled simazine[23]. Resistant corn, intermediately susceptible cotton and susceptible soybean all formed appreciable amounts of $^{14}CO_2$ when treated with chain-14C-labelled simazine. Nearly 70% of the total radioactivity absorbed by corn as chain-^{14}C-labelled atrazine was released as $^{14}CO_2$ within 6 days[24]. A significant amount of $^{14}CO_2$ was evolved by the fungus *Aspergillus fumigatus* Fres.[25], and other soil fungi[21] from chain-^{14}C-labelled simazine. In animals 50% and 24% of the administered dose of chain-^{14}C-labelled propazine was expired as $^{14}CO_2$ in rats and ruminant sheep respectively[26,27]. Therefore the removal of side chains from 2-chloro-s-triazines seems to be a universal reaction found in plants, animals and micro-organisms.

325

The N-dealkylated metabolite of simazine, 2-chloro-4-amino-6-ethylamino-s-triazine (V) (*Figure 2*) was isolated from *A. fumigatus* Fres. and identified by infra-red, nuclear magnetic resonance and mass spectroscopy[28]. One of the two possible N-dealkylated metabolites of atrazine, 2-chloro-4-amino-6-isopropylamino-s-triazine (IV) (*Figure 2*) was isolated as the predominant

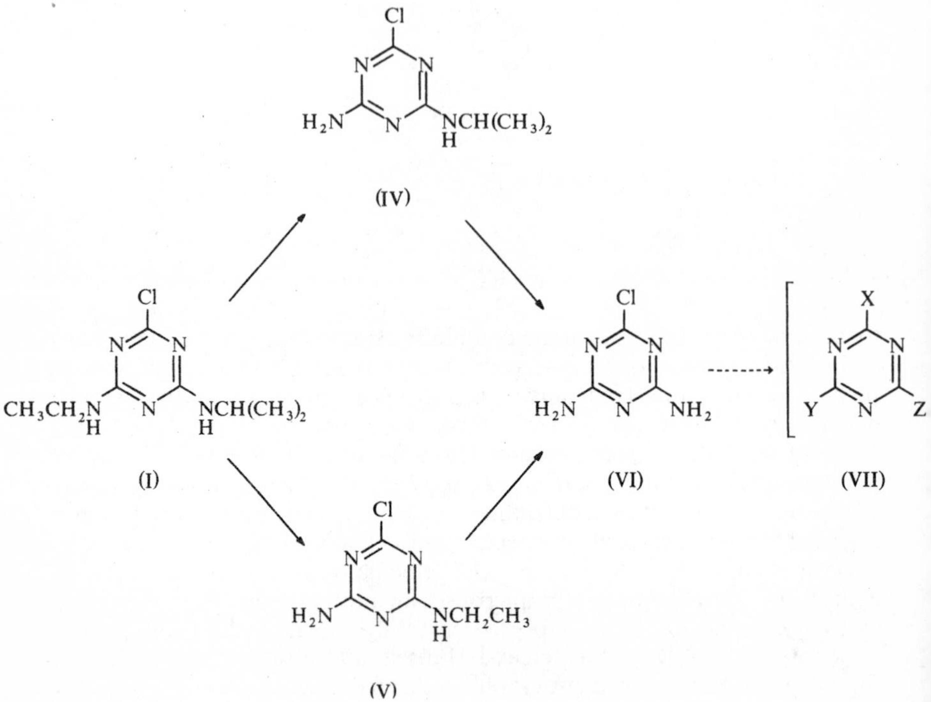

Figure 2. N-Dealkylation of 2-chloro-s-triazine

metabolite from atrazine-treated pea and identified by TLC gas–liquid chromatography and infra-red spectroscopy[29]. Nearly 90% of the total atrazine absorbed by pea plants was present as unchanged atrazine and (IV). The concentration of (IV) was 1.2–2.0 times greater than that of atrazine. Significant amounts of (IV) and (V) were detected by TLC and gas chromatography in atrazine-treated sorghum and lesser amounts of the same metabolites were found in soybean, wheat and corn[17]. The concentration of (V) in sorthum was approximately 50% of (IV), indicating the preferential N-dealkylation *in vivo* of the ethyl side chain. Evidence indicates that N-dealkylation is not limited to resistant species, but may occur to some extent in all higher plants.

Subsequent N-dealkylation of (IV) and (V) in sorghum plants treated with ring-^{14}C-labelled atrazine gave the metabolite 2-chloro-4,6-diamino-s-triazine (VI). It was isolated and identified by TLC, i.r. and mass spectroscopy[30]. This metabolite accounted for 1.8% of the total radioactivity in shoots of sorghum plants after a 5-day treatment period. An unidentified metabolite (VII) accounted for 4.1% of the radioactivity in sorghum shoots. Experiments with ring-^{14}C-labelled and [36]Cl-labelled atrazine indicated that dechlorination had occurred, but the substituent in the 2-position did not appear to be a hydroxyl group[30]. Compounds (V) and (VI) were also detected by aluminium oxide-column chromatography in extracts of *Imperata cylindrica* L. treated with simazine[31].

N-Dealkylation is not limited to the 2-chloro-s-triazines. The N-dealkylated metabolite of hydroxysimazine, 2-hydroxy-4-amino-6-ethylamino-s-triazine (IX) (*Figure 3*) was detected in *Coix lacryma-jobi* L. by ion-exchange chromatography[32] and identified by i.r. spectroscopy from simazine-treated corn[33]. Both 2-hydroxy-4-amino-6-isopropylamino-s-triazine (VIII) and (IX) were identified in corn treated with atrazine or hydroxyatrazine (III) by comparison with authentic compounds on TLC[34].

The formation of hydroxylated metabolites (*Figure 3*) in plants appears to be limited to species such as corn and *Coix lacryma-jobi* L., which contain

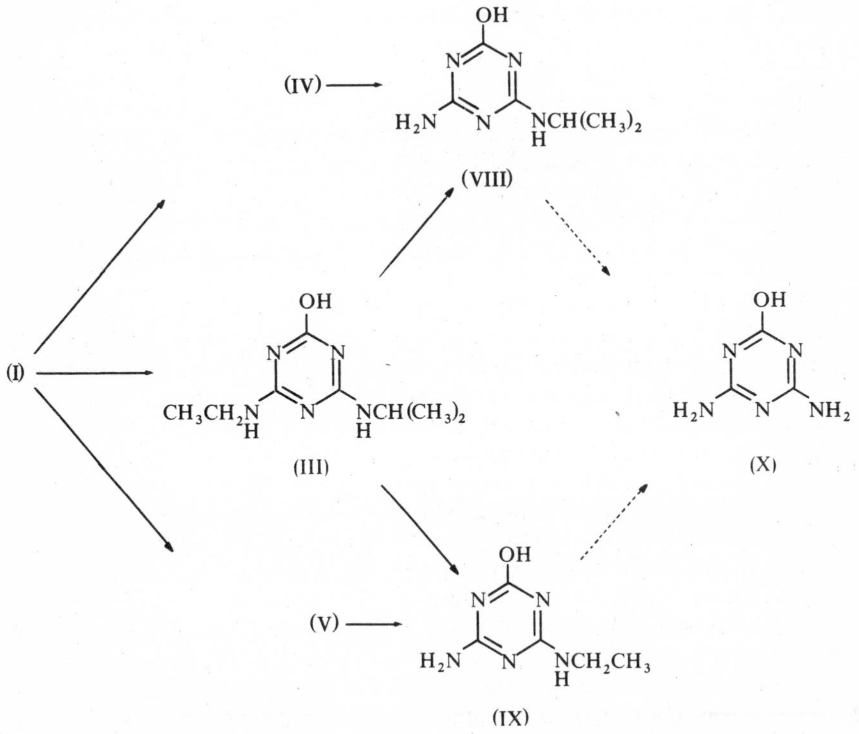

Figure 3. Metabolism of 2-chloro-s-triazine by hydrolysis and N-dealkylation

benzoxazinone. Unlike corn, sorghum produces metabolites (VIII) and (IX) only when this species is treated with hydroxyatrazine[34]. When an extract of sorghum plants containing (I), (IV) and (V) (*Figure 2*) was incubated in a protein-free, crude corn homogenate, the 2-chloro-*s*-triazines were converted non-enzymatically into the 2-hydroxy derivatives (III), (VIII) and (IX) (*Figure 3*)[34]. Therefore in species such as corn, either *N*-dealkylation or hydrolysis may occur first to yield the same end products.

Small amounts of 2-hydroxy-4,6-diamino-*s*-triazine (ammeline) (X) (*Figure 3*) was detected in *Coix lacryma-jobi* L.[32] and corn[33] by ion-exchange and paper chromatography. Partial deamination of ammeline to 2,4-dihydroxy-6-amino-*s*-triazine (ammelide) occurred in *A. fumigatus* Fres.[28]. This reaction has not been reported in higher plants.

Complete dealkylation of 2-hydroxy-*s*-triazines *in vivo* does not seem to occur as readily as with the 2-chloro-*s*-triazines. At least 60% of the extractable radioactivity in ^{14}C-labelled simazine-treated corn plants accumulated as 2-hydroxy-4-amino-6-ethylamino-*s*-triazine after 28 days[33]. Normally the hydroxy derivatives are not found in sorghum. However, when sorghum was treated with hydroxyatrazine, 49.7% of the radioactivity in the roots accumulated as the *N*-dealkylated, hydroxylated metabolites (VIII) and (IX)[34]. Therefore the formation of ammeline by complete dealkylation of (VIII) and (IX) may be a rather slow process. The enzyme catalysing *N*-dealkylation of *s*-triazines has not been isolated from plants, animals or micro-organisms. Many of the observations on rates of metabolism and substrate differences *in vivo* await confirmation by investigations *in vitro*.

Differences in *N*-dealkylation of 2-chloro-*s*-triazines and 2-hydroxy-*s*-triazines also occur in animals[35]. In rats dosed with ring-^{14}C-labelled atrazine, 66% of the radioactivity was excreted in the urine after 72 h. The largest portion of the activity in the urine (30%) was 2-chloro-4,6-diamino-*s*-triazine, identified by mass spectroscopy[35]. No hydroxyatrazine or ammeline was detected. However, in rats dosed with ^{14}C-labelled hydroxyatrazine, 79% was excreted unchanged in the faeces. Only 14% of the radioactivity appeared in the urine. The three major urinary products were hydroxyatrazine and its *N*-dealkylated derivatives (VIII) and (IX). When rats were dosed with (VIII) or (IX) only the unchanged compounds were excreted in the faeces and urine. Ammeline was not formed by complete dealkylation of any of the hydroxylated compounds (III), (VIII) or (IX)[35]. Evidence indicates that in animals as well as plants *N*-dealkylation of the second alkyl side chain is greatly affected by the substitution of the hydroxyl group in place of the chlorine in the 2-position. All of the compounds described above are present as metabolites of atrazine in one or more plants.

Glutathione conjugation. Until recently, the major degradation reaction for 2-chloro-*s*-triazines was believed to be hydroxylation. However, in highly resistant sorghum, atrazine was not converted into hydroxyatrazine but to other major water-soluble compounds[17]. In 7 h, 62% of the absorbed atrazine was converted into water-soluble compounds in sorghum leaf discs[36]. Recently, two of the major metabolites were isolated and identified as S-(4-ethylamino-6-isopropylamino-*s*-triazinyl-2)-glutathione (GS-atrazine) (XI), and S-γ-L-glutamyl-(4-ethylamino-6-isopropylamino-*s*-triazinyl-2)-L-cysteine (XII)[18] (*Figure 4*). The identification of these two metabolites indicated the presence of a third, previously unreported, pathway for 2-chloro-*s*-triazine metabolism in biological systems.

Glutathione conjugation of halogenated xenobiotic compounds is the first of four steps involved in a detoxication mechanism leading to the biosynthesis of mercapturic acid derivatives in mammals[37-39], birds[40]

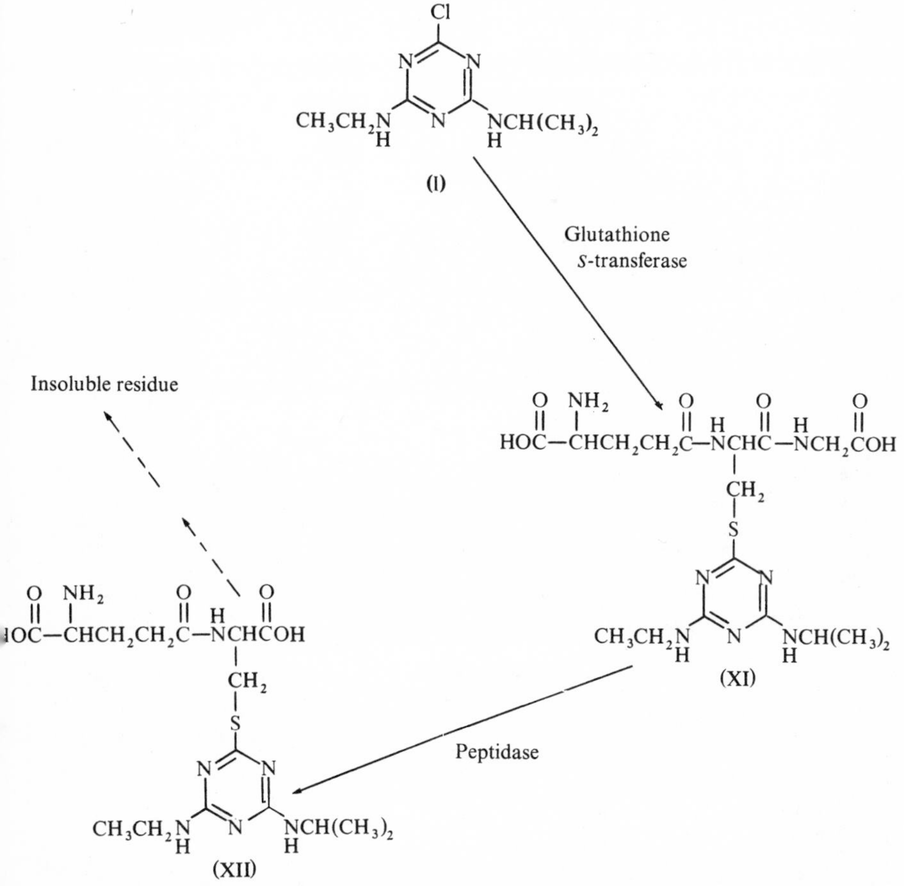

Figure 4. Metabolism of atrazine by glutathione conjugation in plants

and insects[41]. The isolation and identification of GS-atrazine from sorghum leaf sections is the first report indicating that glutathione is involved in the metabolism of pesticides in biological systems[18]. The major metabolite of 2-chloro-4-ethylamino-6-(1-methyl-1-cyanoethylamino)-s-triazine (XIII) in rat urine was identified recently as the mercapturic acid derivative, N-acetyl-S-[4-amino-6-(1-methyl-1-cyanoethylamino)-s-triazinyl-2]-L-cysteine (XVIII) (Figure 5)[42]. The two reports above give direct evidence indicating the presence of a mercapturic acid-type detoxication pathway for 2-chloro-s-triazines in plants[18] and animals[42].

329

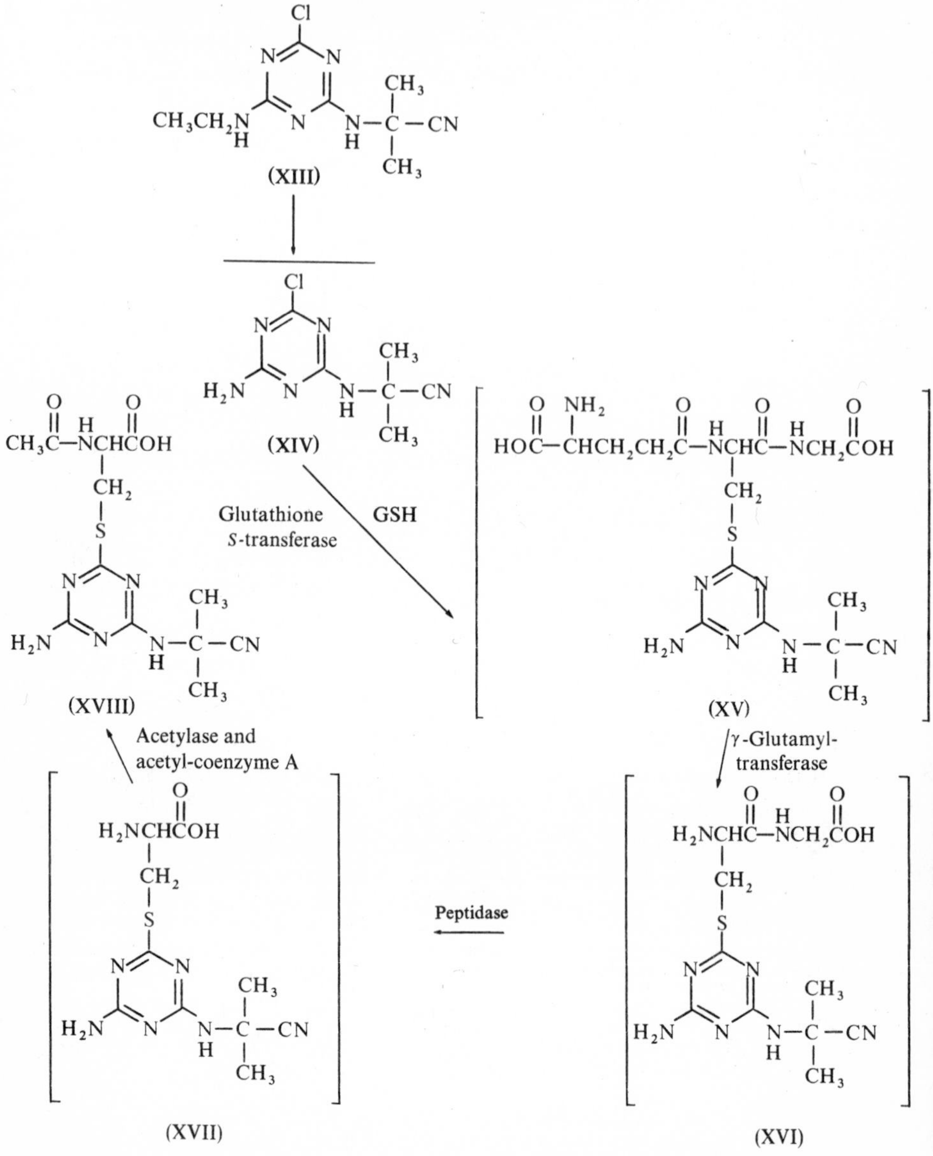

Figure 5. Metabolism of SD–15418 to the mercapturic acid derivative in rats

Figure 4 illustrates the glutathione conjugation pathway of atrazine in sorghum and Figure 5 illustrates the mercapturic acid pathway as it probably applies to the metabolism of (XIII) in rats. In the first step the active halogen is displaced and the substrate is conjugated with glutathione via a sulphide bond. Atrazine was conjugated directly with glutathione in plants (Figure 4) but (XIII) was probably conjugated with glutathione after an initial N-des-ethylation reaction in rats (*Figure 5*). The second step involves the removal of the γ-L-glutamyl moiety of glutathione by γ-glutamyl transferase to yield the dipeptide conjugate (XVI). Glycine is then hydrolytically removed in the third step to yield the cysteine conjugate (XVII), which is enzymatically acetylated at the α-amino group in the final step to give the mercapturic acid derivative. Only the mercapturic acid derivative (XVIII) and the N-des-ethylated metabolite (XIV) were isolated and identified in rats by n.m.r. and mass spectroscopy (*Figure 5*)[42]. The derivatives in brackets are probable intermediates in the pathway that have not been isolated. In plants, the first intermediate, GS-atrazine, and the dipeptide conjugate (XII) have been isolated and identified, but the mercapturic acid derivative of atrazine has not been isolated[18]. The dipeptide conjugate isolated in plants was the γ-L-glutamylcysteine conjugate (*Figure 4*) rather than the L-cysteinylglycine conjugate, which is normally the second intermediate in the mercapturic acid pathway (*Figure 5*). Evidence indicates that a carboxypeptidase in plants catalyses the formation of the dipeptide conjugate (XII)[43].

The peptide conjugates (XI) and (XII) constituted at least 55% of the metabolites in sorghum plants root-treated with atrazine for 48 h[17]. At least ten other water-soluble metabolites were detected in sorghum after 20 days[43]. Three of these metabolites were formed directly from the gluta-thione and γ-L-glutamylcysteine conjugates of atrazine. This was demonstra-ted by injecting sorghum plants with each of the two purified conjugates and extracting the metabolites formed[43]. The same technique also demon-strated that the γ-L-glutamylcysteine conjugate was derived directly from the glutathione conjugate of atrazine *in vivo* and not from a condensation of γ-L-glutamylcysteine with atrazine[43].

Glutathione S-transferases catalyse the initial conjugation of reduced glutathione with organic halide compounds. These enzymes have been

Table 2. Triazine specificity of glutathione S-transferase from corn[48]

Substrate†	Specific activity*
2-Chloro-4-*tert.*-butylamino-6-ethylamino-s-triazine (GS-13529)	6.58
2-Chloro-4-ethylamino-6-isopropylamino-s-triazine (atrazine)	4.50
2-Chloro-4-isopropylamino-6-cyclopropylamino-s-triazine (S-9115)	3.40
2-Chloro-4,6-bis-isopropylamino-s-triazine (propazine)	2.78
2-Chloro-4,6-bis-ethylamino-s-triazine (simazine)	0.36
2-Chloro-4-amino-6-isopropylamino-s-triazine	0.09
2-Hydroxy-4-ethylamino-6-isopropylamino-s-triazine (hydroxyatrazine)	0.07

† The following s-triazine compounds did not react to form glutathione conjugates; 2-methylmercapto-4,6-bis-isopropyl-amino-s-triazine. 2-methylmercapto-4-ethylamino-6-isopropylamino-s-triazine and 2-methoxy-4,6-bis(isopropylamino)-s-triazine.

* Glutathione-s-triazine conjugate formed (nmol/mg of protein per 2 h).

isolated and characterized from several animal tissues and include aryl-transferases, epoxidetransferases, alkyltransferases, aralkyltransferases and alkenetransferases[37-41, 44-47]. The isolation and partial characterization of a soluble enzyme from corn leaves, which catalyses the glutathione conjugation of atrazine and other substituted 2-chloro-s-triazines, is the first report of a glutathione S-transferase in higher plants[48]. This enzyme has been purified over 73-fold from corn leaves and has an estimated molecular weight of 40 000[49]. However, the occurrence of enzyme activity in different protein fractions during purification may indicate that more than one glutathione S-transferase, or multiple molecular forms[50] of the same enzyme, may be present in corn leaves.

Glutathione S-transferase was found primarily in leaves of plants such as corn, sorghum, sugar cane and Johnson grass, which are highly resistant to 2-chloro-s-triazine herbicides[48]. The activity of this enzyme was shown to be a major factor in detoxication and selectivity of substituted 2-chloro-s-triazine herbicides in higher plants[19,51].

Glutathione S-transferase from corn specifically requires reduced glutathione as a substrate. The enzyme also seems to be quite specific for substituted 2-chloro-s-triazine compounds[48] (Table 2). Substitution of methoxy, methylmercapto and hydroxyl groups in place of chlorine in the 2-position resulted in little, if any, enzyme activity[48]. Slight changes in the alkyl side chains at the 4- and 6-positions resulted in significant changes in enzyme activity. The substitution of an isopropyl group (atrazine) in place of an ethyl group (simazine) in the 6-position resulted in over a 12-fold increase in specific activity[48]. N-Dealkylation of one side chain resulted in almost a complete loss of enzyme activity[48]. The metabolism in sugar cane leaves in vivo of several s-triazine herbicides[43] (Figure 6) reflected the specific

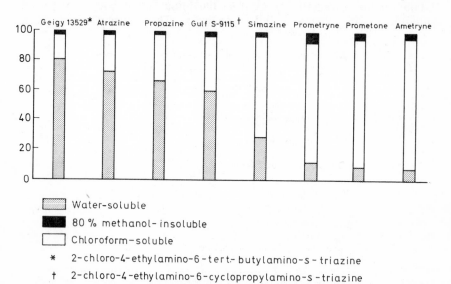

Figure 6. Metabolism of several s-triazines in excised sugar-cane leaves within 6 h. Results are expressed as % of total ^{14}C radioactivity present in leaves

activities obtained *in vitro*[48] (*Table 2*). The water-soluble metabolites of the 2-chloro-s-triazines, atrazine, propazine, simazine, GS-13529 and S-9115 consisted primarily of the γ-L-glutamylcysteine conjugates with lower amounts of the glutathione conjugates[43]. The water-soluble metabolites of the 2-methylmercapto-s-triazines, ametryne and prometryne, and the 2-methoxy-s-triazine, prometone, did not appear to be the peptide conjugates. The relative order of metabolism of the s-triazine herbicides was also similar in excised leaves of sorghum, corn and barley[43].

Inhibition studies with atrazine as the substrate have shown that several s-triazine compounds, prometryne, ametryne and prometone are strong inhibitors of glutathione S-transferase from corn (*Table 3*). However, these

Table 3. Inhibition of glutathione S-transferase by substituted triazines[48]

Inhibitor†	Concn. (mM)	Inhibition (%)
2,4-bis(isopropylamino)-6-methyl-mercapto-s-triazine (prometryne)	0.06	61
2-Ethylamino-4-isopropylamino-6-methylmercapto-s-triazine (ametryne)	0.06	38
2-Chloro-4-(diethylamino)-6-isopropyl-amino-s-triazine (ipazine)	0.05	35
2,4-Dichloro-6-(2-chloroanilino)-s-triazine (dyrene)	0.05	29
2-Methoxy-4,6-bis(isopropylamino)-s-triazine (prometone)	0.06	26

† The following triazine compounds did not inhibit atrazine conjugation with GSH at 0.05 and 0.06 mM levels; 4-amino-6-*tert*.-butyl-3(methylthio)-*as*-triazine-5-(4H)-,one 2-chloro-4-amino-6-isopropylamino-s-triazine, 2-chloro-4-amino-6-ethyl-amino-s-triazine and 2-hydroxy-4-ethylamino-6-isopropylamino-s-triazine.

compounds were not effective substrates of the enzyme[48] (*Table 2*). Prometryne was an especially strong competitive inhibitor of atrazine–glutathione conjugation with an apparent K_i value 2.8 × 10^{-5} M[48]. The N-dealkylated metabolites (IV) and (V) and hydroxyatrazine (III) failed to inhibit glutathione S-transferase (*Table 3*), and were also poor substrates[48] (*Table 2*).

The formation of glutathione conjugates of several aryl and aralkylhalide compounds *in vitro*[48, 49] and *in vivo*[18, 52] suggests either the presence of both aryl and aralkyltransferases[38,39] or a glutathione S-transferase with a broad substrate specificity in corn. Evidence both *in vivo* and *in vitro* indicates the presence of similar mercapturic acid detoxication pathways in plants and animals. However, in plants the pathway may not lead to mercapturic acid as the end product but to insoluble plant residue.

Side chain oxidation. Oxidation of N-alkyl side chains have been reported in animals, but not in plants and micro-organisms. The completely dealkylated metabolite, 2-chloro-4,6-diamino-s-triazine, was detected by t.l.c. as the major metabolite of atrazine, simazine and propazine in the urine of rat and rabbit[53]. However, after initial *N*-dealkylation of the parent compounds, ω-oxidation in the remaining *N*-alkyl side chains gave small amounts of the glycine derivative, *N*-(2-chloro-4-amino-*s*-triazinyl-6)-glycine, for atrazine and simazine, and the alanine derivative, *N*-(2-chloro-4-amino-*s*-triazinyl-6)-alanine, for atrazine and propazine. No 2-hydroxy derivatives of the parent compounds or the metabolites were detected[53].

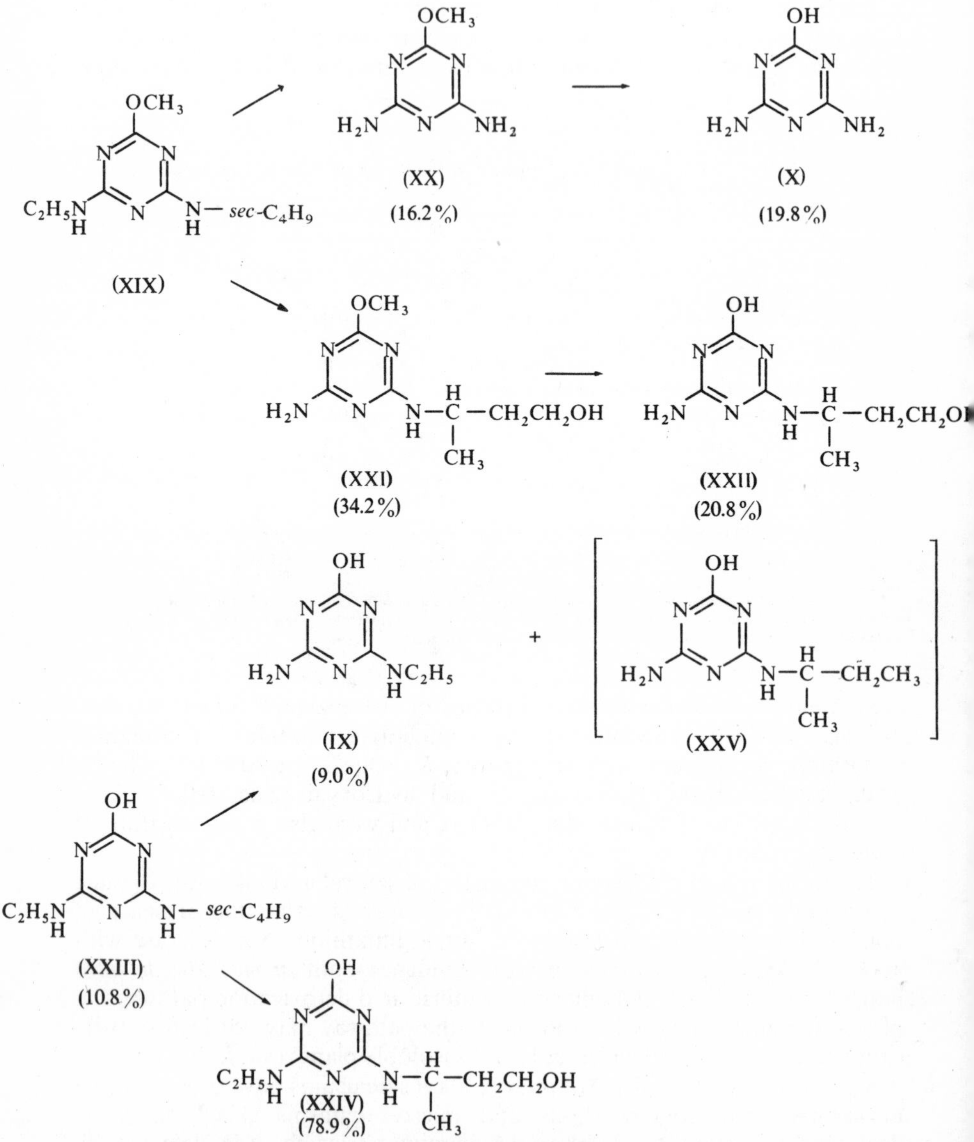

Figure 7. Metabolism of GS–14254 by *N*-dealkylation, ω-oxidation and hydrolysis of the methoxy group in rats

334

Prometryne yielded the same corresponding metabolites with the methyl-mercapto group still intact[53].

A more extensive study with ring- and methoxy-^{14}C-labelled GS-14254 (XIX) demonstrated side-chain oxidation, N-dealkylation and hydrolysis of the methoxy group in the rat[54]. All of the metabolites in *Figure 7*, except (XXV), were isolated and identified by TLC and mass spectroscopy. Rats excreted 67% of a single oral dose of ^{14}C-labelled GS-14254 in the urine as 15 different metabolites. However, four major metabolites identified as (X), (XX), (XXI) and (XXII), accounted for 91% of the radioactivity in the urine. Very little of the parent herbicide was excreted in the urine. The ethyl side chain was removed in all four of the major metabolites. ω-Oxidation of the remaining sec.-butyl side chain to its primary alcohol had occurred in two of the major metabolites, 2-methoxy-4-amino-6(4-hydroxy-sec.-butylamino)-s-triazine (XXI) and 2-hydroxy-4-amino-6(4-hydroxy-sec.-butylamino)-s-triazine (XXII). Ammeline (X) was also identified as one of the major products indicating that hydrolysis of the methoxy group occurred in animals. In plants, hydrolysis of the methoxy group does not appear to be a major reaction[3].

The enzymes involved in the degradation of (XIX) have not been isolated. Therefore the sequential order of the reactions occurring at the alkylamino and methoxy substituents are unknown. However, N-dealkylation and ω-oxidation of the alkyl side chains probably occur before hydrolysis of the methoxy group to give the 2-hydroxy derivatives. When rats were dosed with the hydroxy analogue of GS-14254 (XXIII) (*Figure 7*), its unchanged form and two other metabolites (IX, XXIV) accounted for 99% of the radioactivity excreted in the urine. Dosing of rats with the 2-hydroxy derivatives (IX) and (XXV) resulted in the excretion of only the unchanged compounds. Ammeline was not detected when rats were dosed with any of the hydroxylated analogues described above[54]. These results agreed with the earlier discussion on atrazine metabolism in animals and plants where very little degradation was observed beyond the 2-hydroxy-4-amino-6-alkylamino-s-triazine derivatives of atrazine (VIII, IX)[34,35]. N-Dealkylation of one alkyl side chain and ω-oxidation of the other may occur with either the methoxy or hydroxyl group in the 2-position. However, complete N-dealkylation at a significant rate seems to require substituents other than the hydroxyl group in the 2-position.

Degradation of methylmercapto-s-triazines. Very little is known on the degradation of prometryne and other methylmercapto-s-triazines in biological systems[3]. Following treatment with prometryne, its hydroxy analogue (hydroxypropazine) was detected by paper and thin-layer chromatography in carrot, cotton and broad bean[8,24,55]. Hydroxypropazine may be formed from prometryne by a stepwise oxidation to the sulphoxide, sulphone and hydrolysis as proposed[5]. The sulphone derivative of prometryne was detected by TLC in pea[24]. Prometryne may also be metabolized by N-dealkylation as shown by TLC detection of 2-methyl-2-methylmercapto-4-amino-6-isopropylamino-s-triazine in pea[24]. Unchanged prometryne and its metabolites, 2-methylmercapto-mercapto-4-amino-6-isopropylamino-s-triazinyl-6)-disulphide, were detected in the urine of rats and rabbits dosed with prometryne[53].

Ring cleavage. Several reports have indicated the evolution of $^{14}CO_2$ from ring-^{14}C-labelled 2-chloro-*s*-triazines in plants and micro-organisms[3, 9]. However, the reports on the formation of $^{14}CO_2$ from ring-labelled 2-chloro-*s*-triazines seem to be conflicting. Significant evolution of $^{14}CO_2$ was reported in corn plants treated with ring-^{14}C-labelled simazine and atrazine[56]. Approximately 0.1–2.6% of ring-labelled simazine and atrazine taken up by cucumber and corn plants was metabolized to $^{14}CO_2$[24, 57]. The evolution of $^{14}CO_2$ in corn, cotton and soybean was reported to occur from ring-labelled simazine but not from ring-labelled atrazine[58]. No $^{14}CO_2$ was detected in cotton treated with ring-labelled ipazine[59]. Isolated cultures of soil fungi did not evolve $^{14}CO_2$ from ring-labelled simazine and atrazine[21, 25]. However, a mixed microbial population in non-sterile soil evolved more than 1.0% of the applied ring-labelled simazine as $^{14}CO_2$ within 8 days[57].

A degradation scheme for the cleavage of the heterocyclic ring with an initial oxidation of C-2 to carbon dioxide has been proposed[4]. The first step in ring cleavage requires the hydroxylation of atrazine or simazine in the 2-position. The proposed scheme is based on the assumption that hydroxylation is the major degradation reaction in biological systems. In sorghum, glutathione conjugation was shown to be the major pathway for atrazine metabolism with no 2-hydroxy derivatives being formed. In corn, hydroxylation occurred to a significant extent, but glutathione conjugation was still the major pathway. In both species no $^{14}CO_2$ was evolved from ring-^{14}C-labelled atrazine over a period of seven days[17]. Of the total atrazine applied, 35% was absorbed by sorghum and corn. According to the proposed scheme, sorghum may not evolve $^{14}CO_2$, but some $^{14}CO_2$ evolution would be expected from corn. These results, however, do not preclude other schemes leading to eventual ring cleavage and evolution of carbon dioxide.

Insoluble residue incorporation. Ring cleavage, as the end product of *s*-triazine herbicide metabolism, may not be very significant. Evolution of $^{14}CO_2$ was either not detected or occurred in only small amounts as discussed above. The incorporation of the heterocyclic ring and/or its cleavage products into insoluble plant residues may be a more significant reaction. An increase in insoluble residue occurred with time in ^{14}C-labelled-atrazine-treated sorghum. A pulse treatment of 48 h in 23 μM ^{14}C-labelled atrazine solution with subsequent transfer of plants into fresh solution resulted in more than 50% of the absorbed ^{14}C-radioactivity being incorporated into insoluble residue after 14 days[17]. A continuous exposure of sorghum to a high concentration of ^{14}C-labelled atrazine (100 μM) for a period of 20 days resulted in the incorporation of approximately 21% of the absorbed radioactivity into insoluble residue[60]. Indirect evidence in corn and sorghum indicates that the glutathione–conjugation pathway may lead to eventual incorporation of atrazine derivatives into insoluble residue[43,51]. More than 77% of the leaf surface-absorbed ^{14}C-labelled atrazine in corn was converted into the peptide conjugates within 16 h[51] (*Table 4*). Only 14% was present as the hydroxylated derivatives. The increase in insoluble residue (38%) after 144 h was accompanied by an almost equivalent reduction in the concentration of peptide conjugates. The gradual accumulation of hydroxylated metabolites confirmed a previous observation that metabolism of hydroxylated derivatives beyond the mono-dealkylated derivatives (VIII, IX)

Table 4. Metabolism of leaf surface-absorbed atrazine in corn[51]

Time (h)	Distribution of ^{14}C activity (%)			
	Unchanged atrazine	GS-atrazine	Hydroxylated derivatives†	Methanol-insoluble residue
16	7.9	77.4	13.9	0.8
24	3.9	78.7	15.8	1.6
48	0.4	65.0	27.3	7.2
144	1.9	32.4	28.1	37.6

† Includes metabolites (III), (VIII) and (IX).

occurred very slowly in biological systems.

The chemical nature of the insoluble residue of atrazine is unknown at this time. However, experiments with animals indicate that the residue may be a very stable material, which resists normal digestion in rats and the ruminant sheep[60]. The extracted plant residue of ^{14}C-labelled atrazine-treated sorghum plants was ground and administered to rats and sheep. In rats, after 72 h 2.0–2.8% of the ^{14}C radioactivity was excreted in the urine, 88–92% was excreted in the faeces and less than 1% remained in the carcass. In sheep, after 96 h 93% of the ^{14}C radioactivity was excreted in the faeces and only 7% was found in the urine. The small amounts of radioactivity found in the urine of rats and sheep may be due to incomplete extraction of the plant residue. Very little of the radioactivity from insoluble plant residue was digested and incorporated into body tissue by animals[60].

SIGNIFICANCE OF s-TRIAZINE METABOLISM IN PLANTS

It is quite evident that herbicides, including the s-triazines, may act on more than one biochemically or physiologically sensitive site to cause death in plants[61]. To be effective, a herbicide must reach the sensitive site(s) in its toxic form and at a concentration sufficient to cause severe disruption of normal growth. A number of physical and biochemical factors operating in the environment and plant determine the concentration of the toxic compound which will eventually reach the sensitive site(s)[62]. The primary factor, which determines the tolerance of plants to atrazine and other s-triazine herbicides, seems to be the plant's ability to degrade and detoxify the phytotoxic parent molecule[17]. Atrazine detoxication significantly reduces the concentration of the herbicide that eventually penetrates the chloroplast where the sensitive site (Hill reaction in photosynthesis)[63] is located. Therefore metabolism of s-triazines, as described in the earlier section, is probably the most critical factor in s-triazine resistance and selectivity in higher plants.

Resistance of corn to atrazine and simazine was attributed to the non-enzymatic detoxication of the herbicides to hydroxyatrazine and hydroxysimazine[4, 10-12]. Since the publication of these early results it has become increasingly evident that other pathways, including N-dealkylation and glutathione conjugation, play a significant role in resistance and selectivity. N-Dealkylation was found to be an important pathway in intermediately

337

susceptible species such as pea and cotton[20, 29]. Bioassay indicated that the
N-dealkylated derivatives of atrazine, (IV) and (V), were less toxic than the
parent atrazine[17, 64]. The half-maximal inhibitory concentration (I_{50}) for
the Hill reaction in isolated pea chloroplasts was 23 times greater for the
metabolite (IV) than for the parent atrazine[36]. The conversion of highly
toxic atrazine into its less-toxic N-dealkylated derivatives in the plant
seems to be an important mechanism for intermediate tolerance or susceptibility to atrazine.

The third and most significant atrazine-detoxication pathway in terms of
herbicidal resistance is the recently discovered glutathione-conjugation
pathway[18]. This enzymatic detoxication process was shown to be the primary
factor responsible for atrazine resistance in species such as sorghum and
corn[19, 36, 51]. In resistant sorghum, both N-dealkylation and glutathione-
conjugation pathways are present. In addition to these two pathways, highly
resistant corn also metabolizes atrazine by the non-enzymatic hydroxylation

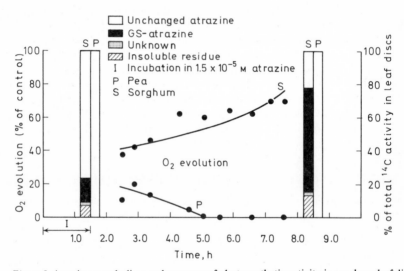

Figure 8. Atrazine metabolism and recovery of photosynthetic activity in sorghum leaf discs

pathway catalysed by benzoxazinone[51]. These different degradation pathways known to exist in higher plants are shown in *Figures 1, 2, 3* and *4*.

Inhibition of photosynthesis by atrazine and rapid recovery within 6 h
occurred in leaf discs of resistant sorghum but not with intermediately susceptible pea[36] (*Figure 8*). The recovery of photosynthesis in sorghum was
accompanied by the conversion of atrazine into GS-atrazine, but in pea
very little metabolism occurred over this short period (*Figure 8*). Corn leaf
discs also showed a similar inhibition and recovery over a 6 h period[51].
Similarly, recovery of photosynthesis was accompanied by a 77% conversion
of atrazine into its glutathione conjugate within 6 h. Hydroxyatrazine
formation in corn leaf discs was negligible over this recovery period[51]. These
results indicated that the glutathione conjugation pathway was responsible

for the rapid recovery of photosynthesis in leaf discs of sorghum and corn.

The hydroxylation pathway, which is quite active in corn, contributed to the total detoxication of atrazine in intact plants, but this pathway, apparently, is not essential for resistance in corn[19]. Hydroxyatrazine was found in significant concentrations in corn plants only when atrazine was absorbed through the roots[19, 65]. The presence of the enzyme glutathione S-transferase in the shoots, but not in roots[48], and the general distribution of

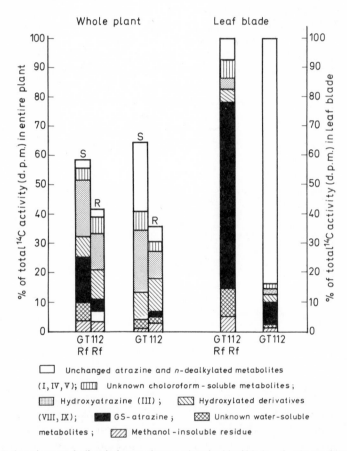

Figure 9. Atrazine metabolism in intact plants and excised leaf blades of resistant (GT112 RfRf) and susceptible (GT112) corn lines

benzoxazinone throughout the corn plant explains the differences in metabolism when atrazine is introduced either through the leaves or roots of corn.

Hydroxyatrazine concentration in root-fed, susceptible inbred corn line GT112 was nearly equal to that of its isogenic resistant line GT112 RfRf (Figure 9)[19]. The shoots (S) and roots (R) were assayed separately after 48 h of treatment. The concentration of atrazine and partially detoxified N-dealkylated derivatives amounted to 28.5% in susceptible GT112 and only

5.4% in resistant GT112 RfRf. The greater accumulation of unchanged atrazine in the susceptible line was undoubtedly due to low glutathione conjugation activity rather than decreased hydroxylation. The differences in the accumulation of unchanged atrazine between the inbred lines were much greater when atrazine was introduced directly into the leaf blades, where glutathione S-transferase activity is present[19, 48] (*Figure 9*; *Table 5*). The specific activity of the critical enzyme was approximately 54 times greater in the resistant line, GT112 RfRf, than in the susceptible line, GT112. The rate of photosynthesis in leaf discs of GT112 RfRf, incubated in atrazine, measured 91–93% of the control rate within 2 h after the incubation period. In leaf discs of GT112, photosynthetic rate measured 34–38% of the control rate with no apparent recovery over a 5 h period[19]. Within 2.5 h, 68% of the atrazine absorbed by leaf discs of resistant GT112 RfRf was converted into

Table 5. Glutathione S-transferase activity in corn leaves[19]

| Corn line | Response to atrazine | Benzoxazinone concn (mg/g dry wt)† | | Specific activity of enzyme* |
		Leaf	Root	
GT112 RfRf	Resistant	—	—	1.63
GT112	Susceptible	—	—	0.03
ND KE47101	Resistant	—	—	2.73
B49	Resistant	2.07	4.56	3.28
CI 31A	Resistant	1.09	3.22	2.31
B52	Resistant	0.48	3.04	1.46
Oh 43	Resistant	0.16	3.19	3.62
WF 9	Resistant	0.10	1.48	2.32

† Data from Klun, Robinson. *J. Econ. Ent.* **62**. 214 (1969).
* Glutathione conjugate formed (nmol per mg of protein per h).

GS-atrazine, whereas only 0.6% conversion occurred in leaf discs of susceptible GT112[19]. Results from other inbred lines of corn with differing concentrations of benzoxazinone (*Table 5*) definitely indicated that most corn plants would be totally resistant to atrazine even if benzoxazinone was absent.

The primary site of atrazine and simazine phytotoxicity seems to be the Hill reaction in photosynthesis[63, 66–70]. The Hill reaction was equally inhibited by simazine in isolated chloroplasts of resistant and susceptible plants[71]. Therefore resistance to atrazine or simazine is dependent on factors outside the chloroplasts. Experiments *in vitro*[72] and *in vivo*[36] indicated that atrazine readily penetrates the chloroplasts and accumulates as an active, reversibly bound concentration[72] in equilibrium with atrazine concentration in the external medium or the cytoplasm[36] of intact cells.

The metabolism of atrazine to its glutathione conjugate by the soluble enzyme glutathione S-transferase reduced the equilibrium concentration of atrazine in the cytoplasm[36]. Consequently, atrazine concentration decreased rapidly in the chloroplasts of sorghum leaves treated with atrazine[36].

Evidence indicates that the ability to metabolize atrazine and effectively reduce the concentration of the active inhibitor at the primary site of action seems to be the basis for selectivity in higher plants.

CONCLUSIONS

Recent research indicates that the *s*-triazine herbicides are metabolized by several pathways in biological systems. Most of our information on *s*-triazine metabolism is based on studies with the 2-chloro-*s*-triazines, atrazine and simazine. Information on the metabolism of 2-methoxy- and 2-methylmercapto-*s*-triazines is limited.

N-Dealkylation of alkyl side chains occurs in plants, animals and micro-organisms. ω-Oxidation of alkyl side chains has been reported only in animals. Glutathione conjugation occurs in plants and animals. No evidence of this pathway in micro-organisms has been reported. Non-enzymatic hydrolysis of 2-chloro-*s*-triazines to the 2-hydroxy-*s*-triazines seems to be significant in only a few selected plant species and in the non-biological mechanism for detoxication in soil.

There is no consistent evidence indicating that plants, animals and soil micro-organisms are capable of cleaving the *s*-triazine ring at a significant rate. In plants the incorporation of *s*-triazine derivatives into insoluble residue is more significant than ring cleavage followed by complete oxidation of the ring carbon atoms. Very little *s*-triazine residues seem to be retained in animal tissue after ingestion of parent *s*-triazine compounds or its soluble and insoluble plant metabolites. The nature of the terminal residues of *s*-triazines in plants is still unknown. The results on the metabolism and disposition of *s*-triazine compounds in plants and animals strongly suggest that the final disposition of *s*-triazine residues will ultimately depend on soil factors and soil micro-organisms.

REFERENCES

[1] A. Gast, E. Knuesli and H. Gysin. *Experientia*, 11, 107 (1955).

[2] J. Neumeyer, D. Gibbons and H. Trask. *Chem. Week*, part I, April 12 (1969).

[3] E. Knüesli, D. Berrer, G. Dupuis and H. Esser. In *Degradation of Herbicides*, Ed. P. C. Kearney and D. D. Kaufman. Marcel Dekker: New York (1969).

[4] H. Gysin and E. Knüesli. *Advan. Pest Control Res.* 3, 289 (1960).

[5] H. Gysin. *Chem. & Ind. Lond.* p. 1393 (1962).

[6] A. S. Crafts. *The Chemistry and Mode of Action of Herbicides*. Wiley (Interscience): New York (1961).

[7] V. H. Freed and M. L. Montgomery. *Residue Rev. e*, 1 (1963).

[8] M. L. Montgomery and V. H. Freed. *J. Agr. Food Chem.* 12, 11 (1964).

[9] C. R. Swanson. *Metabolic Fate of Herbicides in Plants, ARS* 34–66, U.S. Dept. of Agr. (1965).

[10] P. Castelfranco, C. L. Foy and D. B. Deutsch. *Weeds* 9, 580 (1961).

[11] R. H. Hamilton and D. E. Moreland. *Science*, 135, 373 (1962).

[12] W. Roth. *C.R. Acad. Sci., Paris*, 245, 942 (1957).

[13] R. H. Hamilton, R. S. Bandurski and W. H. Reusch. *Cereal Chem.* 39, 107 (1962).

[14] W. Roth and E. Knuesli. *Experientia*, 17, 312 (1961).

[15] Ö. Wahlroos and A. I. Virtanen. *Acta Chem. Scand.* 13, 1906 (1959).

[16] R. H. Hamilton. *J. Agr. Food Chem.* 12, 14 (1964).

[17] R. H. Shimabukuro. *Plant Physiol.* 42, 1269 (1967).

[18] G. L. Lamoureux, R. H. Shimabukuro, H. R. Swanson and D. S. Frear. *J. Agr. Food Chem.* 18, 81 (1970).

[19] R. H. Shimabukuro, D. S. Frear, H. R. Swanson and W. C. Walsh. *Plant Physiol.* **47**, 10 (1971).
[20] R. H. Shimabukuro and H. R. Swanson. *Weed Sci.* **18**, 231 (1970).
[21] R. W. Couch, J. V. Gramlich, D. E. Davis and H. H. Funderburk, Jr. *Proc. Southern Weed Conf.* **18**, 623 (1965).
[22] P. H. Plaisted and M. L. Thornton. *Contrib. Boyce Thompson Inst.* **22**, 399 (1964).
[23] H. H. Funderburk, Jr., and D. E. Davis. *Weeds*, **11**, 101 (1963).
[24] P. W. Müeller and P. H. Payot. *Proc. IAEA Symp. Isotopes Weed Res., Vienna*, p 61 (1966).
[25] D. D. Kaufman, P. C. Kearney and T. J. Sheets. *J. Agr. Food Chem.* **13**, 238 (1965).
[26] J. E. Bakke, J. D. Robbins and V. J. Feil. *J. Agr. Food Chem.* **15**, 628 (1967).
[27] J. D. Robbins, J. E. Bakke and V. J. Feil. *J. Agr. Food Chem.* **16**, 698 (1968).
[28] P. C. Kearney, D. D. Kaufman and T. J. Sheets. *J. Agr. Food Chem.* **13**, 369 (1965).
[29] R. H. Shimabukuro, R. E. Kadunce and D. S. Frear. *J. Agr. Food Chem.* **14**, 392 (1966).
[30] R. H. Shimabukuro and W. C. Walsh. Unpublished data.
[31] J. Hurter. *6th Intern. Congr. Plant Protection, Vienna*, p 398 (1967).
[32] J. Hurter. *Experientia*, **22**, 741 (1966).
[33] M. L. Montgomery, D. L. Botsford and V. H. Freed. *J. Agr. Food Chem.* **17**, 1241 (1969).
[34] R. H. Shimabukuro. *Plant Physiol.* **43**, 1925 (1968).
[35] J. E. Bakke. Unpublished data.
[36] R. H. Shimabukuro and H. R. Swanson. *J. Agr. Food Chem.* **17**, 199 (1969).
[37] J. Booth, E. Boyland and P. Sims. *Biochem. J.* **79**, 516 (1961).
[38] E. Boyland and L. F. Chasseaud. *Advan. Enzymology*, **32**, 173 (1969).
[39] E. Boyland and L. F. Chasseaud. *Biochem. J.* **115**, 985 (1969).
[40] J. G. Wit and P. Leeuwangh. *Biochim. Biophys. Acta*, **177**, 329 (1969).
[41] A. J. Cohen, J. N. Smith and H. Turbert. *Biochem. J.* **90**, 457 (1960).
[42] D. H. Hutson, E. C. Hoadley, M. H. Griffiths and C. Donninger. *J. Agr. Food Chem.* **18**, 507 (1970).
[43] G. L. Lamoureux. Unpublished data.
[44] M. Ishida. *Agr. Biol. Chem.* **32**, 947 (1968).
[45] P. L. Grover and P. Sims. *Biochem. J.* **90**, 603 (1964).
[46] S. Al-Kassab, E. Boyland and K. Williams. *Biochem. J.* **87**, 4 (1963).
[47] D. Jerina, J. Daly, B. Witkop, P. Zaltzman-Nirenberg and S. Udenfriend. *Arch. Biochem. Biophys.* **128**, 176 (1968).
[48] D. S. Frear and H. R. Swanson. *Phytochem.* **9**, 2123 (1970).
[49] D. S. Frear, H. R. Swanson and F. S. Tanaka. *Advan. Phytochem.* (In the Press) (1971).
[50] D. E. Kramer and J. R. Whitaker. *Plant Physiol.* **44**, 1560 (1969).
[51] R. H. Shimabukuro, H. R. Swanson and W. C. Walsh. *Plant Physiol.* **46**, 103 (1970).
[52] G. L. Lamoureux, L. E. Stafford and F. S. Tanaka. *J. Agr. Food Chem.* (In the Press) (1971).
[53] C. Böhme and F. Bär. *Food Cosmet. Toxicol.* **5**, 23 (1967).
[54] J. D. Larson, J. E. Bakke and V. J. Feil. *Joint Conf. Chem. Inst. Can.—Am. Chem. Soc., Abst. Pest* **8**, *Toronto* (1970).
[55] H. C. Sikka and D. E. Davis. *Weed Sci.* **16**, 474 (1968).
[56] M. L. Montgomery and V. J. Freed. *Weeds* **9**, 231 (1961).
[57] M. T. H. Ragab and J. P. McCollum. *Weeds* **9**, 72 (1961).
[58] D. E. Davis, J. V. Gramlich and H. H. Funderburk, Jr. *Weeds*. **13**, 252 (1965).
[59] R. H. Hamilton and D. E. Moreland. *Weeds* **11**, 213 (1963).
[60] J. E. Bakke. Unpublished data.
[61] D. S. Frear and R. H. Shimabukuro. *First FAO Int. Conf. Weed Cont., Davis, Calif.* (June 1970).
[62] W. C. Shaw, J. L. Hilton, D. E. Moreland and L. L. Jansen. *ARS* 20–9, U.S. Dept. of Agr. p 119 (1960).
[63] D. E. Moreland, W. A. Gentner, J. L. Hilton and K. L. Hill. *Plant Physiol.* **34**, 432 (1959).
[64] R. H. Shimabukuro. *J. Agr. Food Chem.* **15**, 557 (1967).
[65] L. Thompson, Jr., F. W. Slife and H. S. Butler. *Weed Sci.* **18**, 509 (1970).
[66] B. Exer. *Weed Res.* **1**, 233 (1961).
[67] B. Exer. *Experientia*, **14**, 136 (1958).
[68] N. E. Good. *Plant Physiol.* **36**, 788 (1961).
[69] N. I. Bishop. *Biochim. Biophys. Acta*, **57**, 186 (1962).
[70] N. I. Bishop. *Biochim Biophys. Acta*, **27**, 205 (1958).
[71] D. E. Moreland and K. L. Hill. *Weeds*, **10**, 229 (1962).
[72] S. Izawa and N. E. Good. *Biochim. Biophys. Acta*, **102**, 20 (1965).

METABOLISM OF THE ACYL ANILIDE HERBICIDES

Shooichi Matsunaka

Department of Physiology and Genetics,
National Institute of Agricultural Sciences, Konosu, Saitama, Japan

ABSTRACT

Acyl anilide herbicides usually are hydrolyzed into corresponding anilines by special higher plants and soil micro-organisms. The processes are dependent upon the selectivity of each plant species and the specificity of their enzymes. The hydrolysis is inhibited by organophosphate or carbamate insecticides. Produced aniline compounds will form complexes with sugars, lignin and others, and especially by micro-organisms or by photochemical reactions they can be condensed to form azobenzenes or triazenes. In the case of 2-chloroacetamide herbicides, they could not be hydrolyzed, but form complexes with intracellular compounds. These metabolisms and interactions have practical meanings in the utilization of the herbicides.

1. INTRODUCTION

The acyl anilide herbicides and related compounds are shown in *Figure 1*. They may be subdivided into three groups: (1) true acyl anilides having the —NH—CO—radical: (2) 2-chloroacetamides: (3) related compounds. Among them, propanil is the best known herbicide, which can be used for rice culture and shows a remarkable selectivity between rice plants and weeds, especially barnyardgrass (*Echinochloa crusgalli*)[1, 2]. Solan also has high selectivity between tomato plant (tolerant) and eggplant (susceptible)[3, 4]. NPA, naptalam, is also used for cucumber or water melon as a selective herbicide. CMPT (5-chloro-4-methyl-2-propionamide thiazole) is not acyl anilide, but has a propionamide radical on the thiazole ring. This analogue of propanil shows high selectivity on wheat[5]. Wheat and some kinds of barley are very tolerant to CMPT.

2-Chloroacetamides are also a unique group, probably having almost the same mode of action on weeds.

One of the characteristics of acyl anilide herbicides may be their unique selectivities.

In this report the metabolism of these chemicals in higher plants and in soils will be described with some comments relating to the residue problem.

2. METABOLISM OF PROPANIL

Metabolism in higher plants[6]
Selectivity of propanil

Nakamura *et al.*[7] showed that, after application of propanil to rice plants

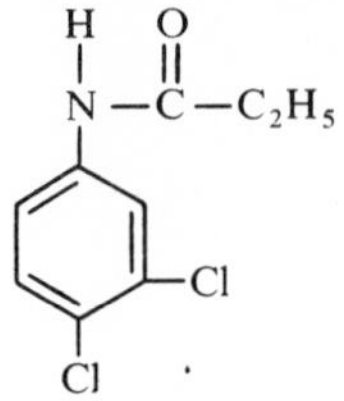

propanil

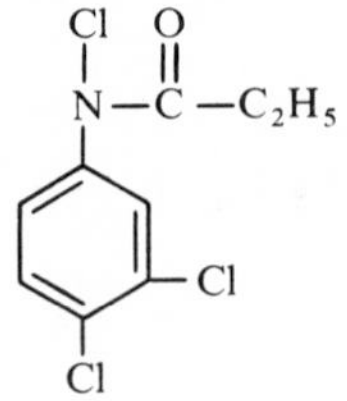

N-Cl-propanil

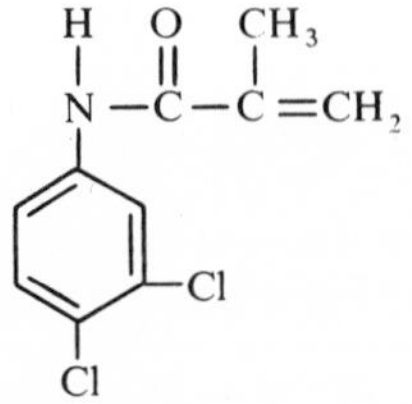

dicryl

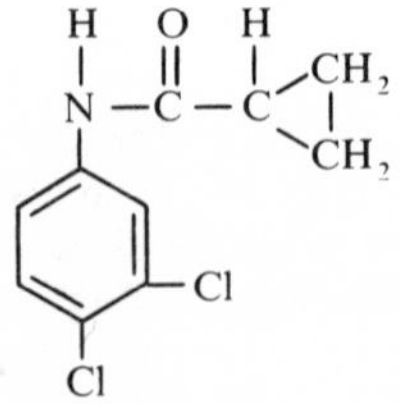

cypromid

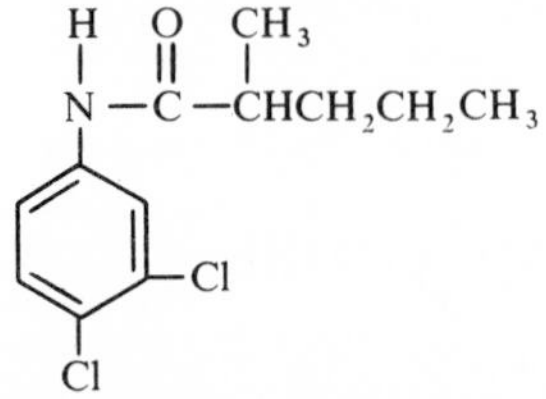

Karsil

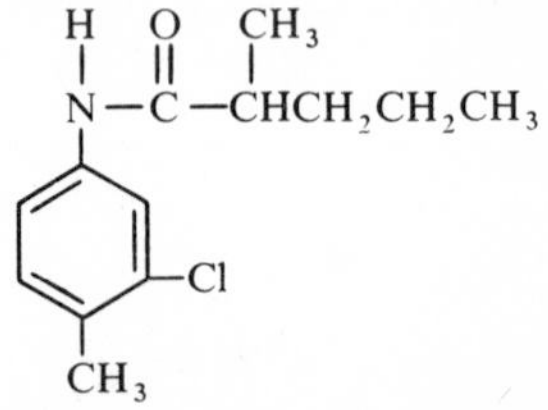

solan

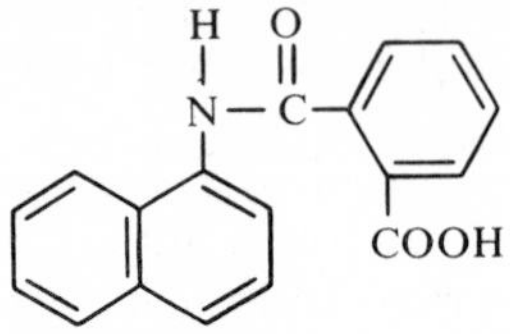

NPA, naptalam

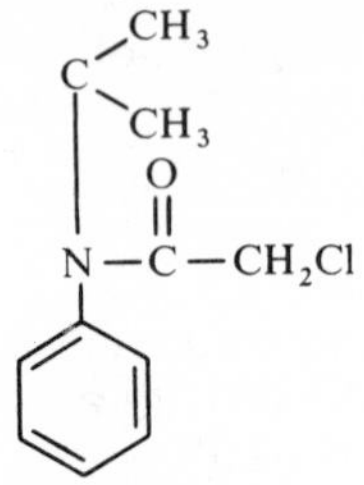

propachlor

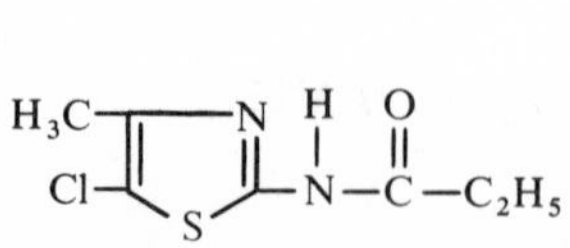

CMPT (TO-2)

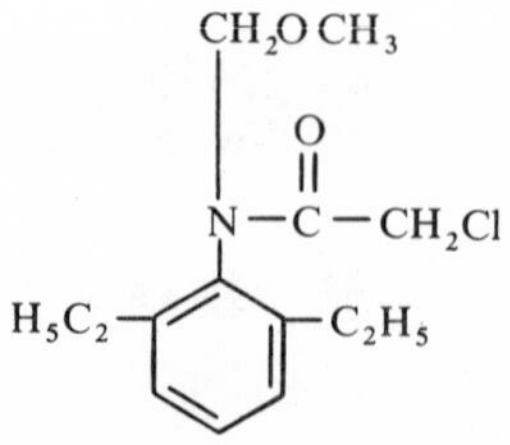

alachlor

344

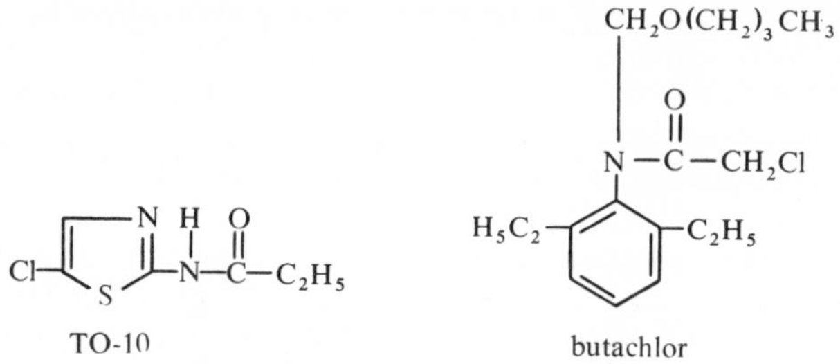

Figure 1. Acyl anilide herbicides and related compounds.

or barnyardgrass, the photosynthesis of both plants was completely inhibited. However, carbon dioxide assimilation in rice plants recovered gradually and was normal 5 days after the treatment; barnyardgrass did not show any recovery and died about 4 days after the treatment. This suggested to us that rice plants have some kind of detoxication mechanism.

As shown in *Figure 2*, one of the mechanisms of tolerance of rice plant against propanil is detoxication, which may be by a specific enzyme, propanil hydrolysing enzyme: rice aryl amidase (EC 3.5.1.a, aryl acylamine amido-hydrolase)[8]. Homogenates or partially purified enzyme preparations can hydrolyse propanil to 3,4-dichloroaniline (DCA).

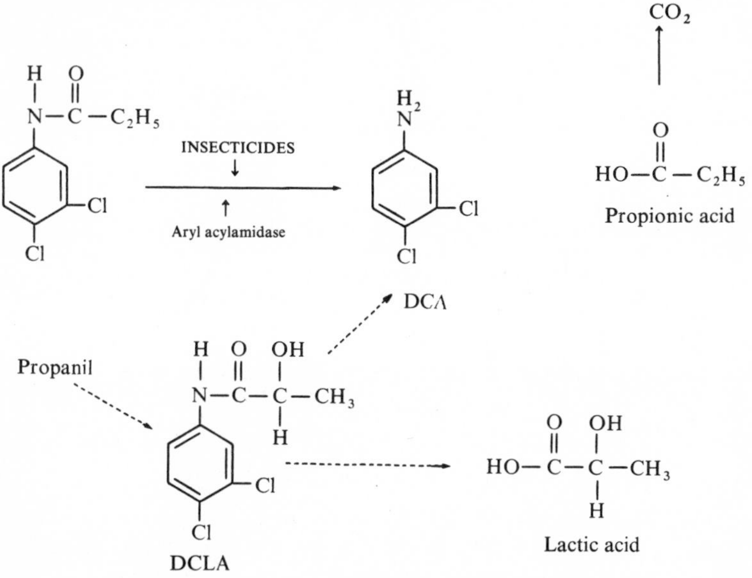

Figure 2. Detoxication of propanil in rice plants.

Propanil-hydrolysing enzyme (rice aryl acylamidase)

The existence of the enzyme in the rice plant has been reported by several workers[1, 9], and its purification attempted[8, 10]. It was found to be a particulate enzyme. Very recently Akatsuka purified the enzyme by centrifugation, sonic treatment, salting out by ammonium sulphate, and Sephadex column

345

chromatography to a single band purity by disc electrophoresis. Frear and Still[8], and Akatsuka's group[10] reported the properties of the partially purified enzyme. Yih *et al.*[12] reported that propanil hydrolysis is not a direct one-step hydrolysis but rather an oxidative metabolism of propanil to 3′,4′-dichlorolacetanilide (DCLA) followed by hydrolysis to DCA and lactic acid, as shown as an alternative pathway in *Figure 2*. Akatsuka and others reported that partially purified enzyme having 15-fold specific activity did not require cofactors or any other enzyme system. Unlike the results of Yih *et al.*, other work seems to show a simple hydrolysis of propanil into 3,4-dichloroaniline and propionic acid, but these discrepancies should be clarified in future.

The pH optimum for propanil hydrolysis by partially purified rice aryl acylamidase was found to be pH 8.4 by Adachi *et al.*[13] and between pH 7.5 and 7.9 by Frear and Still[8], and to be temperature-dependent by Akatsuka's group.

The apparent K_m for propanil was found to be 2.93×10^{-3}M for Frear and Still's enzyme and 3.3×10^{-4}M for Akatsuka's preparation.

As to the substrate specificity, the effect of ring substitution on aryl acylamidase activity is summarized in *Figure 3*. The results by both groups[8, 10]

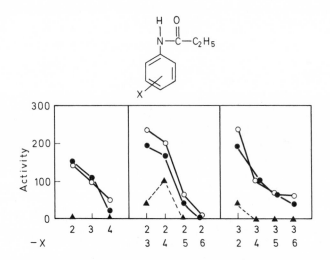

Position of chlorine atom(s) on the ring

Figure 3. Substrate specificity of aryl acylamidase (ring-substitution of propionanilides). Rice plants: ○—○. Frear and Still[8], ●—●. Akatsuka *et al.*[10]. Crabgrass: ▲—▲. Akatsuka and Hattori[14].

showed a real similarity to each other for rice plants. The larger the number position of the chlorine atom in mono-substituted chloropropionanilides, or of another position of the second chlorine atom in di-substituted compounds, the lower the activity: 2,3- and 2,4-substituted compounds have about twice the activity shown by propanil itself (3,4-dichloro substitution).

346

Akatsuka and Hattori[14] found another aryl acylamidase in crabgrass (*Digitaria sanguinalis*), which was specific for 2,4-dichloropropionanilide but had almost no activity for propanil itself as shown in *Figure 3*.

The effect of mono-substituted chloropropionanilides on enzyme activity appears to be opposite to those observed by Nimmo-Smith[15] with a particulate chicken kidney aryl acylamidase and mono-substituted chloroacetanilide substrates.

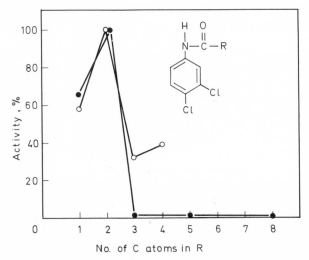

Figure 4. Substrate specificity of rice aryl acylamidase (side-chain substitution of 3',4'-dichloro-anilide). ○—○, Frear and Still[8], ●—●, Akatsuka *et al.*[10].

Various alkyl analogues of 3',4'-dichloroanilide yielded the substrate specificity shown in *Figure 4*. In both sets of data, variation in the carbon chain length showed that 3',4'-dichloropropionanilides were the preferred substrates. A similar substrate preference for the straight C_3 alkyl group was reported by Nimmo-Smith[15] with chicken enzyme.

Alkyl branching at either α- or β-position to the carbonyl carbon atom resulted in almost complete loss of activity, which means that dicryl or Karsil could not be the substrate of the rice enzyme[8].

Acetanilide was shown to be a good substrate for rice enzyme, in which the effect of the ring substitution was the same as in propionanilides although the absolute activity was somewhat lower than that of the corresponding propionanilides[8, 10].

Crabgrass enzyme showed some activity on 3',4'-dichlorocapronanilide and also on 3',4'-dichloropelargonanilide[14]. Of course it had affinity to 2',4'-dichloroacetanilide, and the effect of ring substitution in acetanilides was similar to that in the propionanilides.

Ishizuka *et al.*[16] reported that barnyardgrass had another aryl acylamidase, which showed very low activity on propanil itself but relatively high activity on 3',4'-dichloro-substituted longer side chain anilides, and they concluded that the mechanism of selectivity of propanil between rice plant and barnyardgrass would be explained from a standpoint of substrate specificity, not by the presence or absence of a specific aryl amidase.

The N-chloro-substituted derivative (N-chloro-propanil), which was developed in Japan, showed a potent herbicidal activity and selectivity between rice plant and barnyardgrass, and it easily produced probably 3,4-dichloroaniline by the incubation with rice plant homogenates. From an analysis of infra-red-region absorption curves, the reaction from N-Cl to N-H may proceed easily, when N-chlorine-substituted propanil showed almost the same activity and selectivity as propanil[17].

N-Methyl-substituted propanil also showed herbicidal activity and selectivity between rice plants and weeds[18]. By our experiments[17], both rice plant and barnyardgrass showed recovery from photosynthesis inhibition by N-methyl propanil, but the hydrolysis of this herbicide by plants is still unknown.

In addition to above-described two herbicides, dicryl and Karsil, cypromid, solan, swep[17], chloropropham (CIPC) and monuron[8] were not hydrolysed to the corresponding aniline under standard assay conditions by rice aryl acylamidase.

Inhibition of rice aryl acylamidase by insecticides

In paddy fields the combination of certain insecticides with propanil causes injury to rice plants[19, 20]. Both organophosphate insecticides and carbamate insecticides strongly enhance the herbicidal activity of propanil against the rice plant. Since propanil is used as a selective herbicide on rice plants as described above, the enhancement of toxicity by insecticides used to protect the rice from pest insects is a very severe problem in crop management.

Adachi *et al.*[13] and McRae *et al.*[1] found that these insecticides could inhibit the hydrolysis of propanil by rice enzyme. Matsunaka[21] compared the inhibitory activities of four organophosphate insecticides both on cholinesterase and on the rice propanil-hydrolysing enzyme (aryl acylamidase) (*Table 1*). In insects, the conversion of parathion into the more toxic paraoxon is a very important activation reaction, and in general the P=O

Table 1. Effect of organophosphate insecticides on aryl acylamidase and cholinesterase

Insecticides	Concentration of 50% inhibition (M)		
	Cholinesterase	Aryl acylamidase*	
		Matsunaka[21]	Akatsuka[22]
Phenitrothion†	2.3×10^{-4}	3.4×10^{-4}	5.0×10^{-6}
Oxophenitrothion	1.2×10^{-7}	1.5×10^{-6}	1.9×10^{-6}
Parathion	2.0×10^{-5}	2.4×10^{-5}	5.9×10^{-5}
Paraoxon	2.0×10^{-9}	2.4×10^{-7}	7.2×10^{-7}

* Rice propanil-hydrolysing enzyme.
† Sumithion.

348

type has more toxic activity than the corresponding P=S type. In the case of rice enzyme, such a relationship was observed in both combinations, parathion–paraoxon and phenitrothion–oxophenitrothion. Akatsuka[22] surveyed the inhibitory activities of 61 organophosphate insecticides on rice aryl acylamidase and found a close relationship between the effects on cholinesterase and on rice enzyme. The results showed that the inhibitory patterns for the propanil-hydrolysing enzyme in rice plants and the acetylcholine esterase in insects are very similar. It is speculated that the propanil-detoxifying enzyme and the cholinesterase may resemble each other.

Akatsuka et al.[10] surveyed the effect of about twenty phenyl N-methylcarbamates on the rice aryl acylamidase and found that monochloro-, monomethyl- or dimethyl-substituted ones showed strong inhibitory activity, and such difference as was found for cholinesterase inhibition was not observed. Some of them are cited in Table 2. With a solution culture

Table 2. Effect of carbamate insecticides on aryl acylamidase and cholinesterase

Insecticides	Concentration of 50% inhibition		
	Cholinesterase	Aryl acylamidase*[10]	Growth with 2.5 p.p.m. propanil[23]
	(M)	(M)	(p.p.m.)
Carbaryl	9.0×10^{-7}	1.0×10^{-8}	—
2,5-Dimethyl-PMC†	9.0×10^{-6}	6.0×10^{-8}	0.20
3,4-Dimethyl-PMC	2.6×10^{-5}	2.4×10^{-7}	—
2,4-Dimethyl-PMC	1.3×10^{-4}	7.2×10^{-8}	0.25

* Rice propanil-hydrolysing enzyme.
† PMC: phenyl-N-methylcarbamate.

method, Kawamura[23] tested the synergistic action on the herbicidal activity of propanil by two isomers of dimethylphenyl N-methylcarbamate, the inhibitory activities of which on cholinesterase were quite different from each other: 2,5-dimethyl (more active) and 2,4-dimethyl derivatives. As shown in Table 2, almost no difference was observed in rice growth inhibition with the two treatments. These data show that with carbamate insecticides the similarity between cholinesterase and rice aryl acylamidase is somewhat imperfect.

Frear and Still[8] also found that the apparent K_i for carbaryl was 1.51×10^{-8} M. The very low value for carbaryl and the strong inhibition observed with other insecticides shown in these figures may explain the strong synergistic effects observed in rice fields between propanil and various insecticides. Apparently the insecticidal carbamates are potent inhibitors of propanil hydrolysis and block its normal detoxication pathway in rice plants.

In the case of aryl acylamidase of crabgrass, Akatsuka and Hattori[14] showed similar strong inhibition of hydrolysis of 2.4-dichloropropionanilide by organophosphate or carbamate insecticides. In Japan, a combination of propanil (3',4'-dichloropropionanilide) with carbaryl is being used practically for the control of crabgrass in citrus orchards[24]. However, the relationships between these facts are unexplained.

Propanil-susceptible mutant of rice[25, 26]

Very recently the author fortunately found a rice plant mutant susceptible to propanil. Artificial mutants of rice induced by chemicals or isotopic radiation have been created in the 3rd Laboratory of Genetics of our institute. Using their nursery beds, the author tried to select propanil-susceptible mutants from their stocks. Among about 700 lines of mutants, only one mutant, no. 408, was found to be susceptible after spraying of a practical concentration of propanil.

The susceptibility of the mutant to propanil is very high and the grade resembles that of barnyardgrass. At a concentration of propanil that produces no effect on the original variety, both the mutant and barnyardgrass were killed and withered.

The effect of the treatment of 0.3% propanil emulsion on the photosynthetic activity of the mutant and the original variety is illustrated in *Figure 5*.

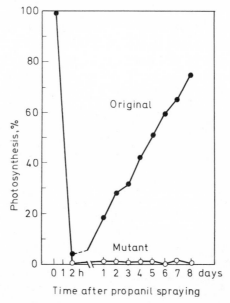

Figure 5. Effect of propanil on the photosynthesis of the original variety (●) and mutant (○) of rice plant.

As described above[7], the carbon dioxide fixation of the original rice plant variety was at first inhibited by the treatment but it recovered gradually. On the other hand, in the propanil-susceptible mutant no recovery was found, as in barnyardgrass.

In the homogenates from the original variety the concentration of propanil in the reaction mixture decreased along with the increase of 3,4-dichloroaniline. However, in the homogenates from the mutant, no decrease of propanil concentration and no production of dichloroaniline were observed in the reaction mixture[26].

From these data the mutant could be supposed to have no propanil-hydrolysing enzyme. In addition to propanil, 2,3-, 2,4-, 2,5-, 2,6- and 3,5-dichloropropionanilides also could not be hydrolysed by homogenates of the mutant; thus it may be concluded that the mutant does not have aryl acylamidase itself.

In order to survey the fundamental properties of the mutant or the original, a genetical approach was made by crossing the mutant with the original variety.

F_1 plants, both mutant × original and original × mutant, were also tolerant to propanil and capable of hydrolysing propanil into DCA.

F_2 plants segretated into a ratio of 3:1. For instance, when 20 plants were tested, five rice plants were killed by propanil and 15 plants survived.

Relationships between tolerance to propanil and existence of the enzyme were analysed by using the same individual F_2 plants. The third leaf was sampled from the intact plant, and its activity of propanil-hydrolysing enzyme was assayed. The remaining plants were sprayed with propanil emulsion. Two weeks afterwards, survival or death of the individual rice plants was checked. All F_2 plants having no aryl acylamidase were killed, whereas F_2 with the enzyme survived.

All results are summarized in *Table 3*. From these data it may be concluded that a gene which controls the formation of aryl acylamidase was attacked

Table 3. Genetic properties of propanil-susceptible rice mutant

	Propanil-hydrolysing enzyme		After propanil-spraying	
	Presence (%)	Absence (%)	Survival (%)	Death (%)
Original variety Norin no. 8	100	0	100	0
Propanil-susceptible mutant	0	100	0	100
F_1	(15)† 100	0	(40) 98	2
F_2	(83) 75	25	(299) 74	26

† Numbers of used grains are shown in parentheses.

by the ^{60}Co radiation and the susceptible mutant was created. The tolerance corresponding to the existence of the enzyme shows genetically a dominant epistasis. These facts would provide direct evidence to show that the propanil-hydrolysing enzyme system in rice plants is genetically controlled.

Fate of 3.4-dichloroaniline (DCA)

Free DCA converted from propanil in rice plants forms several DCA metabolite complexes. Still[27] reported three metabolites, M-1, M-2 and M-3. M-3 was identified as N-(3,4-dichlorophenyl)glucosylamine. Yih *et al.*[29] also independently found four metabolites, soluble aniline–carbohydrate

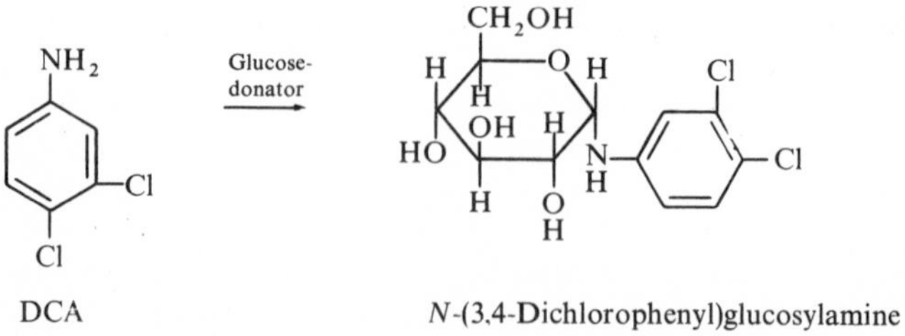

Figure 6. Formation of N-(3,4-dichlorophenyl)glucosylamine.

complexes. One of them was also identified as N-(3,4-dichlorophenyl)-glucosylamine. Other metabolites by both groups were sugar complexes with 3,4-dichloroaniline.

On the other hand, Yih *et al.* also reported that the major portion of the 3,4-dichloroaniline moiety is found in a complex with polymeric cell constituents, mainly lignin. The aniline is lignin-bound as 3,4-dichloroaniline and not as 3'-4'-dichloropropionanilide.

The authors preliminarily tried the further fate of 3,4-dichloroaniline in homogenates of several higher plants[30]. Disappearance of DCA from the reaction mixture could be observed in two steps: one was an instant reaction at zero time and the other proceeded gradually. Conversion from propanil into DCA occurred only in rice plants as described above, but DCA disappearance by homogenates was observed in all plants tested, crabgrass, tomato, barnyardgrass, rice plant, maize, cucumber and spinach. UDPG (uridine diphosphate glucose) had almost no effect on these reactions.

Fate of the side chain of propanil

Yih *et al.*[12] treated rice plants with carbonyl-^{14}C labelled propanil and tried to recover labelled lactic acid and/or propionic acid. With liquid–liquid extraction and thin-layer chromatography, the labelled organic acid recovered had R_j 0.72, whereas the R_j for lactic acid was 0.66 and that for propionic acid was 0.94. The authors wrote: 'it is apparent from these results that the presence of lactic acid was not clearly and consistently established'. If propanil metabolism in the rice plant passes through 3'.4'-dichloroacetanilide as shown by Yih *et al.*[12], the first metabolite of the side chain should be lactic acid, not propionic acid (*Figure 3*).

Before the publication of the reports by Yih *et al.*, Still[27] examined and reported the metabolic fate of the propionic acid moiety. He applied ^{14}C-labelled propanil, labelled in either the C-1 or C-3 atoms of the propionic acid moiety, to the roots of pea and rice plants in nutrient solution. None of the metabolic products which contained aniline was radioactive, suggesting that the plants split the propionic acid moiety from propanil. The time-course of the $^{14}CO_2$ production showed that the intact propionic acid was cleaved from the propanil and subsequently catabolized by the β-oxidation mechanism.

Metabolism of propanil in soils

Hydrolysis of propanil in soils

Bartha[31] reported that propanil was transformed by soil micro-organisms, and suggested that the aliphatic side chain of the molecules was oxidized in part to carbon dioxide and that the aromatic moiety was liberated as a toxic residue that depressed soil respiration. Such easy degradation of propanil in soils may be one of the reasons for the unsuitability of this herbicide for soil treatment.

After incubation of 500 g of soil (Nixon sandy loam moistened to 60% of capacity) with 1.0 g of propanil at 28°C for 17 days, two decomposition products of the herbicide were isolated and characterized chemically as 3.4-dichloroaniline (DCA) and 3.3'.4.4'-tetrachloroazobenzene (TCAB)[32]. The cleavage of the propanil molecule into DCA and propionic acid may be catalysed by an aryl acylamidase of microbial origin.

Kaufman and Miller reported that the soil fungus, *Fusarium solani* (Martius) Appel and Wollenweber, was most effective in degrading propanil. The CIPC degrading enzyme isolated from *Pseudomonas striata* by Kearney[33] can also convert propanil into DCA.

Azobenzene formation in soils

The condensation mechanism that produces another product, TCAB, from DCA as shown in *Figure 7* may be a direct oxidative condensation of two molecules of DCA, or DCA may be first transformed in part into

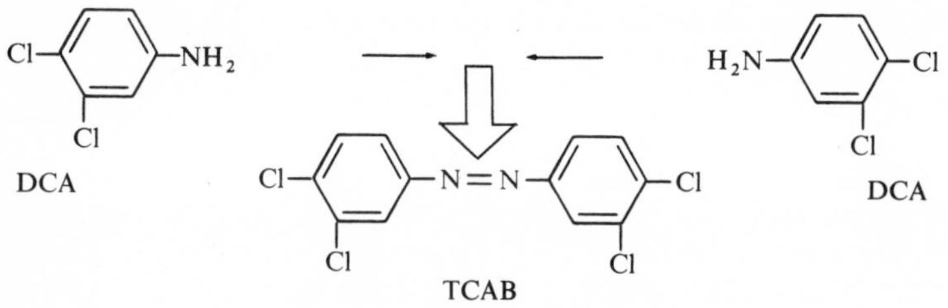

Figure 7. Formation of TCAB.

3.4-dichloronitrosobenzene, after which a spontaneous condensation of one molecule of the aniline compound with one molecule of the nitroso compound may occur.

Bartha *et al.*[34] suggested that a peroxidatic mechanism may be responsible for the production of azo-compounds in soil. The origin of this suggestion was a report by Daniels and Saunders[35] showing the catalysis by peroxidase of the synthesis of 4.4'-dichloroazobenzene from monochloroaniline, and from their findings that horseradish peroxidase could produce TCAB from

DCA with hydrogen peroxide at pH 5.0 and that Nixon sandy loam had peroxidase activity.

Still[36] reported that rice plants supplied with propanil or 3,4-dichloro-aniline in liquid culture were free from any detectable TCAB. As rice plants have highly active peroxidase, the peroxidatic mechanism for TCAB formation could not be generalized.

Bartha and Pramer[32] followed the time-course of propanil, DCA and TCAB in soil, and showed that about 90% of propanil disappeared in 5 days; the concentration of DCA reached a maximum within 10 days and then declined, but TCAB continued to accumulate for the duration of the experiment. In 30 days, 46% of the aromatic moiety of the added propanil was recovered as TCAB.

Chisaka and Kearney[37] tried to find differences in the metabolism of propanil among five different types of soil brought from Japan. Soil type influenced propanil disappearance and TCAB formation.

Triazene compound formation in soils

Kearney's group[38] found a new product having three nitrogen atoms in a Chikugo light claysoil, treated with propanil during the above described studies.

Its chemical structure was determined as 1,3-bis-(3,4-dichlorophenyl)-triazene. The first contribution of soil nitrite probably came from nitrogen

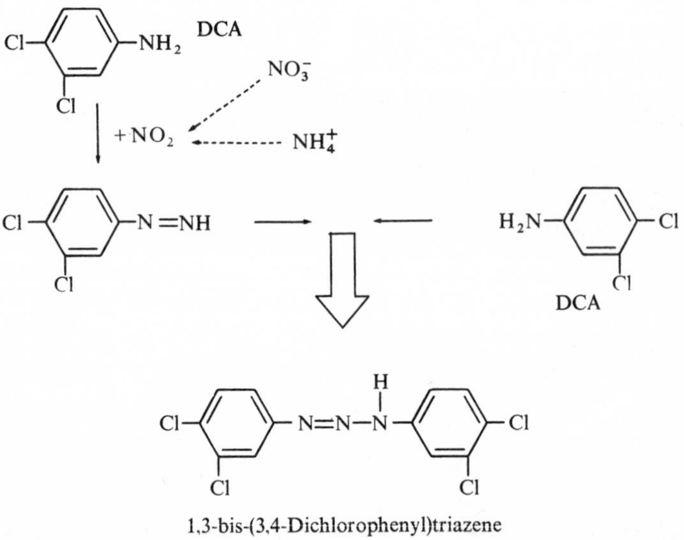

1,3-bis-(3,4-Dichlorophenyl)triazene

Figure 8. Formation of 1,3-bis-(3,4-dichlorophenyl)triazene.

fertilizers, to form an intermediate diazonium cation from 3,4-dichloroaniline. Subsequent coupling of the diazonium cation produced with another DCA molecule may produce the triazene compound.

The fact is very interesting from the standpoint that the fertility of the soil could affect the course of metabolism of certain pesticides.

Hybrid residue formation in soils

Bartha[39] found an unexpected residue, asymmetric 3,3',4-trichloro-4'-methylazobenzene (TCMAB) in the soil treated with propanil and solan in combination. Propanil can produce 3,4-dichloroaniline (DCA) and solan produces 3-chloro-4-methylaniline (CMA); the two aniline compounds produced an asymmetric azobenzene, the middle compound shown in *Table 4*, called by Bartha the 'hybrid residue'.

Table 4. Residues in 100 g of soil treated with both propanil and solan[39]

Compounds	Initial	3 weeks after incubation
Propanil	50	0.80
Solan	50	35.00
DCDMAB	--	0.50
TCMAB	--	1.43
TCAB	--	4.86

From the soil treated with solan only, 3,3'-dichloro-4,4'-dimethylazobenzene (DCDMAB) was isolated. All three azobenzenes, DCDMAB, TCMAB and TCAB, were produced in nearly equal quantities from the same amount of both aniline compounds, CMA and DCA. When the same amount of both anilide herbicides, solan and propanil, was taken, the proportions of the azobenzene residues were not the same, as shown in *Table 4*. The aniline moieties were liberated from the parent herbicides at different rates, and this influenced the proportions. TCAB was the dominant azobenzene residue in this soil, as propanil was degraded more rapidly than solan.

Kearney's group[40], independently of Bartha, also found mixed chloroazobenzene formation in soil. They found the condensation of 3-chloroaniline and 3,4-dichloroaniline to form 3,3',4'-trichloroazobenzene in addition to 3,3'-dichloroazobenzene and TCAB. Simultaneous application of both herbicides, propanil and CIPC, in soil will produce such hybrid residue.

Transformation of 3,4-dichloroaniline by photoreactions

Plimmer and Kearney[41] reported the formation of TCAB and 3,3',4,4'-

tetrachloroazoxybenzene from DCA in benzene solution with a supply of light energy and with benzophenone as the photosensitizer.

Rosen et al.[42] also obtained TCAB and 4-(3,4-dichloroanilino)-3,3',4'-trichloroazobenzene by exposing DCA in aqueous solution with riboflavin 5'-phosphate (FMN) to sunlight.

In practical use, in fields exposed to sunlight, there is the possibility of formation of these azobenzenes, anilinoazobenzene, and azoxybenzene.

Problems of propanil residues

Our knowledge of the metabolism of propanil in general may be summarized as shown in *Figure 9.* Here 3,4-dichloroaniline (DCA) occupies an

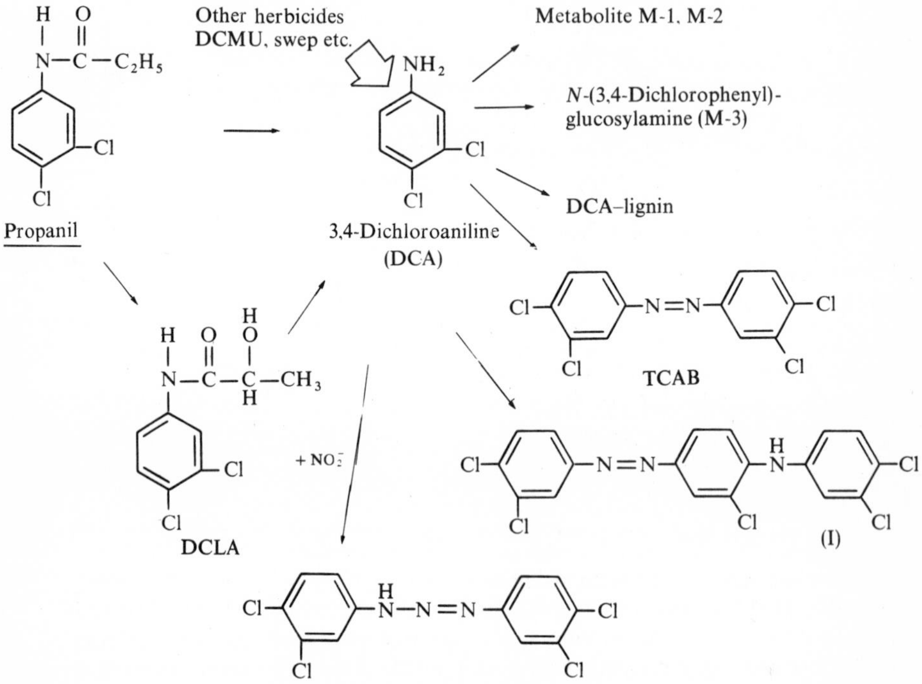

Figure 9. Metabolism of propanil in higher plants and in soils.

important position. Other herbicides, for example DCMU (diuron), swep, dicryl, Karsil etc., will also produce DCA.

DCA itself would be more toxic to humans than propanil, but their condensed compound TCAB should be borne in mind from a standpoint of toxicology. In addition to TCAB, compound (I) [4-(3,4-dichloroanilino)-3,3',4'-trichloroazobenzene][42] or compound (II) [1,3-bis-(3,4-dichloro-phenyl)-triazene][41] were detected as products from DCA.

Residue amounts of DCA or propanil in rice grain were assayed by Still and Mansager[43]. They found DCA in the hydrolysate of the following rice:

rough rice or head rice produced at Stuttgart, Arkansas, commercial brown rice packaged in Texas and two brands of white rice packaged in Texas and Minnesota; but, from rough rice harvested in 1958, 3-chloroaniline was detected. The last one had been treated with CIPC (chloropropham), which contains the 3-chloroaniline moiety not 3,4-dichloroaniline.

DCA was found also in the Stuttgart grain hydrolysate, which was not treated with propanil, and this may reflect the movement of propanil or its soil metabolites in the flood water.

Certain azobenzene compounds, for instance butter yellow (structure shown in *Figure 10*), are known to be carcinogenic, and the Technical Panel on Carcinogenesis in the Secretary's Commission on Pesticides and

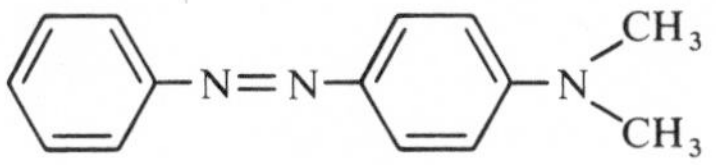

Butter yellow

Figure 10. Butter yellow.

Their Relationship to Environmental Health, U.S. Department of Health, Education and Welfare, judged azobenzene itself to be classified into the Priority Group C_1[44]. The compounds which belong to this group yielded an increased tumour incidence significant at the 0.01 level but were considered less tumourigenic than the mean of a group of positive controls. These compounds have first priority for additional testing.

On the other hand, Bartha and Pramer[45] reported that rats fed with TCAB at a level of 4 mg/week for an initial 3-weeks period and at 10 mg/week for an additional 37 weeks had produced no tumours when the animals were killed at the sixtieth week.

TCAB itself has not been found in plant tissues treated with propanil[36]. On the other hand, DCA, material for the production of TCAB, was found in rice plants, so that the rice plant seems to have no activity to condense DCA into TCAB.

However, TCAB which is produced in soils by the action of micro-organisms can be absorbed and translocated by rice plants. Still[36] found that 20-day-old rice plant seedlings treated for 12 days with saturated TCAB nutrient solution contained TCAB at concentrations of 65.02 p.p.m. (dry weight basis) in root tissue and 0.73 p.p.m. in shoot tissue. These amounts correspond to only 5.37% of the total applied TCAB in the nutrient solution, and only 3.2% of absorbed TCAB was translocated to the shoots. Still stated that it seemed highly unlikely that a concentration of chloroazo-benzene could be reached which would present a problem in the foliar tissues of rice plants.

The solubility of TCAB is 3.13×10^{-1} p.p.m. in water and 8.8×10^{-3} p.p.m. in one-half strength Hoagland's solution[36]. In field surveys conducted on rice-producing soils in Stuttgart, Arkansas, TCAB was detected only at low concentrations less than 0.1 p.p.m.[46].

From these investigations, problems with TCAB in propanil application do not seem to be so severe. However, accumulation of TCAB in paddy

357

fields or production of new compounds such as triazenes, anilinoazo-benzenes or azoxybenzenes, the toxicities of which are unknown, necessitates further study of the production, fate and toxicity of these compounds produced in paddy fields treated with propanil.

3. SOLAN AND OTHER ACYL ANILIDE HERBICIDES

Metabolism in higher plants

Solan (3-chloro-2-methyl-p-valerotoluidide) shows high selectivity between tomato plants and eggplant. Colby and Warren[4] reported that differences in penetration, persistence and metabolism of solan by tomato and eggplant were insufficient to account for the differential susceptibility. If metabolic detoxication of solan occurs in tomato plants, the detoxified product(s) should be chemically distinguishable from solan. Likewise, if solan were activated to a phytotoxic form in eggplant, the activated form should be detectable. No radioactive component other than solan appeared on chromatograms of extracts from ^{14}C-labelled solan-treated plants of either species. These results indicate that solan is not rapidly metabolized or converted into a detoxified or an activated form in plants.

Shirakawa and others[47] reported that crude enzymes extracted from tolerant plants, tomato, Japanese honewort (more tolerant than tomato), carrot and strawberry did not decompose solan as well as a susceptible plant cucumber.

Possibly the 2-methyl grouping on the side chain of solan hinders the occurrence of such hydrolysis of solan in tomato as occurs with propanil in rice plants. Frear and Still[8], as described above, reported that alkyl branching resulted in almost complete loss of hydrolytic activity by rice aryl acylamidase.

Shirakawa and others also found that some injuries were observed even on tolerant plants when phenitrothion dimethoate or carbaryl are sprayed before or after spraying with solan[48]. This discrepancy between the absence of hydrolysis of solan and the presence of synergism with insecticides in tolerant plants is unexplained.

Nakamura and Matsunaka also showed that homogenates from rice plant leaves could not hydrolyse solan or cypromid and that almost no recovery of photosynthesis occurred in intact rice plants treated by these two herbicides.

In the case of tolerant plants, tomato or Japanese honewort, after spraying of solan the photosynthesis recovered to the initial level after a tentative small inhibition.

Shirakawa[49] indicated an instant formation of solan complex with chloroplasts of several plants including tolerant and susceptible ones. The author speculates that solan may form a complex within the intact tolerant plant.

Metabolism in soil

Behaviour of solan in soil was also investigated by Shirakawa's group[50]. Decomposition of solan to 3-chloro-4-methylaniline (CMA) in soil could be expected from the results of the above-described experiment to make hybrid residues (Bartha[39]). Shirakawa[50] confirmed that the decomposition of solan in soil occurred simultaneously through the primary reaction (producing CMA) and the secondary reaction (disappearance of CMA).

Shirakawa also reported that the decomposition of solan was partly prevented by the treatment with a fungicide [N-(phenylmercury)-p-toluene-sulphonanilide] or an insecticide, phenitrothion, and strongly prevented by treatment with another insecticide, carbaryl, before treatment with solan on soil. In *Figure 11*, the effect of carbaryl on the degradation of solan in

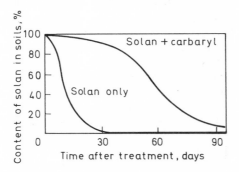

Figure 11. Effect of carbaryl on the degradation of solan in soil[50].

soils is shown. Delay in the degradation of solan was estimated as 20 days for phenitrothion and as over 60 days for carbaryl.

One of the further fates of 3-chloro-4-methylaniline (CMA) may be the formation of azobenzene compounds, for instance, 3,3'-dichloro-4,4'-dimethylazobenzene (DCDMAB). As with propanil, triazenes or other condensed compounds would be produced from CMA in soils.

As to other herbicides, both dicryl and Karsil are also metabolized by the microbial population in soil[31]. The aliphatic moieties of these molecules are oxidized and, in each case, a substantial portion of the liberated 3,4-dichloroaniline is condensed to TCAB.

In general, all acyl anilide herbicides having the —NH—CO— radical could be hydrolysed and condensed to the corresponding azobenzenes and other compounds in soils, in contrast to the findings with higher plants.

Chloroacetamide

Chloroacetamide herbicides can be divided into two sub-groups: aliphatic and aromatic compounds. 2-Chloro-N-alkyl-acetanilides form the latter group.

One of them, 2-chloro-N-isopropylacetanilide, propachlor, the structure of which is shown in *Figure 1*, was designed as a pre-emergent herbicide for use in corn and soybeans to control a broader spectrum of broadleaf weeds, as well as to control barnyardgrass, foxtail, bromegrass, cheatgrass and crabgrass[51,52]. Jaworski and Porter[53] studied the uptake and metabolism of uniformly ring-³H-labelled 2-chloro-N-isopropylacetanilide in corn and soybeans. Both plants were very tolerant to this herbicide and a continued dilution of the amount of radioactivity in the plants (fresh weight basis) was observed. Residues of radioactivity in corn decreased from 46 p.p.m. in plants harvested 5 days after planting to 0.79 p.p.m. in plants harvested 74 days after planting. In soybean a similar dilution of radioactivity from 12.8 p.p.m. to 1.4 p.p.m. was noted.

These workers concluded that propachlor was rapidly metabolized by corn, soybeans and a variety of other resistant crop plants to a water-soluble acidic metabolite, but the absolute structure of this metabolite has not been defined. The metabolite contains essentially the entire structure of the original herbicides, with the exception that the chloro group appears to have been displaced, probably by some nucleophilic endogenous substrate in the plant[54].

Bartha[31] also investigated propachlor metabolism in soil, but obtained no evidence for production of an aniline or azobenzene from propachlor under the same conditions in which DCA and TCAB were produced from propanil, dicryl or Karsil.

Ring-substituted 2-chloro-N-alkyl-acetanilides are now becoming important herbicides. After alachlor, butachlor is registered in Japan as a useful herbicide for the culture of transplanted rice. However, the fate of these new herbicides is unknown.

4. METABOLISM OF CMPT

CMPT (5-chloro-4-methyl-2-propionamide thiazole), was developed in Japan as a selective herbicide for wheat. Wheat and some kinds of barley are very tolerant of this herbicide.

As shown in *Figure 12*, it strongly inhibits the Hill reaction by spinach chloroplasts, and photosynthesis in susceptible plants, for instance, tomato

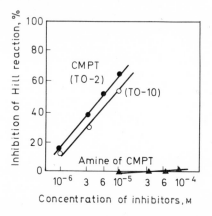

Figure 12. Effect of CMPT on the Hill reaction of spinach chloroplasts.

plant. However, the corresponding amine of CMPT has no inhibitory activity towards the Hill reaction nor herbicidal activity on weeds[5].

As shown in *Figure 13*. the photosynthesis of tolerant plants was completely inhibited by spraying of CMPT for two days, but a recovery was

360

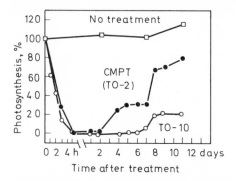

Figure 13. Effect of CMPT and TO-10 on the photosynthesis of wheat.

observed almost to the original level of photosynthesis ten days after the treatment.

From these data in wheat or barley, as shown in *Figure 14*, hydrolysis of CMPT to the corresponding amine, 2-amino-5-chloro-4-methyl thiazole and propionic acid could be assumed. Enzymatic evidence for such hydrolysis could not be obtained.

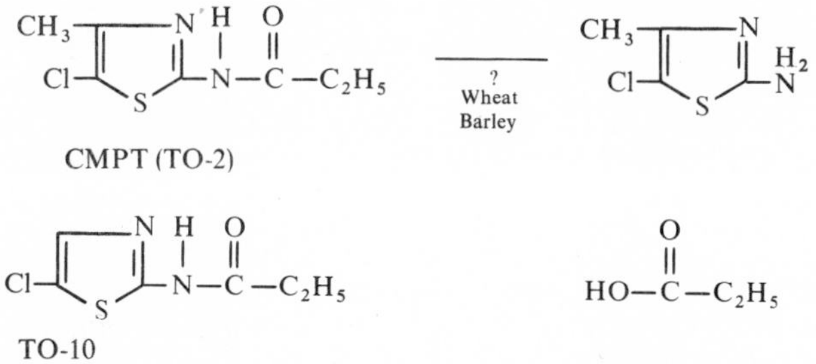

$$CH_3 \underset{Cl}{\overset{}{\bigwedge\limits_{S}}} N\text{-}\overset{H}{\underset{}{N}}\text{-}\overset{O}{\underset{}{C}}\text{-}C_2H_5 \qquad \xrightarrow[\substack{?\\ \text{Wheat}\\ \text{Barley}}]{} \qquad CH_3 \underset{Cl}{\overset{}{\bigwedge\limits_{S}}} N\overset{H_2}{\underset{}{N}}$$

CMPT (TO-2)

$$Cl \overset{}{\underset{S}{\bigwedge}} N\text{-}\overset{H}{\underset{}{N}}\text{-}\overset{O}{\underset{}{C}}\text{-}C_2H_5 \qquad\qquad \overset{O}{\underset{}{HO\text{-}C}}\text{-}C_2H_5$$

TO-10

Figure 14. Speculated detoxication mechanism of CMPT in wheat or barley.

Another related herbicide, TO-10 (5-chloro-2-propionamide thiazole), has less selectivity to wheat than CMPT, which is explained by the lower activity in recovery of inhibition of photosynthesis.

In the case of tolerance of wheat to CMPT, simultaneous application of organophosphate or carbamate insecticides with CMPT could cause injury on wheat itself, as with insecticides in the application of propanil on rice plants.

5. METABOLISM OF SWEP

Chin *et al.*[55] investigated the fate of swep (methyl-3,4-dichlorophenyl-carbamate) in rice plants. They concluded that swep was not readily hydrolysed in rice; instead, it was metabolized without hydrolysis to a stable lignin complex. In contrast to the results obtained with swep, with propanil there was no incorporation of the intact anilide and incorporation occurred after hydrolysis to 3,4-dichloroaniline.

Chin et al.[55] could detect only limited amounts of free 3,4-dichloroaniline. Nakamura and Matsunaka[17] found that homogenates from rice leaves produced almost no DCA from swep.

In practical use in fields, however, swep could be used selectively for the weed control of direct-seeded rice culture in dry conditions. It should be applied before the one-leaf stage of rice seedlings.

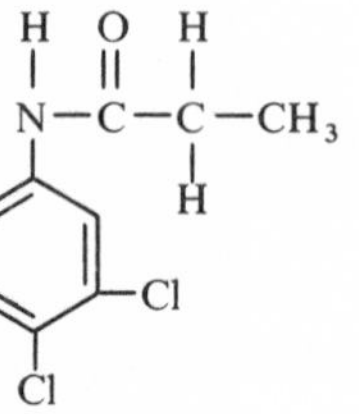

$$
\begin{array}{ccc}
\text{H} & \text{O} & \text{H} \\
| & || & | \\
\text{N} & -\text{C} - \text{C} & -\text{CH}_3
\end{array}
$$

Propanil

$$
\begin{array}{cc}
\text{H} & \text{O} \\
| & || \\
\text{N} & -\text{C} - \text{O} - \text{CH}_3
\end{array}
$$

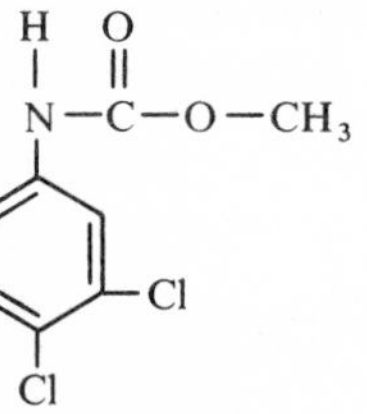

Swep

Figure 15. Similarity of the structures of propanil and swep.

Similarity of chemical structure between swep and propanil, as shown in Figure 15, suggests the hydrolysis of swep by the same enzyme as in propanil hydrolysis in rice plants. The author tried to examine the susceptibility of above-described propanil-susceptible rice mutant to swep. As shown in

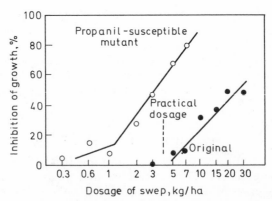

Figure 16. Susceptibility of the propanil-susceptible rice mutant to swep.

362

Figure 16, propanil-susceptible mutant was found to be more susceptible to swep than was the original variety Nōrin no. 8[26]. At the practical dosage, 4 kg a.i./ha, the original variety showed no injury whereas the mutant showed over 60% inhibition of growth.

Contents of swep in top parts of rice plants in soil treated with swep were determined after clean-up and by gas chromatography. The time-course of swep content is shown in *Figure 17.* In the original variety, resistant to

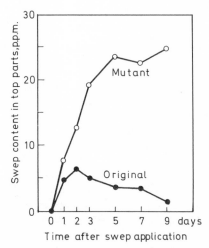

Figure 17. Content of swep in the top parts of rice plants soil-treated with swep.

swep, a small peak on the content curve appeared two days after application, then the content declined gradually. On the other hand the mutant showed gradual increasing of swep content with saturation 5 days after application. With swep, some kinds of insecticides show synergistic injury on rice plants.

From these data, swep seems to be hydrolysed to some extent in the intact rice plant. If a large amount of swep was sprayed over rice plants, for instance, just as with the application of the practical dosage after the two-leaf stage of rice plants, the low hydrolytic activity could not lower the internal swep content to a level without toxicity to the rice plant, so that the selectivity of swep to the rice plant may disappear.

6. CONCLUSION

An outline of the reactions of the acyl anilide herbicides is shown in *Figure 18.*

In higher plants, some acyl anilides could be hydrolysed to corresponding anilines. The processes are dependent upon the selectivity of each plant species and specificity of their enzymes. Aniline compounds will form complexes with sugars, lignin and other compounds. Some of them, especially 2-chloroacetamides, could not be hydrolysed in higher plants, but form a complex with intracellular components.

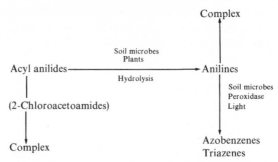

Figure 18. Outline of the metabolic reactions of the acyl anilide herbicides in higher plants and soils.

In soils, micro-organisms can hydrolyse almost all acyl anilides, except 2-chloroacetamides, and the produced anilines can be condensed to azobenzenes. Such condensation of anilines would be done in several ways, depending upon the conditions; for instance, nitrite-rich conditions will increase the amounts of triazene compounds. No hydrolysis of 2-chloroacetamides was observed even in soils.

It is a special characteristic of the acyl anilide herbicides in both higher plants and soils that their hydrolysis is inhibited by organophosphate or carbamate insecticides. These metabolic changes and interactions in acyl anilide herbicides have an important relationship with the herbicidal activity in weeds, injury to crop plants and persistence in soils of the residues and metabolites.

REFERENCES

[1] D. H. McRae, R. Y. Yih and H. F. Wilson. *Abst. 1964 Meeting Weed Soc. Amer. Chicago*, p 87 (1964).
[2] N. Yamada and H. Nakamura. *Proc. Crop Sci. Soc. Japan*, **32**, 69 (1963).
[3] S. R. Colby and G. F. Warren. *Weeds*, **10**, 308 (1962).
[4] S. R. Colby and G. F. Warren. *Weeds*, **13**, 257 (1965).
[5] S. Matsunaka and H. Nakamura. *Abst. 8th Meeting Weed Soc. Japan*, *Tokyo*, p 23 (1969).
[6] S. Matsunaka. *Residue Rev.*, **25**, 45 (1969).
[7] H. Nakamura, J. Koizumi and S. Matsunaka. *Weed Res.*, *Japan*, **7**: 100 (1968).
[8] D. S. Frear and G. G. Still. *Phytochemistry*, **7**, 913 (1968).
[9] M. Adachi, K. Tonegawa and T. Ueshima. *Pesticide Tech.* (*Tokyo*), **14**, 19 (1966).
[10] T. Akatsuka, K. Suzuki and S. Kuwatsuka. *Sci. Rep. Fac. Agric. Ibaraki Univ.* **17**, 45 (1969).
[11] T. Akatsuka. Personal communication.
[12] R. Y. Yih, D. H. McRae and H. F. Wilson. *Plant Physiol.* **43**, 1291 (1968).
[13] M. Adachi, K. Tonegawa and T. Uejima. *Pesticide Tech.* (*Tokyo*), **15**, 11 (1966).
[14] T. Akatsuka and M. Hattori. *Sci. Rep. Fac. Agric. Ibaraki Univ.* **17**, 49 (1969).
[15] R. H. Nimmo-Smith. *Biochem. J.* **75**, 284 (1960).
[16] K. Ishizuka, Y. Inoue and S. Mitsui. *U.S.–Japan Seminar on Biochemical Approaches to Weed Control*, Raleigh, N.C., U.S.A. (1969).
[17] H. Nakamura and S. Matsunaka. *Weed Res.*, *Japan*, **8**, 33 (1969).
[18] T. Toyosato, H. Hagimoto and M. Watanabe. *Weed Res.*, *Japan*, **4**, 123 (1965).
[19] S. Konnai. *Proc. Crop Sci. Soc. Japan*, **30**, 361 (1962).
[20] C. C. Bowling and H. R. Hudgins. *Weeds*, **14**, 94 (1966).
[21] S. Matsunaka. *Science*, **160**, 1360 (1968).
[22] T. Akatsuka. *Sci. Rep. Fac. Agri. Ibaraki Univ.* **18**, (in press) (1970).
[23] Y. Kawamura. *Plant Protection*, *Japan*, **23**, 71 (1969).

[24] T. Hisada. *Proc. 1st Asian-Pacific Weed-Control Interchange*, p 107 (1967).

[25] S. Matsunaka. *U.S.–Japan Seminar on Biochemical Approaches to Weed Control*, Raleigh, N.C., U.S.A. (1969).

[26] S. Matsunaka. *Abst. Ann. Meeting Soc. Chem. Regulation Plants*, p 89 (1970).

[27] G. G. Still. *Science*, **159**, 992 (1968).

[29] R. Y. Yih, D. H. McRae and H. F. Wilson, *Science*, **161**, 376 (1968).

[30] S. Matsunaka and S. Takano. *Abst. 9th Meeting Weed Soc. Japan*, p 39 (1970).

[31] R. Bartha. *J. Agr. Food Chem.* **16**, 602 (1968).

[32] R. Bartha and D. Pramer. *Science*, **156**, 1617 (1967).

[33] P. C. Kearney. *J. Agr. Food Chem.* **13**, 561 (1965).

[34] R. Bartha, H. A. B. Linke and D. Pramer. *Science*, **161**, 582 (1968).

[35] D. G. H. Daniels and B. C. Saunders. *J. Chem. Soc., London*, 833 (1953).

[36] G. G. Still. *Weed Res.* **9**, 211 (1969).

[37] H. Chisaka and P. C. Kearney. *J. Agr. Food Chem.* **18**, 854 (1970).

[38] J. R. Plimmer, P. C. Kearney, H. Chisaka, J. B. Yount and U. I. Klingebiel. *J. Agr. Food Chem.* **18**, 859 (1970).

[39] R. Bartha. *Science*, **166**, 1299 (1969).

[40] P. C. Kearney, J. R. Plimmer and F. B. Guardia. *J. Agr. Food Chem.* **17**, 1418 (1969).

[41] J. R. Plimmer and P. C. Kearney. *Abst. 158th Meeting Amer. Chem. Soc.*, New York City (1969).

[42] J. D. Rosen, M. Siewierski and G. Winnett. *Abst. 158th Meeting Amer. Chem. Soc.*, New York City (1969).

[43] G. G. Still and E. R. Mansager. *Weed Res.* **9**, 218 (1969).

[44] U.S. Department of Health, Education and Welfare. *Rept. Secretary's Comm. Pesticides and their Relationship to Environmental Health*, p 473 (1969).

[45] R. Bartha and D. Pramer. *Advan. Appl. Microbiol.* (in press) (1970).

[46] P. C. Kearney, R. J. Smith Jr, J. R. Plimmer and F. B. Guardia. *Weed Sci.* **18**, 464 (1970).

[47] N. Shirakawa, H. Tomioka and K. Togashi. *J. Jap. Soc. Horti. Sci.* **38**, 74 (1969).

[48] N. Shirakawa, H. Tomioka and K. Togashi. *Weed Res., Japan*, **6**, 84 (1967).

[49] N. Shirakawa. *J. Jap. Soc. Horti. Sci.* **39**, 95 (1970).

[50] N. Shirakawa. *Weed Res., Japan*, **10**, 32 (1970).

[51] D. D. Baird, R. F. Husted and C. L. Wilson. *Proc. Southern Weed Conf.* **18**, 653 (1965).

[52] G. W. Selleck, P. L. Berthet, D. M. Evans and P. M. Vincent. *2nd Symp. New Herb.*, Paris. pp 277, 287 (1965).

[53] E. G. Jaworski and C. A. Porter. *Abst. 148th Amer. Chem. Soc. Meeting*, Detroit (1965).

[54] E. G. Jaworski. In *Degradation of Herbicides*, p. 165. Ed. by P. C. Kearney and D. D. Kaufman. Marcel Dekker Inc. (1969).

[55] W. T. Chin, R. P. Stanovick, T. E. Cullen and G. C. Holsing. *Weeds*, **12**, 201 (1964).